evolve

To access your Student Resources, visit the web address below:

http://evolve.elsevier.com/Greene/kinesiology

- ### Interactive Exercises, Animations, and Movies
  These animated activities expand on concepts learned in the main text.

- ### Animations and Video Clips
  Goniometry and range-of-motion are explored in these pages.

- ### Crossword Puzzles
  Test your knowledge of the vocabulary.

- ### Review Questions and Answers
  Self-tests provide extra resources for understanding the chapters.

- ### Lab Manual
  An online version of the lab manual included in the text.

KINESIOLOGY

Movement in the Context of Activity

KINESIOLOGY

Movement in the Context of Activity

Second Edition

David Paul Greene, PhD, MS, OTR

Associate Professor,
Department of Occupational Therapy,
Colorado State University,
Fort Collins, Colorado

Susan L. Roberts, MDiv, OTR

Changes Occupational Therapy
Tucson, Arizona

With 1 Contributing Author

Includes 298 illustrations

Illustrations by
David Paul Greene, PhD, MS, OTR

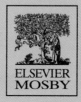

ELSEVIER
MOSBY

ELSEVIER
MOSBY

11830 Westline Industrial Drive
St. Louis, Missouri 63146

KINESIOLOGY: MOVEMENT IN THE CONTEXT OF ACTIVITY   0-323-02822-5
Copyright © 2005, Elsevier Inc.

Previous edition copyrighted 1999

International Standard Book Number 0-323-02822-5

Publishing Director: Linda Duncan
Editor: Kathy Falk
Developmental Editor: Melissa Kuster Deutsch
Publishing Services Manager: John Rogers
Senior Project Manager: Kathleen L. Teal
Senior Designer: Kathi Gosche

Printed in the United States of America

Last digit is the print number: 9 8 7 6 5 4 3 2 1

Contributor

John Martin, MS, OTR

Hand and Upper Exremities Specialist

Orthopedic Center of the Rockies

Fort Collins, Colorado

Foreword

Occupation is the foundation of the practice of occupational therapy. Work and productive activities, play and leisure, and activities of daily living are all occupational performance areas comprising occupation. Understanding the meaning of occupation greatly contributes to its use as a therapeutic mechanism for change. In occupational therapy, change is what the process is all about. Occupational therapy practitioners advocate change in others. We talk about change as transformation.

Kinesiology: Movement in the Context of Activity provides a wonderful resource for better understanding one component integral to occupation—human movement. What David Greene and Susan Roberts have achieved in their text is to provide the occupational therapy student and practitioner with an engaging approach to the understanding of human movement in a person-environment context. The authors have explored the kinesiology of the upper and lower extremities in this text and have included clear explanations of both normal kinesiologic function and pathokinesiology of the wrist and hand. Learning kinesiology and biomechanics is made more comprehensible through the incorporation of clinical problems throughout the text in the form of ongoing vignettes. The authors also have demystified and de-emphasized algebra and trigonometry without compromising understanding—no easy feat!

I believe this textbook will be especially successful in facilitating the student's understanding of kinesiology and biomechanics. Each chapter includes a Content Outline, a list of Key Terms, and Problem-Solving Exercises. "A Closer Look" boxes provide an in-depth look at more complicated and difficult-to-understand topics. In addition, the material in each chapter is brought to life through numerous illustrations.

The rigor required to become a competent, ethical, and skilled occupational therapy practitioner seems to increase daily as we face an ever-changing and complex health-care environment and evolving occupational therapy theories and models that support evidence-based outcomes. I applaud the authors for providing us with *Kinesiology: Movement in the Context of Activity*. This text is an important addition to the student's library and will support the practitioner's lifelong continuing competency.

Karen Jacobs, EdD, OTR/L, CPE, FAOTA
Clinical Associate Professor,
Department of Occupational Therapy,
Boston University,
Boston, Massachusetts

Preface

Kinesiology and biomechanics help practitioners carefully analyze human activity. In this book, we explore the intricacies of kinesiology as it relates to the practice of occupational therapy with an intention in every lesson to maintain a perspective in which the relative significance of the details are viewed in the context of the larger life experience. We present practice-relevant problems throughout the book as experience encountered by *individuals*. Although the biomechanical aspects of the problems provide an immediate and initial focus, our ultimate concern lies with the individual's contextual experience of encountering biomechanical problems.

Appendix H, summarizes these individuals' situations in brief, narrative form. We have attempted to present some diversity of age, race, and ethnic background in this cast of characters. The "characters" are fictional compilations of people we have known, and many appear more than once throughout the course of the book. Alphabetical listings by first name allow quick reference to the "bigger picture" in each case.

The clients and practitioners presented in the book reflect a variety of OT settings. Occupational therapists alternate with assistants in the vignettes and portray realistic clinical roles. In most instances the roles are interchangeable, but evaluation activities usually feature therapists rather than assistants because evaluation is chiefly a therapist's role. Although we often refer to assistants as *OT assistants,* the term *OT practitioner* is used to refer to individuals, both therapists and assistants, who engage in OT practice.

Overview of Chapters

Five chapters comprise Section One of this book providing background information from other fields pertaining to philosophical issues and contributions to the kinesiologic aspects of occupational therapy. Chapter 1 defines the role of kinesiology and biomechanics in current OT practice and attempts to provide some perspective as to their important role in the scope of practice. Chapter 2 introduces new interactive animations, providing basic vocabulary and concepts for discussion of the human musculoskeletal system and mechanical physics. These animations facilitate learning of concepts in the following chapters as well. Chapter 3 looks at how gravity affects movement, whereas Chapters 4 and 5 explore linear and rotary forces and movement.

The final four chapters of the book comprise Section Two, in which concepts presented in the first half of the book provide a basis for more complex, intervention-based thinking about regions of the human musculoskeletal system. Chapter 6 explores the head and torso. Chapters 7 and 8 look at the upper extremity, both proximal and distal, and Chapter 9 introduces the lower extremity. Section Two of this new edition brings forth a wealth of practice-relevant evaluative information in the same accessible Closer-Look-Box format used in the first edition.

Each chapter begins with an outline and a list of key terms. In addition to "A Closer Look" boxes, look for multiple references to animations (on the CD ROM and

Evolve website) that expand on various topics presented in the book. Each chapter concludes with applications in the form of questions to be answered or problems to be solved. All answers and related discussions are included in Appendix C. We encourage you to work through each application before consulting Appendix C for the answers.

There are 11 Appendixes at the end of the book. In addition to the listing of characters (Appendix H) and answers to the chapter applications (Appendix C) already mentioned, these Appendixes include a conversion table from English to metric equivalents, a diagram of body segment parameters, a brief review of mathematics, a table of trigonometric functions, a listing of commonly used formulas in biomechanics, a journal article, an illustrated review of muscle anatomy, instructions for the creation of finger and wrist models and learning objectives. A Glossary also is provided to aid in the understanding of complex terminology.

How We Solve Problems Based on Kinesiology

Talk to any practitioner about their kinesiology course in school and stories abound about sines and cosines, multi-step mathematical solutions, and conversions to unfamiliar units of measure. Typically, practitioners wonder why they "did what they did" in school in their kinesiology courses – for they certainly don't approach problem solving "that way" in practice!

Our text is quite different in its approach to solving biomechanical and kinesiologic problems in human activity performance. Each scenario follows a logical progression, presenting information in much the same order an OT practitioner would follow to solve a clinical problem. We've employed pictorial (graphic) solutions throughout this text, and only absolutely necessary mathematics. Our attempt to teach clear conceptual thinking centers around presenting problems and solutions without letting unfamiliar units and processes get in the way. For example, while it is correct to convert kilograms to Newtons in determining the absolute value of torque, the conversion confuses practitioners accustomed to referring to kilograms in their every-day practice. Further, the conversion proves unnecessary when comparing one scenario to the other – a comparison emphasizing relative difference and not absolute value.[1]

We trust our nontraditional approach will provide tools for clear thinking and problem solving. These are concepts and thought processes important to our full understanding of real client situations on a daily basis in practice. This is *not* something you do "only in school."

David Paul Greene
Susan L. Roberts

---

[1]For those practitioners considering working with engineers to design complex adaptive equipment, orthotics, and ergonomic industry tools, the more complete, multi step solutions to problems are included in Appendix C. Understanding how mathematics works in biomechanics can help OT practitioners identify the relevant data needed to solve clinical problems that may require teamwork with bioengineers or orthotists.

Acknowledgments

Many people were helpful to us in writing this book. Without their assistance and support, writing would have been more difficult and far less enjoyable.

Our acquisitions editor, Kathy Falk served as an energetic facilitator and was forever open to unique formats for material for the new edition. She was a true encourager of further development of our ideas for interactive animations and the inclusion of the CD ROM for instruction in goniometry and manual muscle testing. Our development editor, Melissa Kuster assured that frequent and continuous communication would be "the order of the day," and provided a seamless network for transfer of ideas, files, and clarifying information in every aspect of development and writing. She attended to our project as if it were her only concern!

Our desire to expand readers' views beyond mere biomechanics, yielded the addition of fictional clients. These clients were fortunate enough to have a very real team of people who were not only interested in the client's progress but willing to accept phone calls at home, often late at night. All these people shaped the lives of the fictional clients and ensured that this book would look at more than just body parts and principles of physics.

Barbara E. Brown, OTR, offered a wealth of treatment suggestions for almost every character, especially those clients with spinal cord and hand injuries. Ellen Buenaventura, MD, considered how particular diagnoses and complications might affect various clients, especially children. Melissa Price, PhD, suggested that if one of our characters, Eduardo Ybarra, taught his son carpentry, this may help him recover from depression. Sharon Kutok, SLP, provided the essential information that allowed Bernice Richardson, another character, to resume her singing career. Mary Raye Hestand, MBA, provided detailed consultation on the character Xavier Morales and would have been happy to shoot a few baskets with him on the court if he had been a real person. Finally, Joel Cannon, PhD, served as our contact in the world of theoretical physics, ensuring the integrity of the information as we attempted to explain basic but complicated concepts in understandable terms.

Linda Larson, COTA, and Noelle Everhart, COTA, made it possible for Susan to spend time concentrating on the book without worrying that students were going without OT services. Ellen Buenaventura kept the house running and provided meals when writing consumed entire days.

Over the years, students in David's biomechanics classes unknowingly contributed to this second edition through thoughtful questions and comments derived from their dedicated studies of the assigned readings in the first edition. David's sons, Josh and Jonah provided endless entertainment and a few finger tricks for photographs. Donna Wills Greene handled her own job, took up the slack managing the increasing activities and adventures of two growing boys, and consistently provided an attentive ear.

David Paul Greene
Susan L. Roberts

List of Electronic Resources on CD-ROM

INTERACTIVE EXERCISES

ANIMATIONS

MOVIES

Contents

Multidisciplinary Basis for the Understanding of Human Movement

SECTION**OUTLINE**

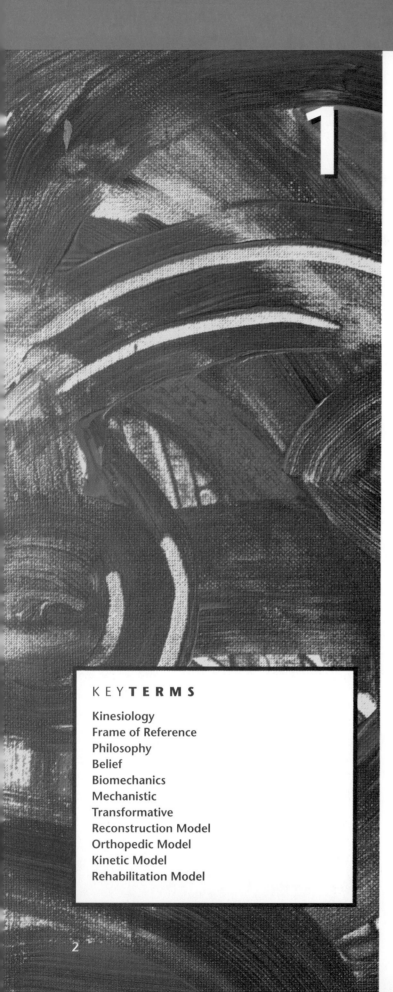

1

Biomechanics, Kinesiology, and Occupational Therapy

A Good Fit

KEY**TERMS**

Kinesiology
Frame of Reference
Philosophy
Belief
Biomechanics
Mechanistic
Transformative
Reconstruction Model
Orthopedic Model
Kinetic Model
Rehabilitation Model

The 8-year-old third grader with cerebral palsy struggles to raise his head when introduced to the occupational therapy (OT) assistant visiting his classroom to make equipment modifications. He presses his head against the back of his wheelchair and holds it there unsteadily while the teacher explains, "Jason's* biggest problem is that he won't pay attention and keeps ignoring us. He's always looking down at his lap tray. We've been giving him a sticker when he holds his head up and pays attention for 5 minutes. If he can get five stickers in one day, Jason can go on our weekly field trip, but so far he just hasn't tried hard enough." Reminded of his failures, Jason begins to cry.

"I don't care what you people in rehab say about Mrs. Smith being a one-person transfer; it takes two of my CNAs (certified nursing assistants) to get her on and off the toilet!" complains the head nurse at the weekly review of residents in Maple Grove Skilled Care Facility.

The OT practitioner remembers Mrs. Smith was fearful of falling and had difficulty leaning forward when standing for transfers from her wheelchair. It took a lot of coaxing and reassurance to get her up.

"Why don't we bring her into therapy for a few weeks and see if we can get her into our dance group, as well as work with your aides to show them some ways to get her to stand up more easily," the OT practitioner suggests.

Kinesiology provides the best means of solving these problems because of the unique blend of fields that converge in this area of study. Kinesiology is the study of movement from the perspective of three physical sciences: musculoskeletal anatomy, neuromuscular physiology, and biomechanics. The complexity of these three fields often makes their introduction into activity analysis an exercise in examining details to the extent that we lose sight of the meaningful activity behind the movement (A Closer Look Box 1-1).

As OT practitioners, we must recognize that although kinesiology presents concrete and solvable solutions, it never tells the whole story. We may focus on a specific movement or adaptation and even perfect it in the clinic, only to find it falls apart in the context of our client's natural environment. An understanding of movement only leads to successful adaptations when we integrate these solutions into real-life activity and apply them to individual environments.

An OT practitioner who saw Jason could write two very different evaluation notes. Focusing primarily on kinesiology, the OT practitioner may write the following:

This 8-year-old boy with cerebral palsy has limited head and neck extension secondary to severe spasticity. Abnormal tone has resulted in flexion contractures of the elbows and wrists. Spasticity and fluctuating muscle tone limit control of the head, as well as neck and wrist extension.

A change of focus, based on performance in the school environment, might lead to a very different evaluation:

Jason, an active 8-year-old boy, attends third grade in a regular classroom. He has difficulty in class because of poor head control secondary to cerebral palsy. His inability to lift his head from the lap tray interferes with his ability to participate in class. Jason also experiences flexion contractures of the elbow and wrist secondary to severe flexor spasticity, making it difficult for him to use his upper extremities to reach and grasp as his classmates do.

BOX 1-1

A CLOSER LOOK

Defining Kinesiology and Biomechanics

People often confuse the terms kinesiology and biomechanics. The biomechanical frame of reference commonly referred to in treatment settings involves aspects of kinesiology that include functional anatomy of the musculoskeletal system, neuromuscular physiology, and biomechanics. OT educational programs offer courses that typically blend content from these three areas into courses called kinesiology, biomechanics, and human movement.

The following definitions from Stedman's Medical Dictionary[7] may clarify an understanding of the interdependence of these two sciences:

Kinesiology: The science of the study of movement and the active and passive structures involved

Biomechanics: The science of the action of forces, internal or external, on the living body

Kinesiology studies movement. Biomechanics focuses on the forces that affect movement. Biomechanics provides one perspective for the study of movement.

Both evaluation notes contain the important details. The first demonstrates a keen sense of biomechanics and kinesiology, but the document shows little insight into the significance of these problems. The latter evaluation represents a bigger picture, a view that embraces the importance of meaningful activity leading to successful role function. An OT practitioner's point of view affects the way we conduct assessments and perform treatments. Understanding this **frame of reference** forms an essential part of professional development for every OT practitioner.

Beliefs and Definitions

Perspective shapes the way we define the limitations and possibilities of any problem. The combination of our philosophy about life and the way we integrate these beliefs into OT models of practice gives us our perspective. **Philosophy** affects an individual's perceptions of experience by providing a broad-based view of life. Related theories, models, and frames of reference add structure to our perceptions, but each of these gets consciously or unconsciously filtered through an overall philosophy.

OT practice evolves from a **belief** that purposeful activity (occupation), including its interpersonal and environmental components, can serve to improve one's functional ability or prevent dysfunction by promoting maximum functional adaptation. Kinesiology, the study of movement influenced by active and passive structures, includes **biomechanics**, the study of internal and external forces. Together, they represent two restricted views of purposeful activity and adaptation, helping OT practitioners to understand movement in the context of the musculoskeletal system but not necessarily in the broader context of life activities.

Because kinesiology and biomechanics restrict our frame of reference, OT practitioners must question how these approaches fit within the philosophy and definition of the profession. When we base our interventions solely on scientific collections of techniques and protocols, they become therapeutic only in the narrowest sense. Effective practice demands a broader view of therapy than range of motion, strength, and endurance.

As OT practitioners, our focus goes far beyond movement for movement's sake (for example, flexing the arm to move through full range of motion). Our focus also goes beyond functional movement when that involves nothing more than completing a specific action with a particular joint. Our primary concern for movement involves movement within the context of activity.

Supports, barriers, specific skills, and occupational demands in real-life environments have tremendous effects on individual performance. Kinesiology fits when its more restrictive viewpoint for intervention is anchored in the context of meaningful activity and the effect of activity on role function. Then kinesiology becomes a powerful tool for assessment and treatment of any individual with movement-related difficulties.

The practice of occupational therapy requires us to understand the fundamental details of a situation. We must know, for example, the specifics of splinting, including the necessity of a perpendicular force and the danger of forces applied at angles other than 90 degrees. The ultimate value of this intervention includes both accurate biomechanics and understanding the reason why this splint will facilitate individual adaptation. Every detail must help the individual to perform the necessary and desirable role functions that are meaningful to that individual's life. Biomechanics provides the means to the end.

To understand how we use kinesiology in OT practice, we need to define it and understand its place in our beliefs about human movement. Kinesiology, and even more so biomechanics, has its roots in a branch of physics based on the belief that individuals function like complex machines. This belief system, mechanistic philosophy, shaped the study of science and medicine for many centuries. In the twentieth century, a newer system, transformative philosophy, gained precedence over mechanistic philosophy. Transformative philosophy made many new discoveries and theories possible. How do these philosophies continue to affect our understanding of functional activity?

Mechanistic and Transformative Philosophies

Aristotle and his contemporaries recorded an interest in the analysis of human motion in the fifth century, BC. They developed a view of the human musculoskeletal system as a mechanism involving levers, forces, and a center of gravity. In the early part of the sixteenth century, Galileo, considered the father of modern science, combined his observations of the world with mathematics. Descartes, his contemporary, outlined a mechanistic philosophy that separated mind from matter. These radical ideas upset the way people viewed the world and earned Galileo a decade of house arrest and threats of torture. Ultimately Galileo renounced his belief that the Earth revolved around the sun. Descartes published his work more quietly to avoid similar persecution.

Nonetheless, the work of both Galileo and Descartes influenced Sir Isaac Newton. In the latter half of the sixteenth century, he constructed a system of mechanics that became the foundation of classical physics. In 1703, Newton earned knighthood for his work. The science and technology that grew out of this mechanistic world view spawned the Industrial Revolution of the nineteenth century.[2,5,12]

Mechanistic philosophy separates mind from body. Subscribers to this viewpoint see human beings as compositions of interrelated components. Time is linear and evolutionary. The past becomes a focus for management of future events. Relationships between people and objects interface like parts of a larger machine. When the machine is managed and maintained, it functions at peak efficiency. Conflict, trauma, and other difficulties cause systemic breakdowns. People, communities, or objects at the center of these breakdowns become victims requiring removal or restoration for the good of themselves and the system. Those who choose to intervene with a mechanistic philosophy use a managerial style to coordinate the isolated parts.[1,8,9] The outcomes of their intervention reflect this out-of-context perspective, resulting in poor coordination between "therapy," activity performance, and role completion in their clients' everyday lives.

Newtonian physics remained unchallenged until Einstein's work in the twentieth century. Einstein's theories, coupled with the advent of nuclear technology and quantum physics, caused major upheavals in both science and philosophy. As a result, new sciences and philosophies developed.[5]

For example, scientists trying to understand the chaotic phenomena of both weather and cardiac rhythms developed a new field of mathematics. The mathematics of chaos provided a means for understanding previously unpredictable events. They found that relatively insignificant changes at particular moments produced global changes later; it was as if a butterfly flapping its wings in China could produce rainstorms in Iowa.[6]

The mathematics of chaos reflected and influenced **transformative** philosophy as it emerged from radical changes in the twentieth century. Individuals who subscribe to a transformative philosophy see others as integral members of a large and interdependent organic system. The relativity of time means that new emerges from old and that both are changed. Human relationships form dynamic, infinitely unique patterns and harmonies. Conflict, trauma, and difficulty serve as catalysts for creative adaptation. Individuals and communities who adapt and change behave like artists creating dynamic new niches for their environment.[1,8,9]

A Biomechanical Frame of Reference

Although OT practice evolved in the mechanistic model of medical management, most contemporary OT practitioners define problems in terms of creative adaptations. Nonetheless, OT models of practice based on biomechanics have an important place in the history of the OT profession.

In 1918, psychologist Bird T. Baldwin organized an OT department at Walter Reed General Hospital in Washington, DC. He began routine measurements of joint motion and muscle strength to develop a method of evaluation and treatment. From these measurements, he developed a set of problem-solving steps known as the **reconstruction model.** Baldwin believed that voluntary activities, graded and adapted to specific muscles and joints, would result in a return of function. Whenever contemporary OT practitioners increase resistance or complexity in an activity, they use the knowledge this model provided.

In the first half of the century, OT practitioner Marjorie Taylor used anatomy, physiology, pathology, and kinesiology to develop the **orthopedic model.** She devised treatment activities specific to muscle and joint problems. OT practitioners use this model whenever they tailor an activity to strengthen a specific muscle group or increase the movement in specific joints.[11]

In 1950, physicians Sidney Licht and William R. Dunton, Jr. wrote an OT textbook outlining the **kinetic model.** Licht believed that OT practitioners needed to become more scientific. To this end, he developed many valuable working definitions of OT. He promoted activity analysis and reported on many kinds of adaptive equipment.[11]

OT models based on biomechanics have provided practitioners a means to do the following:

1. Outline and define musculoskeletal problems
2. Develop exercises and activities that restore and maintain function
3. Design and fabricate adaptive equipment to meet functional activity goals
4. Measure functional musculoskeletal progress in treatment

Biomechanics can be used to research the effects of activity on the musculoskeletal system. It provides a useful approach in hand clinics, centers for physical rehabilitation, work-hardening clinics, and ergonomics. Biomechanics at its best becomes a lens for focusing treatment approaches, only when practitioners remain aware of its corresponding tendency to reduce and isolate problems.

LIMITATIONS OF BIOMECHANICAL APPROACHES

Biomechanics emphasizes the mechanics of the musculoskeletal system. It does not address the cognitive, emotional, and social aspects of human occupation.

Kinesiology, although it encompasses the psychomotor aspects of movement, still falls short of balancing performance components of individual function with the environment in which a person operates. Kinesiology has not provided a comprehensive framework for OT practice. The confusion of OT with physical therapy has resulted from a single-minded focus on using activities, including exercise, to improve and maintain musculoskeletal function only.

OT practitioners must use kinesiology to fuel their problem-solving engines and then move on to the next step. An individual's improved musculoskeletal function, made possible through biomechanical applications, should contribute to a functional occupational role. Improved musculoskeletal function isolated from the occupational contexts of self-care, work, and play* has no place in OT practice. Because our profession stresses a holistic approach, we must use biomechanics within other models of practice.

Integration of Biomechanics with Models of Practice

Kinesiology provides a structured way of evaluating movement in activity. Movement generally involves the musculoskeletal system, and some evaluation of movement belongs in every OT assessment. Biomechanics provides a means for examining movement in activities. If necessary it can guide an OT practitioner to provide interventions that emphasize remediation of specific body parts. Although this focus may lie tangential to an individual's occupational function, biomechanics, blended and used within current models of practice, remains essential to contemporary OT practice.

OT theorists have developed many models of practice more closely related to transformative philosophy. Jean Ayres' theory of sensory integration postulated that small changes in the processing of sensory input produce global adaptive responses. Lorna Jean King elaborated on Ayres' work to develop a model of adaptive responses for understanding patterns of change and growth. Mary Reilly and Gary Kielhofner used open system models to describe human activity. These models assumed that growth and change involve interdependent, not linear, progress. Their belief in the uniqueness of individual experience resulted from a transformative rather than mechanistic philosophy. Yet, even in these

transformative models of practice, an understanding of movement depends on principles of biomechanics.

The **rehabilitation model** highlights adaptations toward function in meaningful activity, not remediation of specific body parts. Anne Fisher's Occupational Therapy Intervention Process Model[3] identifies four domains of function: level of independence, level of effort, degree of efficiency, and degree of safety, providing a broader range of information for the understanding of motor and processing skills. Under this model, mechanistic frames of reference, like biomechanics, occur in the context of solving problems associated with meaningful activities.

Summary

Biomechanics provides a key to understanding levels of independence, effort, efficiency, and safety. As a part of kinesiology, an understanding of biomechanics better equips the OT practitioner to solve problems and offer suggestions leading to improved function in relevant contexts.

Kinesiology equips OT practitioners with tools to formulate a problem and arrive at a solution. That solution must stay relevant to an individual's everyday life. For example, a device that improves hand grip will work brilliantly only if it gives an individual a functional grasp at work. OT practitioners have responsibility not just for solving a problem but also for ensuring that these solutions get incorporated into daily life. The latter responsibility offers our profession its greatest challenges and rewards.

OT practitioners use kinesiology to design and modify adaptive equipment, evaluate the safety of home and work environments, or create therapeutic activities and exercise programs. Effective OT practitioners further determine how a piece of equipment, modified work station, or trip to the mall enables an individual to participate more fully in their community. Like the butterfly in China that sets off a weather pattern leading to rain in Iowa, OT practitioners expect their little bit to go a long way.

REFERENCES

1. Cannon K: *Katie's cannon: womanism and the soul of the black community*, New York, 1995, Continuum.
2. *The concise Columbia encyclopedia*, New York, 1995, Columbia University Press.
3. Fisher AG: Uniting practice and theory in an occupational framework: 1998 Eleanor Clarke Slagle Lecture, *Am J Occup Ther*, 52, 509-521, 1998.
4. Florey LL: An approach to play and play development, *Am J Occup Ther* 25:275-280, 1971.

---

*Play encompasses a broader range of human occupation than recreation. "Under Reilly's leadership, the 'play lady'[4] was taken out of the closet, and a new generation of leaders and scholars in the profession were inspired to reclaim play as a fundamental concept in OT practice and to make it an object of research."[10]

5. Fritjof C: *The Tao of physics*, New York, 1984, Bantam.

6. Gleick J: *Chaos: making a new science*, New York, 1987, Viking.

7. *Illustrated Stedman's medical dictionary*, ed 24, Baltimore, 1982, Williams & Wilkins.

8. Levine RL, Fitzgerald HE: *Analysis of dynamic psychological systems, vol 1: basic approaches to general systems, dynamic systems, and cybernetics*, New York, 1992, Plenum Press.

9. Mead GH: *Movements of thought in the nineteenth century*, Chicago, 1936, University of Chicago Press.

10. Parham LD, Fazio LS: *Play in occupational therapy with children*, St Louis, 1997, Mosby.

11. Reed K: *Models of practice in occupational therapy*, Baltimore, 1984, Williams & Wilkins.

12. Trager J: *The people's chronology*, New York, 1995, Henry Holt.

13. World Health Organization: International Classification of Function, Disability and Health (ICF). Available from: http://www3.who.int/icf/onlinebrowser/icf.cfm found on 3-1-04 [Cited 03-01-2004].

LAB BOX

Find applied activities exploring concepts in Chapter 1 in the following laboratory exercises:

Topic	*Laboratory*
Movement of the human musculoskeletal system	Lab 1 Kinematic Chain, Human Musculoskeletal Movement, Shoulder Model of Joint Movement

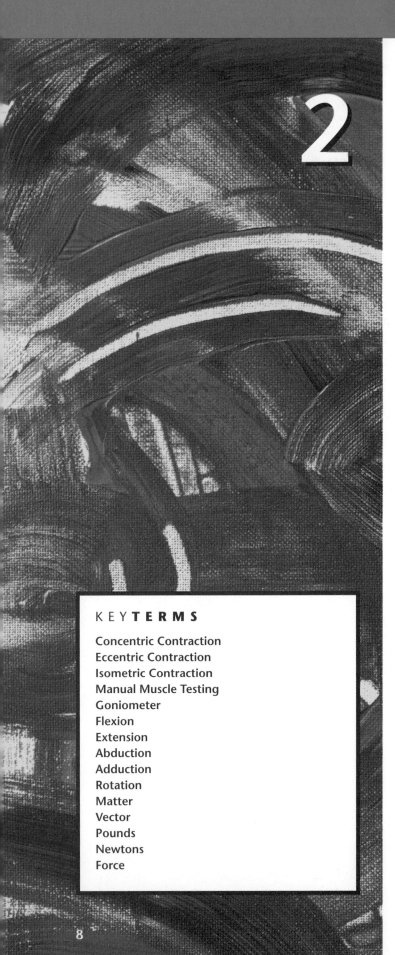

2

The Study of Human Movement

Concepts from Related Fields

edicine and physics converge in the study of biomechanics and kinesiology. Each discipline has its own perspective and language. An OT practitioner must learn vocabulary and concepts from both disciplines to combine and apply this knowledge to functional activity.

The rich language of medicine uses words derived from Greek, Latin, and a variety of other languages to describe unique physiologic conditions and minute areas of anatomical geography. Although medical terms often confuse the uninitiated, one word often communicates concepts that would otherwise require several phrases. This chapter explores terms commonly used to describe human movement and diagnoses characterized by abnormal biomechanics and kinesiology.

Terms from physics serve an equally valuable purpose as those in medicine. Physics describes the world and its relationships with mathematics. These relationships help explain the past and predict the future. Classical physics communicates the study of motion in gases, liquids, and solids, concepts essential for understanding biomechanics.

Although you probably know many of the terms relating to the musculoskeletal system, we may apply them in new and unfamiliar ways. We will review the gross anatomy, neuroanatomy, motor control, and muscle physiology necessary for solving the problems presented in this text. This book presents problems so that readers can solve them without resorting to mathematics, but OT practitioners who enjoy mathematics can find these solutions in Appendix C. Further reading and study of physics will help those practitioners who need to apply mathematics to human motion more precisely. The brief summary of concepts that follows provides a guide. It is not a comprehensive list.

Concepts from Medicine

Identifying specific areas of the human body forms the groundwork for practicing any of the medical arts. As a common point of reference we envision the body in anatomical position, that is, upright with the face, feet, and palms facing forward. The head lies superior to the shoulders because the head is above, or higher than, the shoulders. The shoulders are inferior to the head because they lie below the head when the body is vertical. Those parts closer to the front of the body are anterior, and those near the back are posterior. Medial body parts lie near the middle of the body, and lateral parts lie near the right or left sides of the body. Arms and legs

are extremities, and they connect to the trunk at their proximal ends. Fingers and toes are located at the distal ends of the extremities. Tissues close to the surface are superficial to underlying, or deep, tissues.

THE CENTRAL NERVOUS SYSTEM

The brain and spinal cord comprise the central nervous system (CNS), which controls all the body's activities. The brain is divided into three major anatomical parts: the cerebrum, cerebellum, and brain stem. The cerebrum receives sensory information and processes it to produce body responses, including movement. The cerebrum forms two hemispheres. Fibers that transmit impulses from each hemisphere cross from one side to the other in the corpus callosum and other smaller pathways, allowing one side of the brain to communicate with the other. Generally, each hemisphere receives sensory information from and controls movement of the opposite side of the body. The cortex makes up the superficial layer of the cerebrum and processes information for all tasks that require conscious thought. Two strips of cells run from ear to ear over the superior part of the cortex. Each strip contains a functionally separate cell population—one for processing of sensory information and one for direction of motor performance.

The final common pathway for motor signals generated in the motor cortex is comprised of neurons whose cell bodies are located in this motor area and whose axonal projections exit the cortex through the brain stem and spinal cord. These neurons are referred to as upper motor neurons as they synapse at lower levels of the cord onto lower motor neurons. These lower motor neurons are called such because they begin (their cell bodies are located) lower than the upper motor neurons, in the ventral area of all levels of the spinal cord. Their axonal projections exit the spinal cord, travel as peripheral nerves, and connect with skeletal muscles, completing the circuit to result in voluntary movement. Although lower motor neurons begin in the CNS, they travel in and connect to the periphery (outside of the CNS); therefore they are considered part of the peripheral nervous system (discussed below). (The role of upper and lower motor neurons in clinical syndromes is discussed in A Closer Look Box 2-1.)

The cerebrum contains other important centers for processing of sensory information and organization of the subcortical motor responses, which do not require conscious thought. The cortex and corpus callosum

Upper versus Lower Motor Neuron Syndromes
In practice, two basic syndromes are identified as pathological movement patterns based on the upper–lower motor neuron scheme. Upper motor neuron syndrome (for example, stroke, spinal cord injury, traumatic brain injury) involves damage to motor neurons originating in the motor cortex. It results in paralysis (lack of voluntary motion) accompanied by abnormally high muscle tone (spasticity). Lower motor neuron syndrome (for example, polio myelitis and peripheral nerve damage) involves damage to the lower motor neuron originating in the spinal cord; it results in paralysis accompanied by abnormally low muscle tone (flaccidity).

surround the limbic lobe and basal ganglia. Cells in the limbic lobe govern behavior and emotion. In the basal ganglia, cells coordinate complex motor responses to environmental stimulation.

The brain stem connects the cerebrum to the spinal cord. It contains a number of differentiated cellular structures. The thalamus and hypothalamus regulate breathing, digestion, alertness, hormonal balance, and temperature control.

The cerebellum rises out of the brain stem to form a separate structure. The cerebellum chiefly regulates muscle tone and equilibrium, or balance, reactions. It also coordinates voluntary motor acts.

The spinal cord carries information to the brain from the body and to the body from the brain. Cells that carry specific kinds of information group together to form pathways, which are known as *tracts*. The reflex arc, moving directly through synapses in the spinal cord, can carry out motor responses to some external stimuli before those sensory impulses reach the brain.

THE PERIPHERAL NERVOUS SYSTEM

Nerve fibers that have cell bodies in the spinal cord or in special structures called *ganglia* carry information to and from the body to the CNS. (Ganglia are collections of nerve-cell bodies that lie outside the brain or spinal cord). This peripheral nervous system (PNS) extends from the CNS, and the two systems operate interdependently. Anatomists and physiologists studying the body differentiate these systems to understand how they work.

Afferent nerve fibers carry impulses from the body tissues to the spinal cord and brain. Efferent fibers carry information from the brain and spinal cord to muscles and glands. Somatic nerves carry impulses to and from muscles. Visceral nerves transmit impulses to and from organs and glands.

Spinal nerves branch out from the spinal cord in an organized pattern. Their organization makes it possible to identify the segments of the spinal cord responsible for specific areas of sensation and muscle movement. In several locations, spinal nerves group into a network that forms a plexus composed of motor and sensory fibers that innervate various structures. The cervical plexus, located in the neck, innervates structures in the neck and shoulder. The brachial plexus, located under the shoulder joint, in the axilla, supplies the upper extremities. Lumbar and sacral plexuses supply the lower extremities.

The 12 pairs of cranial nerves branch out directly from the brain and brain stem. All these nerves except the tenth cranial nerve innervate structures in the head and neck. The tenth nerve, the vagus nerve, primarily innervates organs and other structures in the thorax and abdomen.

The CNS controls organs and glands through a system of visceral efferent fibers and ganglia known as the *autonomic nervous system* (ANS). Nerve fibers that carry messages from the body's organs are not considered part of the ANS. These visceral afferent fibers run alongside the nerves of the ANS and go directly to the brain or spinal cord, not to autonomic ganglia. The CNS interprets sensory information and directs a response. The ANS then carries these reaction messages back to the organs and glands.

The ANS balances control of bodily functions through the sympathetic and parasympathetic systems. Parasympathetic (craniosacral) fibers originate in the brain and lower portion of the spinal cord and connect with secondary fibers in ganglia located throughout the viscera. These fibers transmit impulses that conserve energy to calm the body, for example, by slowing the heart rate and facilitating digestion. The sympathetic (thoracolumbar) fibers and ganglia emerge from the middle position of the spinal cord. They respond to environmental crises and produce an excitatory effect on the body known as the *fight-or-flight* reaction.

CONTROL OF MOVEMENT

The nervous system controls movement in the head, neck, trunk, and limbs through impulses generated in the brain's motor centers. These impulses, initiated by a conscious intention to move or in response to incoming sensory impulses, depend on sensory receptors in the skin, muscles, and related tissues.

Skin contains an assortment of sensory end organs that produce withdrawal responses when stimulated. Skeletal muscles contain muscle spindles. These sensory organs react to prolonged muscle stretch (tonic response) and rapid changes in length (phasic response). Stimulation of a muscle spindle through stretch to the muscle most commonly results in contraction of the muscle. However, tension-sensitive golgi tendon organs protect muscles from tearing by inhibiting muscle contraction when stimulated by very forceful contractions during extreme muscle stretch.

Under certain conditions, motor responses to muscle spindle stimulation appear exaggerated. Too much muscular activity occurs, and skeletal muscles cannot relax. An unyielding contraction of the muscle on one side of a joint limits desired movement in the opposite direction. These types of imbalance or movement disturbances, called *abnormal muscle tone*, sometimes respond to pharmacological or physical interventions that allow an individual to regain normal motor control and movement.

Responses to sensory receptors can occur without conscious thought. They follow reflexes, which are subcortical pathways that make a complete sensory-to-motor connection without involving parts of the brain that control volitional movement. Spinal reflexes make a simple sensory to motor synapse in the spinal cord that provides an immediate protective response to noxious stimuli or muscle spindle stretch. Brain stem reflexes make connections in the brain stem and regulate muscle responses to gravity acting on the body. Brain stem reflexes also regulate head movements that affect the entire body.

More complex interconnections that travel pathways to higher levels of the brain stem, called righting reactions, involve positioning the head in relation to gravity. They respond to stimulation of the semicircular canals, or labyrinths, and the visual pathways. Equilibrium reactions require connections between the cortex, basal ganglia, and cerebellum. They involve adjustments of the entire body to changes in its center of gravity.

Bones

More than 200 bones compose the skeletal system. Although rigid, dynamic bone tissues constantly respond to physiologic and environmental changes throughout life. The most obvious of these changes occurs during a child's early years as cartilage becomes bone. An infant skeleton has a smaller percentage of bone than a child or an adult because epiphyseal plates, centers of cartilaginous growth, permit bones to grow. This process occurs throughout childhood and into an individual's early 20s. Stress from carrying weight, movement, or trauma all stimulate bony tissue growth. Bone continually remodels itself throughout life because the skeleton provides both structure and storage for calcium. The body absorbs bone to harvest calcium for use along with (or in the absence of) dietary calcium as needed for various physiological processes including nerve transmission and muscle contraction.

Joints

A joint connects (articulates) adjacent bones. Diarthrodial joints have a fluid-filled space between two or more bones enclosed in a strong ligamentous capsule. Smooth hyaline cartilage covers articulating surfaces of the bones in the numerous diarthrodial joints. Elbow, knee, hip, shoulder, finger, and toe joints owe their mobility to their diarthrodial construction. This mobility provides a basis for the study of movement and our understanding of it through biomechanics and kinesiology.

Amphiarthrodial joints, composed of adjacent bones connected by cartilage, such as the symphysis joints located between vertebral bodies and the temporary epiphyseal plates, allow only slight movement. Synarthrodial joints, such as the suture joints of the skull, involve a fibrous interface between bones that does not move at all.

Muscles

Muscle tissue has the unique ability to contract. Three varieties exist: smooth, cardiac, and skeletal. Muscle fibers are the cellular units that make up muscles. Their measurements increase or decrease depending on the intracellular buildup or removal of contractile proteins (A Closer Look Box 2-2).

Skeletal, or striated, muscle interests students of biomechanics and kinesiology most. Skeletal muscle strength depends on the thickness of the muscle's cross section. Genetics determines the number of fibers contained in a muscle. Strengthening a muscle results in thicker fibers, not a greater quantity of fibers.

The length of the muscle fiber determines the distance a muscle can contract to a shorter length or stretch to a longer length. Shorter muscles (shorter fiber lengths) contract less distance (excursion) than longer muscles. Generally, muscle fibers can contract or stretch 50% of their resting lengths. A muscle with 10-centimeter fibers can contract or shorten to a length of 5 centimeters or be stretched by an outside force to a length of 15 centimeters.

Skeletal muscles vary greatly in shape and fiber configuration. The attachment of muscles to bones via either broad, fleshy attachments or concentrated, tendinous insertions determines the gross shape of the muscle and its force for movement. The biceps brachii and the lumbricals in the hand are fusiform muscles. All the fibers in fusiform muscles run from the origin to the insertion.

BOX 2-2

A**CLOSER**LOOK

Contractions versus Contractures

Contractions and contractures are two words with almost identical spellings, but they describe two very different concepts. A contraction occurs in a skeletal muscle. This process depends on the expenditure of energy. In a concentric contraction the muscle fibers shorten, but in an eccentric contraction an opposing force pulls the muscle longer as it contracts to slow or stop the effect of the opposing force. A contracture describes a state of being, not a process. In a contracture, the resting length of the tissue has become physically shorter than at a previous time. Contractures occur in muscle and joint ligaments that are inadequately stretched over time or in skin scarred by second- and third-degree burns. A contraction produces a normal muscle movement, but a contracture limits movement through a pathological process.

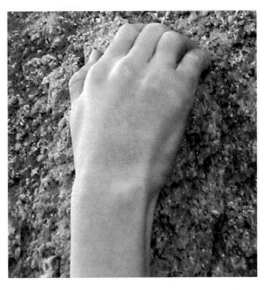

FIGURE **2-1**
A rock climber's handhold often consists of four fingertips or less supporting the weight of the entire body.

Pennate and bipennate muscles have fibers that course from a flattened, fleshy proximal attachment to a central tendon, bridging the gap between the fibers' end and the muscle's distal attachment yielding the appearance of a feather. Pennate and bipennate muscles such as the interossei and the long flexors of the digits have short excursions because of their short lengths. However, while their excursion may be limited, their large cross section provides impressive strength. Imagining a rock climber pulling up the weight of his body with one small "handhold" comprised of four fingertips helps one understand the way these short, thick cross sections provide impressive strength (Figure 2-1).

Muscles may spread out in broad sheets like the pronator quadratus and trapezius or assume unique shapes like the deltoid and serratus anterior. Some muscles, like the latissimus dorsi and pectoralis major, twist 180° at their distal attachments.

Muscles connect intimately to the skeletal system through tissue called fascia. Fascial sheaths surrounding bundles of muscle fibers and entire muscles continue along the tendons that attach muscle to bone.

Muscle fibers contract through a chemical process involving oxygen and adenosine triphosphate (ATP). Myoglobin provides the primary source of oxygen in muscle tissue. Like hemoglobin in the blood, myoglobin contains oxygen bonded to iron, which produces a characteristic red color. Red muscles contain fibers with high concentrations of myoglobin. These slow-twitch fibers

rely on high concentrations of myoglobin and a rich blood supply. Red postural muscles with slow-twitch fibers must work for prolonged periods without becoming fatigued. White muscles, composed of fast-twitch fibers, contain lower concentrations of myoglobin. These fibers can contract rapidly, like the flight muscles of birds. Fast-twitch fibers contract quickly for limited amounts of time because of their lower concentrations of myoglobin.

Muscle Activity

All skeletal muscles have several types of contractions in common. When a muscle contracts, one attachment usually remains stationary while the other attachment moves. **Concentric contractions** cause muscles to shorten (Figure 2-2). **Eccentric contractions** occur when muscles attempt to shorten but are stretched by an overpowering external effort. The opposing force pulls the contracting muscle to a longer length. Eccentric contractions often are used to control or slow down the effect of an external force. In Figure 2-3 the weight is controlled; that is, it is let down slowly through an eccentric contraction to protect the joint from being forced into rapid extension by the weight. In **isometric contractions** the contractile mechanisms are activated, but no appreciable change in fiber length or movement results. Isometric contractions occur when some force in the opposite direction equally balances the effort of the contraction.

Different contraction types generate different amounts of force. When we move weight we can easily

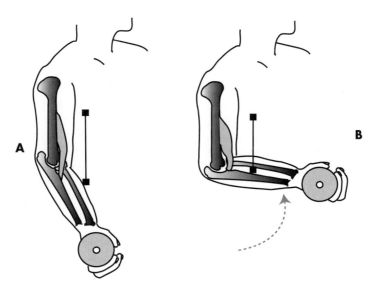

FIGURE **2-2**
Concentric contractions result in muscle shortening. The muscle begins the contraction at a longer length **(A)** than the length at completion **(B)**. We call the distance traveled by the moving end of the muscle *muscle excursion.*

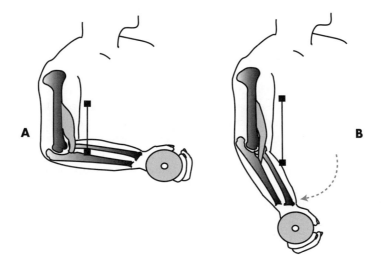

FIGURE **2-3**
In eccentric contractions, the muscle is able to control the effect of an external force and protect the joint from damage by forced, rapid motion. Here the elbow flexors slowly lower the weight instead of letting it drop rapidly. The muscle achieves this by attempting to shorten against an opposing force, creating just enough upward force that the weight overcomes the contraction and the contraction serves to slow the descent of the weight. The muscle begins in its shortened length **(A)** and, while attempting to shorten, experiences lengthening due to the overwhelming effect of the opposing force **(B)**.

control, the greatest force involves a concentric contraction, then an isometric contraction, and finally an eccentric contraction. This follows the reasoning that to lift (concentric), we must overcome; to hold (isometric), we must balance; and to lower with control (eccentric), we must let the weight overcome the muscle by creating an upward pull that is slightly less than the downward pull of the weight we are lowering.

If a weight reaches or exceeds the maximum limit of our control, the ratio changes. Then the greatest force is associated with eccentric contractions and the least with concentric contractions; isometric contractions remain in the middle. It is best to think of this scenario as a series of weights being lifted. Imagine you are getting wood for a fire and are trying to carry as much as possible. You stand with your arms at your sides, elbows slightly flexed, for your friend to load each log into your arms. With the first few logs, you can flex both elbows, lifting the load slightly to adjust the weight (concentric—least force). As she adds more logs, you can hold it, but no longer can you lift the load (isometric—moderate force). Finally she adds one too many logs, and the load begins to pull your arms down into elbow extension, even as you try to hold the load up (eccentric—greatest force). In sum we can lower more weight (eccentric) than we can hold (isometric) and hold more than we can lift (concentric).

Every action involves more muscles than those primarily responsible for a particular movement. Prime movers, or agonists, act to produce a specific movement. Antagonists oppose prime movers. Antagonists must relax before an agonist can move. Cocontraction of agonists and antagonists stabilizes joints through simultaneous activity on opposite sides of the joint as in isometric exercise. Antagonists slow and stop movement at the end of a range of motion to protect joints. This occurs through eccentric contraction of the antagonist. When gravity initiates movement as the primary force, antagonists control that movement through eccentric contraction.

Muscles that act together to produce specific movements are working in synergy. If a muscle performs more than one action, another muscle must neutralize one of those actions via stabilization. Imagine someone grasping a door handle as he pulls open a heavy door. If the wrist extensors did not stabilize the wrist in extension, the finger flexors would flex both the fingers and the wrist, diminishing the strength of the grip.

When a person's hand holds a bar tightly, finger flexors act as agonists for grasp, wrist extensors stabilize the wrist as synergists, and finger extensors relax as antagonists. Other muscles function as supporting muscles that hold the trunk, arms, and legs in advantageous positions. For example, while opening a heavy door, the back may extend, shoulders adduct and extend, elbows flex, and the legs alternately stand firm and step backward to pull the door open.

Slow, active movement involves continuous muscle tension throughout a range of motion. Ballistic movements produce strong, rapid contractions completed primarily through momentum. Antagonistic muscles slow these movements at the end of the range. Uncontrolled ballistic movements stop passively through the limitations of muscles, ligaments, and other joint tissues at the end of a range of motion. Uncontrolled ballistic movements put joints at more risk for injury than ballistic movements actively controlled by eccentric contractions of antagonistic muscles.

Often adolescent baseball pitchers put themselves at risk for elbow injuries because a good fastball requires ballistic elbow extension. When *Zachary Larson* returned to middle school baseball practice after spending months the previous year in a bivalve cast while recovering from surgery to repair his right ulnar nerve, his coach asked the school therapist for advice on how to make sure that Zachary did not reinjure himself.

Muscle Strength

We can measure muscle strength with force gauges (grip and pinch strength dynamometers) or by the application of graded resistance in **manual muscle testing (MMT)**. MMT evaluates muscle groups responsible for pure motions and isolates single muscles when possible.

An individual moves through a specified range of motion against the resistance of gravity, that is, the weight of the body part moved. If this motion is complete, the evaluator adds resistance at the endpoint of the range; if the motion is incomplete, the evaluator has the subject attempt to move again after minimizing the effects of gravity through positioning. In this way, the evaluator determines grades above and below fair strength, respectively.

MMT uses a 6-point measuring scale of 0 to 5, with 0 as no movement (no palpable contraction) and 5 as normal strength. A measure of 1 is trace, or palpable contraction; is poor, or insufficient strength to move the body part through the entire active range of motion with gravity's effect minimized; 3 is fair, or the ability to lift the weight of the body part through its active range of motion against gravity; and 4 is good, or the ability to move through complete range of motion against gravity and hold the contraction against some but less than maximum resistance.

The school therapist used MMT to evaluate Zachary's arm strength. She found that Zachary could move his left arm through complete range of motion at all joints and could withstand considerable resistance at each muscle group. On the right side Zach's shoulder muscles all stood up to "normal" resistance, the same as the left shoulder muscles. Zachary could not flex or extend his right elbow as forcefully as the left one. He completed elbow flexion palm up and palm down with "good" resistance (4/5), but not as much resistance as he took on the left side. Zachary extended his elbow enough to place his right hand on his head, but could not quite reach into full elbow extension—hand reaching toward ceiling. The therapist had Zachary put his right hand over his heart and supported his forearm through full extension, moving at chest level out away from his body, to determine that he had "poor" strength (2/5) in his triceps. Zachary rested his forearms palms down on the desk and lifted both hands at the wrist into full wrist extension; but when the OT pushed down across the knuckles Zachary's right hand collapsed down on the desk. She graded Zachary's right wrist extensors as "fair" (3/5).

Practitioners have questioned the subjectivity and consistency of MMT scoring. Some earlier studies indicated a high degree of reliability among experienced practitioners, but more recent work demonstrated otherwise.[*]

Regardless, MMT remains a universally used technique in the assessment of muscle strength; reliability improves with experience. The relatively inexpensive techniques are simple to learn, and a variety of textbooks explain testing in great detail. (Guidelines for the examination of isolated muscle functions are provided in later chapters and on the motion CD.)

The school therapist at Zachary's middle school knew how eagerly he wanted to resume playing baseball. Using information from Zachary's MMT the coach and therapist devised a program to strengthen Zachary's elbow and forearm muscles. In addition they found an athletic brace that would prevent full elbow extension during maximum effort, as in a game. At the therapist's recommendation the coach insisted Zachary avoid using a fastball, and instead they worked to perfect his curveball and "knuckler."

Muscle Tone

Practitioners use observation and palpation (feeling the muscles) to assess muscle tone. Hypertonia, or increased muscle tone, makes muscles feel very firm and causes increased resistance to passive stretching. Although the evaluation of the severity of spasticity has questionable reliability, it is helpful to think of it in terms of a graded response. Severe spasticity causes resistance to quick stretching in the first third of a range of motion. In moderate spasticity resistance occurs during the second third of the range. Mild spasticity results in resistance during the last third of the range of motion. We can also observe hypertonicity as responses to resistance that involve

muscles on the opposite side of the body or muscles located above or below those being tested on the same side. We call uncontrollable resistance throughout a range of motion rigidity.

The classroom aides at *Jason Black*'s school tried teaching him to feed himself by using a "hand-over-hand" technique. They complained to the school OT practitioner that Jason often became "uncooperative" and fought their assistance, especially when he "knew" they had to finish in a hurry. Once the OT practitioner explained how spasticity works, the aides could see that Jason had no control over his ability to "cooperate" with rapid, externally driven movements. They agreed to let Jason feed himself with gentle support at the elbows during relaxed mealtimes, and to put food in his mouth as he opened it on those days when school routines called for shortened lunchtimes.

Hypotonia, or low muscle tone, causes muscles to feel soft and mushy and to give in to sustained resistance. We observe hypotonicity in the postural muscles as individual's slump over a table when sitting or slouch against a wall when standing. Sometimes, but not always, hypotonicity contributes to these postures. Hyper- and hypotonic disturbances in muscles invalidate MMT grades. Most practitioners agree that strength testing in cases of spasticity (as in upper motor neuron syndromes) is an inappropriate assessment. Instead, practitioners assess the severity of spasticity and its impact on function.

MUSCULOSKELETAL MOVEMENT

We can measure joint movement with a **goniometer** (Figure 2-4) by placing it directly over the axis of motion in a joint and aligning the arms of the goniometer with

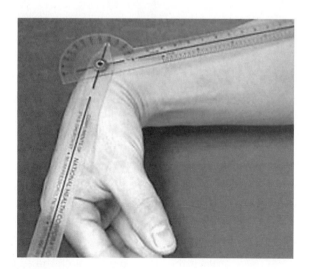

FIGURE **2-4**
Goniometers measure joint position and range of motion.

---

[*]Lawson and Calderon[2] found consistency among practitioners in two of four muscles tested. Freese and others[1] conducted a larger study that demonstrated low consistency in all four muscles tested, even when adhering to a strict testing protocol.

the two musculoskeletal segments extending from the joint. A goniometer measures a full 360 degrees of rotary motion, but most joints exhibit a range of motion within 180 degrees. We typically measure the movement by following the motion of the distal segment in relation to the proximal segment. The proximal segment serves as a nonmoving reference point for the measurement.

In order to accurately communicate with other caregivers, we document movement by reading the goniometer to identify the number of degrees of the arc swept by the distal segment. The segment moves in its circular path along the surface of a plane, around an axis. We measure pure motion in only one plane, although functional motion occurs in a number of planes. [This is most similar to a windshield wiper blade, which sweeps out its arc on the surface of the windshield (plane). The wiper blade moves around an axis located in the "proximal" end of the wiper where it attaches ("articulates") to the base of the windshield.]

Figure 2-5 shows an individual divided into parts by each of the three planes. Each plane exists as a primary plane, but multiple "copies" exist as parallel planes for movements of the various joints. The primary sagittal plane divides the body into right and left halves. Rotary movement in this plane (**flexion** and **extension**) centers on an axis oriented left to right, also referred to as side-to-side. Vertebral flexion and extension occur along the surface of this plane. Flexion and extension of joints such as the shoulder, elbow, and wrist occur in a parallel sagittal plane.

Abduction and **adduction** occur in the frontal plane. This plane divides the body into front and back halves, and movement orients around an axis that runs front-to-back, or anterior-to-posterior. Examples of joints displaying abduction and adduction include the shoulder, wrist, and hip.

Rotation occurs in the transverse, or horizontal, plane, which divides the body into upper and lower halves. The axis for movement in this plane always orients in an up-to-down position. As in flexion and

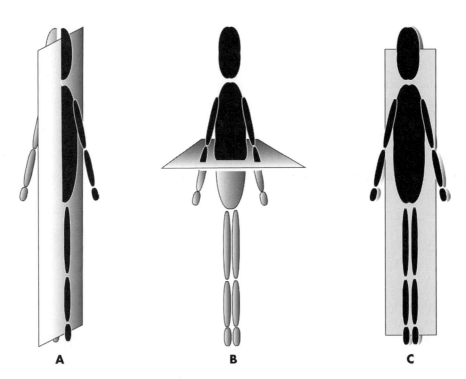

A   **B**   **C**

FIGURE **2-5**
We divide the human body into three anatomical planes, each of which is associated with an axis around which movement takes place. **A** demonstrates the sagittal plane; **B**, the horizontal plane; **C**, the frontal plane. The axis of movement is oriented 90 degrees to the plane of movement, and the movement sweeps out an arc around the axis and on the surface of the plane. In the game "Pin the Tail on the Donkey," the board onto which we attach the tail is the plane, and the pin is the axis. After the pin is stuck into the board (oriented at 90 degrees to the board), the tail swings along the surface of the board (plane) and around the axis (pin).

extension, rotation at various joints including shoulder, hip and knee occurs along transverse planes situated parallel to the primary transverse plane shown in Figure 2-5.

Goniometry measures the extent of active and passive joint motions within these planes. Active motion occurs when an individual uses muscle contractions to voluntarily move a body part. Passive motion occurs when someone or something moves the body part in the absence of muscle contractions across the joints of the part being moved.

MEDICAL DIAGNOSES AFFECTING MOVEMENT

Any pathological condition that affects the nervous system or the musculoskeletal system has some effect on movement. How movement changes varies according to the condition and the individual involved. A brief look at some conditions that can affect movement follows.

Many different pathological processes, from traumatic injuries to illnesses, can affect the CNS. When the head receives severe blows or rocks forward and backward violently, damage to the cerebrum results.*

Physicians diagnose a *cerebral vascular accident* (CVA) or *stroke* when CNS damage occurs after intracerebral bleeding or clotting. A variety of illnesses, such as multiple sclerosis, which affects the myelin sheath covering nerves, also cause damage to CNS tissues.

In all cases, damage to the cerebrum affects voluntary and involuntary movements. Generally, problems that affect one hemisphere restrict movements on the opposite side of the body. Damage to cerebellar structures affects muscle tone and coordination. Spinal cord damage affects muscle use and sensation below the level of the lesion. We can map this damage according to the affected ranges of sensory and motor loss.

Damage to peripheral nerves affects individual muscles and areas of sensation. Peripheral nerves get cut, crushed, or attacked by viruses, bacteria, and the body's immune response system. Peripheral nerve fibers have the ability to regenerate, unlike CNS structures. If the nerve cell body remains intact after injury, recovery of muscle use and sensation often occurs.

Metabolic problems, trauma, and disease often result in skeletal disorders, which affect movement. Some conditions such as scoliosis occur because of abnormally formed but healthy bone tissue. In scoliosis the vertebral bodies form an abnormal spinal curvature. Muscle imbalance, wedge-shaped vertebrae, severe

weakness, or lack of adequate trunk support may lead to scoliosis or scoliosis may have an idiopathic cause (no known reason).

Severe scoliosis can compromise the heart, lungs, and other organs. Although surgery sometimes offers the only permanent solution, careful positioning that provides lateral support to the trunk may slow the progression of spinal curvatures.

Diseases that alter bone development can influence movement. For example, osteogenesis imperfecta affects the metabolic formation of bone tissue and makes the bone more susceptible to fracture and deformity. Fractures or trauma to the epiphyseal plates in growing children may disrupt or halt bone growth. Damage to a bone's blood supply can lead to avascular necrosis and progressive bone deterioration.

Osteoporosis affects bone through a gradual decrease in calcium content. The bone becomes weaker until it fractures during normal shifts in body weight or with muscle contractions. Weakened bones place older adults with age-related osteoporosis at greater risk of fractures from falls.

Both biomechanics and kinesiology play parts in the treatment of fractures. Normal muscle forces can contribute to the misalignment of fractured fragments and deserve consideration in splinting or range-of-motion restrictions, such as those provided after hip fractures, surgical replacement of hip joint components, or total hip arthroplasty (A Closer Look Box 2-3).

Damage to joints also may restrict movement. Fractures that cross the joint line or extend to the joint surface may result in limited joint motion after the fracture has healed completely. Ligaments severely damaged through

---

*Infants in particular are susceptible to this form of trauma. Their neck muscles are insufficient to stabilize the head, and even brief shaking can cause brain damage.

BOX 2-3

A **CLOSER** LOOK

Range of Motion Precautions after Hip Surgery
Hip-replacement surgery, or total hip arthroplasty, repairs the hip joint but leaves it vulnerable. If an individual moves the wrong way, the carefully placed artificial joint can move out of alignment due to the muscle forces acting on it. Hip precautions differ slightly depending on the surgical approach used, but most surgeons usually recommend the following movement modifications after total hip arthroplasty:

- No hip flexion beyond 90 degrees
- No hip internal rotation past the neutral position
- No hip adduction past the neutral position

dislocation may produce chronic joint instability or predispose the joint to stiffening and decreased range of motion from osteoarthritis.

Rheumatoid arthritis, in contrast, causes joints to become loose and unstable. The joints may exhibit subluxation under normal use and muscle pull, causing misalignments such as ulnar drift (Figure 2-6, *A*). Boutonniere misalignment consists of hyperflexion in the proximal interphalangeal joint (Figure 2-6, *B*). Swan neck causes hyperextension of the proximal interphalangeal joint, which may occur with volar subluxation

(Figure 2-6, *C*). Each condition commonly leads to secondary joint contractures involving the distal interphalangeal joints. (We will explore these four conditions more fully in later chapters.)

A pathological condition of the joint also can occur after a CVA when the weight of the affected arm stretches the joint capsule and separates the head of the humerus from the glenoid fossa. In this situation, instead of measuring joint motion with a goniometer, we often describe shoulder subluxation in terms of the distance developed between bony landmarks.

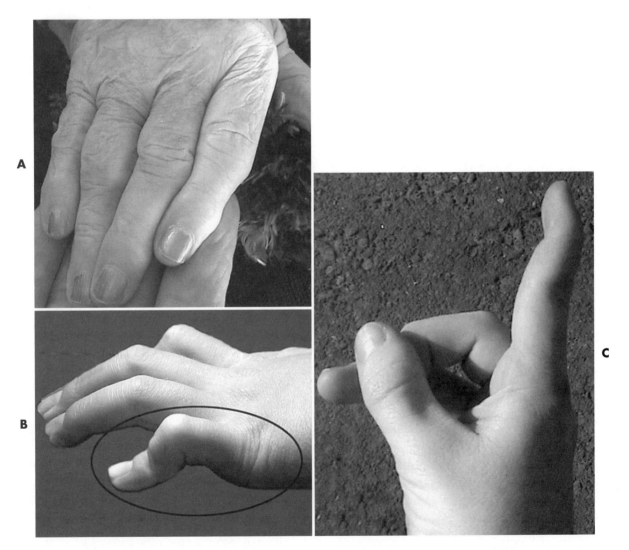

FIGURE **2-6**
A, Ulnar drift occurs after displacement of the extensor digitorum tendon in the ulnar direction. Digits 2 through 5 exhibit a measurable amount of ulnar deviation at the metacarpophalangeal joints. **B**, Boutonniere involves a buttonhole tear in the extensor aponeurosis and inability to actively extend the proximal interphalangeal joint. **C**, Swan neck exhibits hyperextension of the proximal interphalangeal joint and may occur with volar subluxation of the metacarpophalangeal joint. Here it is shown in the long finger.

Tendons and muscles also suffer from movement-related pathological conditions. Boutonniere consists of a buttonhole tear in the elaborate extensor tendon of the extensor digitorum communis muscle. The proximal interphalangeal joint protrudes through this hole as the finger flexes. When the tendon falls from the posterior to the anterior side of the joint axis of motion, further contraction of the extensor muscle causes the finger to bend rather than straighten (see Figure 2-6, *B*).

Imbalances in muscle function make specific movements difficult or impossible. For example, weak or nonfunctioning intrinsic muscles of the hand prevent a strong extensor digitorum communis muscle from extending the fingers completely. When the extensor contracts, the interphalangeal joints extend, but the metacarpophalangeal joint hyperextends. Over time, metacarpophalangeal hyperextension increases and interphalangeal extension becomes less complete. We call the resulting condition *intrinsic minus* (Figure 2-7).

Repeated use of a tendon causes tendinitis, or inflammation of the tendon. Painful swelling usually results and sometimes causes severe crowding of tissues and reduced blood flow. Damage to nearby nerves can follow severe and prolonged episodes of swelling.

Wendy Dabdoub, a fruit packer for a mail order company, acquired tingling in the thumbs and index fingers of both hands after a particularly busy season. Her physician diagnosed carpal tunnel syndrome, caused by long hours of repetitive finger flexion leading to swelling of the flexor tendons and impingement of the median nerve.

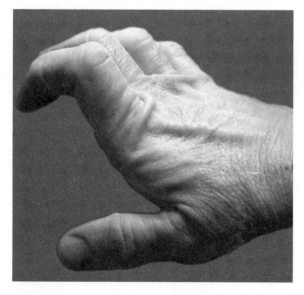

FIGURE **2-7**
The hallmark of intrinsic minus hand ("claw") is metacarpophalangeal hyperextension with incomplete interphalangeal extension.

Concepts from Physics and Engineering

When physicists talk about a body, they refer to a collection of matter. A body may be incredibly small, like protons and electrons, to unimaginably large, like stars. The human body is a specific collection of matter. In physics the generic term body must have specific modifiers to prevent confusion.

Physicists quantify space, time, and mass to describe their relationships with one another. Different systems of measurement develop in different cultures. Most Americans use the English system, but the scientific community worldwide uses the metric system. This book uses both systems in different examples to represent practitioners' typical thinking and problem-solving in various practice settings. (Appendix A contains a complete conversion table for English and metric systems.)

SCALAR QUANTITIES

We call static quantities, measured by an instrument or a scale, scalar. These quantities tend to stay in one place, making them relatively easy to measure.

Measures of Space
Length, area, and volume are spatial measurements. In the metric system, we measure space in millimeters, centimeters, and meters. The English system measures space in inches, feet, and yards. Length has one dimension, so we use a linear measure of distance (centimeters, meters, inches, and miles). Area has two dimensions and uses a planar measure of its flat surface (square centimeters or square feet). Volume has three dimensions requiring a cubic measurement (cubic centimeters, liters, cubic inches, quarts, and gallons).

Measures of Time
Time presents a fourth dimension. Both the metric and the English systems use seconds as the basic unit of measurement for time.

Measures of Mass
Matter consists of the neutrons, protons, and electrons that come together to make up atoms and further collect into molecules. The chemical composition of a substance and the closeness of its molecules determine the quantity of mass. For example, a hydrogen atom has only

1 proton and electron pair, whereas larger atoms like carbon, nitrogen, and oxygen have 6, 7, and 8 proton–electron pairs. Potassium, calcium, and iron have 19, 20, and 26, respectively. As OT practitioners, we rarely consult a periodic table to discover the number of proton–electron pairs in a particular element, but we do encounter matter daily and need to understand this concept.

The arrangements of these elements within solids, liquids, and gases affect the mass of the different substances. Closely packed molecules form solids. In liquids molecules move freely around each other, and in gases they bounce around and keep their distance from everything else. Water behaves in a class by itself.

Hydrogen, carbon, and oxygen compounds form the tissues of the human body in various arrangements. Their slightly different chemical compositions determine their mass. Bone and muscle, which have more calcium and iron in their compositions, have a greater density than fat, for example.

VECTOR QUANTITIES

A **vector** indicates movement. It can be measured only at a specific moment in time because it constantly changes. Arrows that indicate a starting point (point of application), magnitude, and direction represent vectors. A simple arrowhead drawn on the end of a line converts a haphazard mark into a story indicating a specific force, a specific point at which it was applied, and a specific direction in which it is moving.

Measures of Physical Movement

The vector quantity displacement indicates movement from a designated starting point, motion in a specific direction, and distance traveled. A more familiar vector quantity, velocity (v), requires us to divide displacement (s) by time (t). We can express velocity, the rate at which displacement occurs, as an equation:

$$v = s/t$$

When velocity increases, it accelerates; acceleration is the change in velocity over time. Therefore we calculate acceleration (a) by subtracting an initial velocity (u) from a final velocity (v) and dividing the result by time (t).

$$a = \frac{v - u}{t}$$

Measures of Weight

Weight, another familiar vector quantity, reflects both mass and the pull of gravity on that mass. Gravity always pulls toward the center of the Earth. For example,

individuals stand on the Earth's surface with their feet toward the Earth's center and experience gravity as a downward pull, a vector quantity. As long as we stand on the Earth's surface, we must calculate gravity as a constant factor; therefore as mass increases, weight increases. In the English system, we measure weight (a force) in **pounds**. In the metric system, we measure weight in **newtons,** named after Sir Isaac Newton. He first realized that gravity gives mass its direction when an apple landed on his head.

Measures of Force

In physics, **forces** cause objects to deform or move and are represented in their actions as vectors. The force muscles produce is the most common force encountered in this text.

Drawing muscle forces as vectors requires that we understand that a muscle contraction applies force to one segment at one attachment of the muscle and directs the force specifically in the direction of the other attachment. The length of a vector indicates the specific amount of force generated by the muscle contraction. Because the arrow indicates the amount of force, we may draw these vectors longer or shorter than the actual muscle itself. Vectors can originate from the proximal attachment or the distal attachment of the muscle, depending on the direction of movement, but the arrowed line always runs parallel to the direction of muscle fibers (Figure 2-8).

Normal forces act perpendicularly toward or away from a surface area. Compressive normal forces push two surfaces together (Figure 2-9, *A*). Tensile normal forces pull two surfaces apart (Figure 2-9, *B*). In contrast, shear, or tangential, forces act parallel to surface areas (Figure 2-9, *C*).

Gravity is a normal force. Reaction forces, another type of normal force, produce an equal and opposite response to gravity or other forces. Muscle forces producing joint motion often result in joint reaction forces respond in a variety of ways to reaction forces.

Measures of Stress

Unlike force, stress occurs in the material on which forces act. Tensile forces on the knee produce tensile stress in the tissues of the knee joint. We determine the amount of stress produced by dividing the amount of force by the specific quantity of tissue on which it acts. We measure stress in units of Pascals (Pa) or newtons per square meter (N/m^2). Stress also can be measured in pounds per square inch (psi).

Measures of Friction

Similar to stress, friction occurs on surface areas. To determine friction (F), multiply a normal force (N)

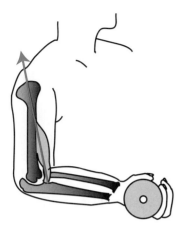

FIGURE **2-8**
A vector representing the pull (force) of a muscle must be drawn from the moving attachment, through the muscle fibers, toward the stationary attachment.

times a coefficient (μ) unique to the material in question:

$$F = \mu N$$

For instance, the coefficient of cartilage in a synovial joint is essentially 0, whereas the coefficient of a crutch tip on rough wood is about 0.70 to 0.75 (Figure 2-10). The closer a coefficient gets to 1.0, the more force we need to move that material across a specific surface.

Measures of Work

We calculate work by multiplying weight by distance by the number of repetitions. For example, to measure the amount of lifting work needed to do a job, use the following formula:

$$L = w \times h \times r$$

Here, L represents lifting work, w represents the weight of the object, h represents the height of objects lifted, and r represents the number of repetitions. To find the amount of hauling work done on a job, use the following formula:

$$H = w \times d \times r$$

H represents hauling work, w is its weight, d is the distance traveled, and r is the number of repetitions.

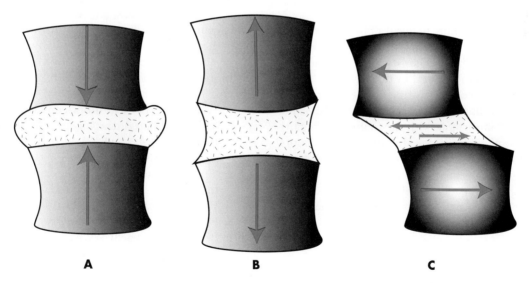

A   **B**   **C**

FIGURE **2-9**
Normal forces act perpendicular to surfaces pushing together as compressive forces **(A)** or pulling apart as tensile forces **(B)**. Shear forces act parallel to the surfaces they affect **(C)**. Stress occurs in the materials on which forces act.

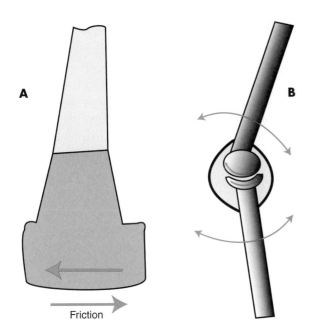

FIGURE 2-10
We determine friction by the nature of the surface material. The friction between a rubber crutch tip and concrete **(A)** is much greater than that between two cartilaginous joint surfaces coated with synovial fluid **(B)**.

Summary

An OT practitioner's ability to accurately analyze functional activity depends on the ability to understand and apply principles of biomechanics and kinesiology. Biomechanics and kinesiology, in turn, require familiarity with the basic concepts of medicine and physics presented in this chapter. Often OT practitioners and students seem comfortable with medicine, but regard physics as strange territory. The physical concepts presented in this chapter form an intrinsic part of every problem presented in the chapters that follow, so that in solving them the reader develops as much comfort applying physics to human activity as he or she may have orienting to the human musculoskeletal system.

Applications

■ APPLICATION 2-1
Appreciating Mass and Gravity

We must begin to think about mass and gravity separately to understand how they operate, especially once we move beyond the confines of this planet. Although our body mass changes throughout life, the Earth's gravity does not. As mass changes so does gravity's effect on it—we experience this as weight. To appreciate mass, we must remove the effect of gravity:

1. Obtain samples of two vastly different elements: lead (a fishing weight) and aluminum (foil).
2. Crumple a piece of aluminum foil to equal roughly the size of the fishing weight.
3. Compare the two weights by feel.

Which is heavier? Because gravity affects both equally, what accounts for the difference in weight?

■ APPLICATION 2-2
Identifying the Active Muscle

To understand which muscles affect movements we must reexamine what we learned studying gross anatomy through books and cadaver dissection. Without realizing it, most of us developed a bias that flexors flex and extensors extend. When we observe elbow flexion as a movement, we often credit elbow flexors as the primary source of power, but in the following case, activation of the elbow flexors to control elbow flexion would lead to disaster.

Imagine slowly lowering a bowling ball from above your head to the top of your head. The elbow moves from extension into flexion. Elbow extensors work hard to control the rate of elbow flexion. *Don't* activate the elbow flexors. The ball will accelerate and hit your head.

Try this activity. Hold a heavy book above your head with your elbow fully extended. Lower it slowly about half the distance to the top of your head. At this point the elbow has flexed through about 45 degrees of motion. Hold it there and think about the active group:

1. Palpate the belly of the triceps and compare this feeling to that of the biceps. Which muscle feels more active? As you hold the book overhead, which muscle gets sore?
2. Now raise the book two times and palpate the two muscles one at a time each time you raise the book. Which muscle feels more active?
3. Now lower the book slowly two times and again determine the active group.
4. Repeat these steps with the opposite hand and measure the origin-to-insertion distance for the long head of the triceps (infraglenoid tubercle to the olecranon). Now move into flexion, stopping at 45 degrees. Again measure origin to insertion. What happened to the distance as you slowly flexed the elbow? Which muscle was active? What kind of contraction takes place?
5. As you hold the book steady with a partially flexed elbow, what happens to the origin-to-insertion

distance for the triceps long head? Which muscle was active? What kind of contraction takes place?

6. As you raise the book back into full elbow extension, what happens to the triceps long head origin-to-insertion distance? Which muscle was active? What kind of contraction occurs?

See Appendix C for solutions to Applications.

REFERENCES

1. Freese F, Brown M, Norton BJ: Clinical reliability of manual muscle testing middle trapezius and gluteus medius muscles, *Phys Ther* 67(7):1072-1076, 1987.
2. Lawson A, Calderon L: Interexaminer agreement for applied kinesiology manual muscle testing, *Percept Mot Skills* 84(2):539-546, 1997.

RELATED READINGS

Behrman RE, Kliegman RM, Jenson HB: *Nelson textbook of pediatrics*, ed 17, Philadelphia, 2003, Saunders.
Fiorentino M: *Reflex testing methods for evaluating CNS development*, ed 2, Springfield, Ill, 1973, Charles C Thomas.
Fritjof C: *The Tao of physics*, New York, 1984, Bantam.
Gowitzke BA, Milner M: *Scientific bases of human movement*, ed 3, Baltimore, 1987, Williams & Wilkins.
Leveau BF: *Williams & Lissner's biomechanics of human motion*, ed 3, Philadelphia, 1992, WB Saunders.
Norkin CC, Levangie PK: *Joint structure and function: a comprehensive analysis*, ed 2, Philadelphia, 1992, FA Davis.
Rasch PJ: *Kinesiology and applied anatomy*, ed 7, Philadelphia, 1989, Lea & Febiger.
Williams PL, Bannister LH: *Gray's anatomy: the anatomical basis of medicine and surgery*, ed 38, New York, 1995, Churchill Livingstone.

LAB BOX

Find applied activities exploring concepts in Chapter 2 in the following laboratory exercises:

Topic	Laboratory
Movements in planes around axes	**Lab 1** Kinematic Chain, Human Musculoskeletal Movement, Shoulder Model of Joint Movement
Goniometry and Manual Muscle Testing	**Lab 3** Overview of ROM & MMT
Vectors drawn to represent muscle contraction force	**Lab 3** Overview of ROM & MMT
Muscle excursion	**Lab 4** Accessory Joint Motions/Muscle Excursion/Active & Passive Insufficiency/Max Assist Transfers
Eccentric muscle contractions controlling gravity; differentiating contractions in activity	Biomechanical Analysis Lab

Gravity

A Constant Force

KEY**TERMS**

Gravity Environment
Center of Gravity
Segmental Centers of Gravity
Percentage Weight
Gravitational Attraction
Rate of Acceleration
Weight
Center of Gravity Height
Base of Support
Center of Gravity Projection
Weight (as a Stability Factor)
Camber

Gravity affects every aspect of movement. We feel its constant tug on our bodies even before birth. From infancy we struggle to stand upright and break free of its pull. We drop toys off our high chair trays to experiment with gravity. It keeps us seated upright in chairs and creates the familiar slouches we assume in sofas and overstuffed chairs. Gravity imposes itself on our system at every turn—sometimes helping, most times hindering. This constant struggle causes us to fall into bed exhausted at the end of the day. In fact, gravity permeates so much of our daily experiences that we know intuitively how it works.

We know that skiers and parachutists move in the same direction—down. If we throw a bowling ball and a baseball out the window at the same time, we expect them to land on the ground at the same time. We know that rockets break free of the Earth's pull of gravity because they have tremendous power. Gravity holds the space shuttle in orbit around our planet, just as the moon orbits the Earth and the Earth orbits the sun. We take these facts for granted.

Yet, if we had stated these beliefs 500 years ago, we could have been persecuted or put to death.* Even 400 years ago, students and professors argued ideas about gravity that seem like common sense to us today.

In the late sixteenth century, Galileo explored movement with a series of experiments in which he rolled objects down ramps. From these experiments, he developed laws of uniform acceleration, which state that objects of differing sizes and weights travel at equal speeds. These "radical" ideas caused the University of Pisa to force his resignation from teaching in 1592.

A mathematician, Galileo wrote these laws of uniform acceleration as mathematics equations. Some 20 years after Galileo's death, Isaac Newton used these formulas not only to explain why objects always fall to the ground but also to extrapolate gravity as the underlying force affecting all movement, celestial and earthbound. Newton's laws of motion help us understand forces and their interactions. These laws have become part of our general experience with gravity. We readily accept that gravity produces a constant force on matter (A Closer Look Box 3-1).

---

*In 1600, authorities burned Italian priest and scholar Giordano Bruno at the stake for speculating on similarities between the stars and the sun. He believed planets might circle the stars as a result of the same forces that cause the Earth to revolve around the sun.

Gravity and the Development of Movement

Gravity exerts physical effects on bodies to the extent that all internal muscle forces respond in one way or another to the **gravity environment.** Voluntary movements are neuromuscular responses to external stimuli; these movements look and feel radically different in the gravity-free environment of space or the gravity-diminished environment of the moon than those same movements do here on Earth.

In early life, gravity acts as both a stimulus and a barrier to movement. Infants must overcome its effects to raise their heads, reach out, crawl, and stand. Gravity also stimulates mechanisms (reflexes) within the body that result in movement. Gravity's tug on muscle stretch receptors (muscle spindles) results in muscle contractions, yielding trunk and limb movements. Gravity makes an infant's environment rich with experience in movement.

When a baby lies in the prone position with her head unsupported, gravity pulls on the head and produces head and neck flexion that stretches the neck extensors. Gravity first stimulates and then resists contractions in the neck extensor muscles. Likewise, a baby lying in a supine position with his head unsupported experiences gravity pulling the head into extension. Gravity stretches, stimulates, and resists the neck flexors. Supporting the back of the baby's head, gravity acts to rotate the head to the left or right, stretching, stimulating, and resisting various neck rotators. Over time infants gain the strength and experience to control their head movements voluntarily.

Development proceeds in response to the environment. Movement caused by gravity in one direction typically leads to movement by muscle contraction in the opposite direction. When an infant begins to support herself with her elbows in the prone position, gravity pulls down on her upper trunk, stretching the shoulder girdle muscles (scapular protractors) and upper back and neck extensors. This stimulus results in responsive contractions, and the baby develops an ability to suspend her upper trunk away from the floor or mat.

As children mature and learn to sit and stand upright, gravity affects the trunk and lower extremity muscles. When the child leans forward, gravity pulls his trunk into more flexion, stretching and stimulating the trunk and hip extensors.

As Jason begins crying the OT assistant reaches out to gently rub and pat his back and neck. "I think the force of gravity

BOX 3-1

A **CLOSER** LOOK

Galileo and Newton

Galileo and Newton explained their ideas with mathematics. Galileo found that whenever he rolled a ball down a ramp, it traveled faster as it reached the bottom of the ramp. He could measure the rate of acceleration (a) by subtracting the initial velocity (u, the distance traveled divided by time, as in miles per hour) from the final velocity (v) and dividing that by time (t). Galileo found that objects always accelerate at the same rate:

$$a = \frac{(v - u)}{t}$$

If objects drop from a tall building, they all experience the same rate of acceleration, 9.8 m/sec².

Newton took Galileo's ideas a step further. He said that all bodies of matter attract one another and that we can measure that force of gravity (F_g) by multiplying a constant (G) times the masses of the two objects (m_1m_2) divided by the square of the distance between them (r^2):

$$F_g = \frac{G(m_1 m_2)}{r^2}$$

Because of the Earth's size, it pulls stronger than any other mass in our environment. This pull is a gravitational constant, 9.8 m/sec². We always measure the force of gravity as mass times acceleration. By considering mass and the acceleration together we come up with weight, the force produced by gravity on mass:

$$F = ma$$

We can determine how gravity affects us when we measure the mass of any object and multiply that by the average rate of acceleration of all objects on Earth, 9.8 m/sec², often rounded to 10 m/sec² for convenience.

If we went to the moon, the average rate of acceleration would change, and we would multiply mass by a different rate of acceleration. We can see this diminished rate of acceleration on video clips from the days of the Apollo explorations as we watch the slow-motion moon walkers. Objects also descend to the moon's surface more slowly due to the smaller pull of gravity in that environment.

We appreciate gravity's effect on us daily when we stand on a scale and read our weight. In this case the multiplication of mass by the constant for the acceleration of gravity has been done in the calibration of the scale. The number value we read in pounds reflects the multiplication of slugs (mass) by the constant, 32 ft/sec² (or 9.8 m/sec² in metric units).

causes Jason's head to drop down and these muscles of his back and neck just don't have enough strength to pull against that force all day long."

"I never considered that," says Jason's teacher. "Is there anything we can do to help him?"

"Actually, we can try a number of things," says the OT assistant. While tapping the long extensor muscles in Jason's neck, the OT assistant wonders whether this added stimulation to his muscle stretch receptors or "hope" has had a greater part in helping Jason raise his head upright again.

Gravity interacts with Jason's impaired motor status to create a disability, although the World Health Organization's International Classification of Functioning, Disability, and Health does not yet consider gravity as an Environmental Factor[4] leading to disability. Sadly, Jason's class has no field trips planned for scuba diving or visits to the moon where Jason could demonstrate increased attentiveness by holding his head up more easily.

Gravity plays a large role in its affect on stretch reflexes, but it also has more subtle effects. The delicate vestibular mechanism of the inner ear (labyrinth) responds to gravity's downward pull on small crystals of calcium carbonate (otoliths) located there. Movements of the head stimulate hair cells in gelatinous material surrounding the otoliths and in the fluid of the semicircular canals. These hair cells transmit messages to the brain, causing awareness of head movement. They also produce a variety of eye, trunk, and limb movements known as *labyrinthine reflexes*.[2,3]

"Do you really think a couple of dance sessions in OT will help Mrs. Smith lose weight?" asks the head nurse. "I think she'd do better walking up and down the halls with PT."

"Well, walking would certainly help, but in our dance group we do a lot of bending and twirling. These movements will stimulate Mrs. Smith's balance systems so hopefully she will have less fear when she leans forward. I think if Mrs. Smith can lean forward more easily she will have enough strength to stand up with only one person assisting her."

In Mrs. Smith's case, everyone understands gravity's role all too well: Mrs. Smith's weight. OT taught her to handle her weight and use gravity to assist in transfers. Successful transfer training for the nursing staff and the added stimulation of dance on Mrs. Smith's vestibular system could reduce her fear of falling (fear of gravity!).

In all these examples, gravity's effect on body segments concentrates around the center of gravity, a central point. We use this point in diagrams to represent the effect of gravity acting on the body or a specific limb segment.

Gravity and the Human Body

Gravity's force acts on a body's **center of gravity** by pulling it down toward the center of the Earth. In uniform bodies like balls and cubes, we find the center of gravity located in the exact center of the object. Bodies have three dimensions; therefore we must locate the exact center of three planes, each of which divides the object into equal halves.

Figure 3-1 shows an orange cut three ways to demonstrate these planes. The first cut from top to bottom divides the orange into front and back pieces; the second divides it into left and right pieces. The third cut is from side to side and divides the fruit into top and bottom sections. Each cut represents the surface of a plane. The two top to bottom planes intersect to form a central line, and the third plane intersects that line at its center. The point where all three cuts (planes) meet is the center of gravity.

The human body lacks uniformity, but we find its center of gravity in much the same way. The body's sagittal plane divides it into left and right halves, its frontal plane separates front from back, and its horizontal plane forms top and bottom sections. Like the orange, a person's center of gravity is the point at which the three planes meet.

We define a body's center of gravity as its *balance point.* Mobiles suspend objects from strings connected to each object's balance point. As the mobile moves, the objects may shift position but remain balanced. The subtle changes in movement make the mobile bodies appear to float. An object suspended from a point other than its center of gravity remains stationary.

For example, in Figure 3-2, *A,* a bicycle wheel hangs by a cord tied around its rim. The part of the rim attached to the cord remains the highest point. We can elevate another part of the rim, but once we release it, the wheel falls back into its original position.

However, once we attach a cord to the wheel's axle (its center of gravity) as in Figure 3-2, *B,* it does not matter how we move the wheel. Wherever we release the wheel is where it stays. A balanced wheel remains at rest in any position.

Any analysis of activity must account for the force of gravity acting on the person and tools or other objects involved. The force of gravity always has its effect at the body's center of gravity. We indicate it with a line drawn straight downward from that point (A Closer Look Box 3-2).

CENTERS OF GRAVITY

Our center of gravity changes when we move. The human body moves constantly, so its center of gravity

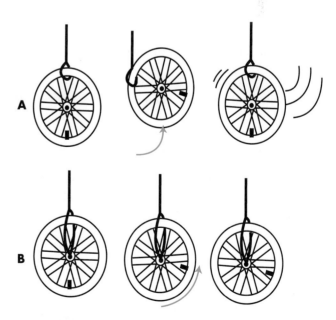

FIGURE **3-2**
A, A bicycle wheel suspended from a point other than its center of gravity falls to its most stable position. **B,** A rotated wheel stays in any position once suspended from its center of gravity.

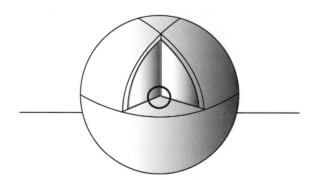

FIGURE **3-1**
The vertical and horizontal planes meet at an object's center of gravity, indicated here by the circle around the point where the three planes meet.

BOX 3-2

A CLOSER LOOK

Vectors Representing the Pull of Gravity

Gravity is a force and must be drawn as a vector. Use these general guidelines to indicate vectors representing gravity when you diagram an activity:

1. Use a small circle to indicate the center of gravity.
2. Draw a line from the circle to indicate the direction of gravity's pull. Always make the line perpendicular (90 degrees) to the ground.
3. Draw an arrowhead on the end of the line to indicate the direction in which gravity pulls. Always put the arrow on the end of the line closest to the Earth so that the *arrow* points toward the center of the Earth.
4. Make the length of the line proportional to the body's weight. It helps to write down the scale so that you do not forget it. For instance, 1 cm = 10 newtons (N). The scale converts distance (1 cm) to a measure of weight/force (10 N).

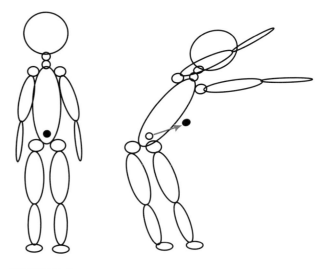

FIGURE **3-3**
Body position influences the entire body's center of gravity. With the arms raised and the trunk arched to the left side, the center of gravity moves upward and leftward. The *arrow* in this figure represents the direction the center of gravity moved when the body position changed.

constantly changes. When we stand upright, our center of gravity lies in the abdominal cavity, about 6 inches above the pubic symphysis. As we move our arms and legs, this center of gravity shifts, and in some instances it becomes located outside the physical body (Figure 3-3).

To determine the center of gravity for the entire human body, we must locate each body segment's center of gravity. Then we tabulate the cumulative effect of these **segmental centers of gravity** to locate a new center of gravity.

OT practitioners also use segmental centers of gravity when analyzing the forces that operate on a specific body part, for instance, when they design orthotic or adaptive equipment. We call diagrams of human body segments free body diagrams. We indicate individual muscles, other forces, and a specific segment's center of gravity with vectors drawn from their respective points of action.

The center of gravity in a nonuniform object lies closer to the end with the greatest mass. For example, the forearm has more proximal bulk; therefore we would expect its center of gravity to lie closer to the elbow than the wrist.

To get more specific than this, we use percentages of total body mass for each body segment; this has already been determined through research.[1] (Table 3-1 gives each body segment's **percentage weight,** and Figure B-1 in Appendix B shows the center of gravity in terms of a percentage of distance from either end of a line running proximal to distal.) This information enables us to draw

a more exact center of gravity for each body segment on a line drawing, a photograph, or an actual person.

School staff asks an OT practitioner to design a piece of equipment that would help Jason eat more independently. To scoop food from a bowl, Jason needs to flex his forearm to about 90 degrees. The OT practitioner determines the center of gravity of Jason's forearm by measuring the distance from his olecranon process to the styloid process of his ulna [25 centimeters (cm)]. She multiplies that distance by the percentage value from

TABLE 3-1
Proportional Percentages of Body Segments to Total Body Weight*

BODY SEGMENT	% OF TOTAL BODY WEIGHT
Head and neck	7.9
Trunk with head and neck	56.5
Upper arm	2.7
Forearm	1.5
Hand	0.6
Thigh	9.7
Lower leg	4.5
Foot	1.4

*Modified from Dempster WT: *Space requirements of the seated operator,* WADC technical report 55-159, Fairborn, Ohio, 1955, Wright-Patterson Air Force Base.

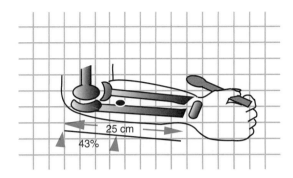

FIGURE **3-4**
Multiply the length of the forearm by the percentage from Figure B-1 to determine the forearm's center of gravity.

Appendix B, Figure B-1 (43% from the olecranon process or 57% from the styloid process). The product of 25 cm and 0.43 cm is 10.8 cm. The OT practitioner starts at the olecranon and measures 10.8 cm down the forearm. She places a dot on the forearm diagram to represent its center of gravity (Figure 3-4). A vector representing the pull of gravity on Jason's forearm would begin at this point.

We can apply this segmental method of determining center of gravity to the entire person in a specific position by taking a photograph and superimposing it onto a graph or by making a scale drawing on a grid.

During the kitchen evaluation for Iris Clark, a 60-kilogram (kg) housewife with a hand injury and multiple sclerosis, a student intern studies the effect of Iris' position on various lower extremity muscle groups and her overall stability. (Figure 3-5, A, shows a scale drawing of Iris standing on one leg reaching into an overhead cabinet.) The student starts by measuring the length of Iris' body segments. Next he multiplies the percentage amount from Appendix B, Figure B-1 to determine each segment's center of gravity. The student marks each bony segment and its center of gravity with small circles that correspond to x and y coordinates on a grid (Figure 3-5, B).

Our total body center of gravity includes the centers of gravity for each body segment. Because x and y coordinates give us specific positions for segmental centers of gravity, we use these coordinates multiplied by each segment's percentage of body weight to calculate a center of gravity for the entire body. Each segment moves the center of gravity of the entire body up or down and left or right in proportion to that segment's weight and position.

The student intern multiplies the proportion of body segment weight (see Table 3-1) by Iris' segmental center of gravity x and y coordinates. (Table 3-2 shows these calculations.) The student locates Iris' center of gravity on x coordinate −1.74 and y coordinate 2.88. He marks this spot with a large dot (see Figure 3-5, B) and draws a vector to represent the force of gravity acting on Iris' total body mass. (Remember, the combination of mass and gravity's effect equals weight.)

Adaptive equipment and tools can alter an individual's center of gravity. Imagine how the use of a reacher might affect Iris' center of gravity. It could allow her to stand on both feet (with greater stability) or encourage her to reach even farther, thus pulling her center of gravity farther from the center of her body (possibly causing her to fall). Another example is forward and upward shift of the center of gravity occurring while sitting in a wheelchair due to hip and knee flexion while sitting (Figure 3-6). A lack of lower extremities shifts an individual's center of gravity rearward. If the wheelchair's design does not accommodate the posterior shift, the chair may tip over.

Xavier Morales, a salesman who lost both legs in the Vietnam war uses several wheelchairs. When making sales presentations he usually wears his prostheses and uses a standard wheelchair. When he plays basketball Xavier wants to move fast (push less weight) and leaves his prostheses at home. Xavier's basketball chair has its larger wheels placed farther toward the rear than a standard wheelchair to accommodate a posterior shift in his center of gravity. (We will explore this scenario when we discuss stability.)

Mass, Weight, and Acceleration

We have considered gravity and its effect on objects. We now turn to gravity's daily effect on us as we move our bodies and use tools.

Newton said all objects gravitate toward each other with an attraction in proportion to their mass. The Earth's large mass overwhelms smaller attractions that occur between objects on the planet. We feel the pull of **gravitational attraction** when we jump. The massive Earth causes all objects on it to move toward its center. This pulling force of attraction changes in proportion to an object's mass, but its **rate of acceleration** remains constant.

Consider standing at windows on various floors of a tall building. If we drop a bowling ball and a billiard ball off various floors, we can observe the following phenomena: When the balls fall from the first floor, they hit the ground in 1 second (sec). When they fall from the fourth floor, they hit the ground in 2 sec. When they fall from the ninth floor, they hit the ground in 3 sec. They take 4 sec to reach the ground from the sixteenth floor.

We will notice that the balls always land simultaneously and the rate of acceleration follows a pattern proportional to the square root of the distance traveled. The average rate of acceleration caused by the Earth's gravitational field is 9.8 meters per second squared (m/sec²), which we can round off to 10 m/sec². We multiply this constant by the mass of an object to calculate the force

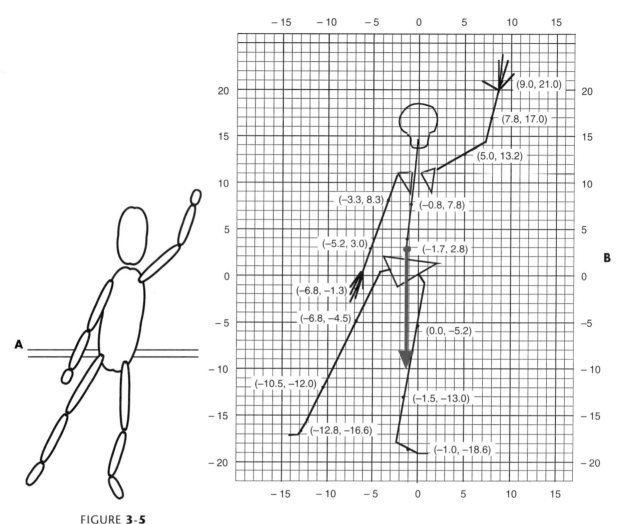

FIGURE **3-5**

A, Iris Clark, 60 kg, stands on her right leg to reach an overhead cabinet. **B**, This motion changes her body's center of gravity in response to the proportion of body weight and its distance from the body's midline. In this case the center of gravity shifts upward. If Iris leaned far enough forward, her center of gravity would fall outside her body and project outside of the base of support.

of gravity's attraction on that object. The **weight** of an object equals the force of gravity's attraction on its mass. In the metric system we measure this force in newtons. One newton equals 9.8 kg-m/sec². To determine an object's weight we multiply its mass (kilograms) by the force of gravity (rate of acceleration, 10 m/sec²).

We might find the difference between weight and mass confusing. At home we read the number that appears on the bathroom scale in pounds, and we understand this unit as a measure of weight. In the clinic we read the numbers written on wrist cuffs and engraved on free weights as kilograms which we likewise interpret as units of weight. But the number of kilograms on weights actually indicates mass, a scalar measurement. To convert kilograms to newtons (a vector measurement), we would have to account for gravity by

multiplying mass (kilograms) by the constant for acceleration (10 m/sec²).

The British system of measurement (which uses pounds as a measure of weight) has a scalar term equivalent to the kilogram, called a slug. Slugs multiplied by the rate of acceleration, 32 ft/sec², give us pounds, a vector force that takes gravity into account. To further confuse things, kilograms (the metric unit of mass) and pounds (the British unit of weight) get used interchangeably to refer to both weight and mass except by scientists and mathematicians, who must make that distinction in their calculations.

The calculations in this text will not require the use of such fine distinctions. We will use pounds or kilograms, the terms most often found in our clinics, to indicate weight (A Closer Look Box 3-3).

	% BODY WEIGHT (EXPRESSED AS DECIMAL)	X COORDINATE	PRODUCT (% BODY WEIGHT × X COORDINATE)	Y COORDINATE	PRODUCT (% BODY WEIGHT × Y COORDINATE)
TABLE 3-2 *The Center of Gravity*					
BODY SEGMENT					
Head and trunk	0.565	−0.8	−0.45	7.8	4.41
Right upper arm	0.027	5.0	0.14	13.2	0.36
Right forearm	0.015	7.8	0.12	17.0	0.26
Right hand	0.006	9.0	0.05	21.0	0.13
Left upper arm	0.027	−3.3	−0.09	8.3	0.22
Left forearm	0.015	−5.2	−0.08	3.0	0.05
Left hand	0.006	−6.8	−0.04	−1.3	−0.01
Right thigh	0.097	0.0	0.00	−5.2	−0.50
Right lower leg	0.045	−1.5	−0.07	−13.0	−0.59
Right foot	0.014	−1.0	−0.01	−18.6	−0.26
Left thigh	0.097	−6.8	−0.66	−4.5	−0.44
Left lower leg	0.045	−10.5	−0.47	−12.0	−0.54
Left foot	0.014	−12.8	−0.18	−16.6	−0.23
Product total*	N/A	N/A	−1.74	N/A	2.86

N/A, not applicable.
*The two product totals serve as the x and y coordinates of the body's center of gravity. x coordinate, −1.74; y coordinate, 2.86.

Factors in Stability

What determines whether an individual falls or maintains balance? Why does an individual fall during a wheelchair or mat transfer? What makes curb-hopping in a wheelchair so difficult? Exploring the factors that affect stability in a gravity-controlled environment provides answers to these questions.

Imagine yourself standing on a thin ledge of rock, high on the face of a mountain. Would you stand tall or crouch down low? Would you place your feet close together or spread them apart? Would you lean forward, backward, leftward, or rightward or plant yourself directly over your feet? Would you take off your belt pack

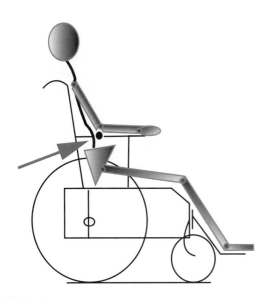

FIGURE **3-6**
The center of gravity for a person seated in a wheelchair lies forward and slightly higher than that of a person standing because of the forward and upward placement of the lower extremities due to hip and knee flexion while sitting.

BOX 3-3

A **CLOSER**LOOK

Daily Encounters with Weight and Mass
In a clinical setting an OT practitioner responds to the question, "How much weight is George lifting?" by reading the number of kilograms marked on the weight. Few OT practitioners carry out the multiplication (for example, 10 kg × 10 m/sec²).

To understand and communicate the forces George uses to lift the weight, we can continue the practical convention and refer to the force of the muscle contraction in kilograms as well. Or we convert the weight and muscle force into true units of force by converting kilogram amounts (mass) into newtons (units of force). To do this, multiply the kilogram amount by 10 m/sec². Keep in mind that weight labeled in pounds requires no multiplication.

or keep its weight around your waist? In each case the second selection represents the most stable choice. These answers demonstrate the four factors that affect stability.

A lower **center of gravity height** gives bodies more stability. Notice that toddlers begin to walk by bending at the knees and hips, lowering their center of gravity. Stability depends on a wide stance, or **base of support**, like the one toddlers adopt. The third factor, the **center of gravity projection**, exhibits interplay with the base of support. Standing straight up on the ledge of rock maintains the center of gravity projection through the base of support. Leaning over projects the center of gravity into dangerous zones.

Balance depends on a center of gravity projection. When this projection falls outside the base of support, we lose our balance. In our efforts to recover we attempt to reposition the center of gravity projection within the base of support. For example, if someone pushes you from behind, you may step forward in the direction of the impending fall, increasing your base of support so that the projection once again falls within it. Alternatively, you may lean backward to place the projection back within the original base of support.

Weight makes the fourth contributing factor in stability. We know that we have a harder time moving a more massive object. Newton stated this as a law: *force equals mass times acceleration (F = ma)*. Simply put, it takes more force to move (accelerate) a larger object. Traditional Japanese Sumo wrestlers demonstrate mastery of stability and weight. High-heeled shoes disregard all four factors (A Closer Look Box 3-4).

UPPER MOTOR NEURON SYNDROME

Stability often becomes a major concern in neurorehabilitation. *When Iris Clark reaches into the overhead cabinet while standing it challenges her stability.* Multiple sclerosis and other upper motor neuron lesions disrupt the normal communication between sensory receptors and motor responses. A cerebral vascular accident (CVA) further challenges balance responses when it results in asymmetrical weight-bearing. Challenges to stability occur on an even more basic level as the individual attempts to sit upright and unsupported on a mat table.

Threats to Balance

Mary Smith has a left-side hemiplegia, the result of a right-side cerebral vascular accident (CVA) several months ago. In the course of her therapy, Mary spends time every day on a mat table in Maple Grove Skilled Care Facility. The area where her

BOX 3-4

A C L O S E R L O O K

High-Heeled Shoes and Stability
High-heeled shoes seem designed to make walking difficult because they violate all four stability factors. High heels raise the center of gravity and shift weight forward onto the toes. Pointed toes narrow the base of support in front, and small heels provide an unnaturally narrow base of posterior support. The higher the heel, the shorter the front-to-back dimension at the base of support. The narrow side-to-side base of support translates into unstable ankles.

Due to the heel height, the center of gravity projection migrates toward the front of an ever-narrowing base of support, concentrating the weight of the body into areas the size of ice-cream cones. Attempting to fight this forward tendency and maintain upright balance, the upper back and shoulders shift to move the center of gravity projection posteriorly into a negligable base of support. Body weight does not change, but its application becomes directed into a small area with an extremely high force. Thus high heels ruin floors and make walking nearly impossible on outdoor surfaces—ever watch the homecoming queen and her court on the football field?

Constant wearing of high heels causes problems in a number of musculoskeletal segments and leads to unhealthy alterations in gait.

buttocks and posterior thighs contact the mat surface forms her base of support (Figure 3-7). Mary's thighs and buttocks make a deep, front-to-back base of support, but the weight of her upper body concentrates at the rear of that base. In other words the projection of Mary's center of gravity lies near the posterior border of her base of support. She must move this inherently unstable projection toward the center of that base for greater stability.

With a posterior location for her center of gravity projection, Mary can sway only a little backward before her upper-body projection falls outside the posterior border of her base of support. As long as Mary's projection remains within that base, the mat's upward push into her body through the base of support balances her upper-body weight's downward pull. Once the projection moves outside that base of support, gravity will pull Mary's upper body down in a place where nothing pushes up to hold her trunk erect. No wonder Mrs. Smith seems fearful of sitting unsupported on the mat.

Normally, projecting the center of gravity backward outside the base of support produces two typical responses. Trunk flexors overcome the extension effect

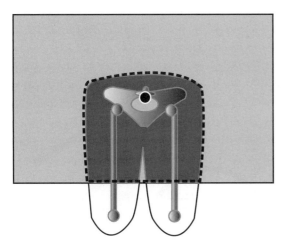

FIGURE **3-7**
Mary's base of support when she sits on a mat table.

of gravity and pull the upper body forward so that the center of gravity projects through the original base; or both shoulders extend to place the hands behind the back, extending the base of support and allowing the center of gravity to project through this new, deeper base.

Mrs. Smith finds these typical responses more difficult because she sustained upper motor neuron impairments after her CVA. Mary's left-side hemiplegia causes her trunk muscles to activate asymmetrically. As the right trunk flexors contract, part of her trunk rotates to the left and flexes laterally to the right instead of flexing forward symmetrically. Attempting the other response, she can extend her right shoulder backward but can move her left arm only minimally to her left side, where it lies with wrist flexed, bearing weight on the dorsal surface. Because of this impairment, her left arm cannot hold its full share of her upper-body weight. Thus she extends the base of support on one side only. The projection of her trunk's center of gravity falls to the left side of her deeper but narrower base of support.

In addition, Mary's altered sensory motor function after her CVA has changed her perception of midline. She tends to lean to the right, shifting the side-to-side dimensions of her base of support and bringing her center of gravity projection closer to the right. This increases her risk of falling. When she leans far enough to the right so that her projection falls outside the base, she loses her balance. Her impaired responses diminish her capacity to recover stability and increase her probability of falling.

Mary has similar difficulties standing because she cannot assume a symmetrical stance even with both feet on the ground. The unreliability of Mary's left lower extremity alters her base of support. Mrs. Smith's functional base of support extends around her right foot only, giving her less than half the normal standing base. This narrow base of support and Mary's impaired ability to shift upper-body weight right-to-left make it difficult for her to maintain a center of gravity projection through her base of support.

Iris Clark's multiple sclerosis affects her sensation and response to weight-bearing, compromising her ability to reach into overhead cabinets. When Iris raises her right hand over her head and forward, her center of gravity moves upward and forward. Her straight-down projection eventually falls outside her base of support, causing her to lose her balance. Iris could put her left hand on the counter, placing it forward to extend her base of support to compensate for her more forward center of gravity projection. She also could use a long-handled reacher, but this too would move her center of gravity, causing it to project downward to a position in front of her base of support. Again she would have to compensate by putting her left hand on the counter.

TRANSFERS

These factors in stability come into play each time someone transfers from a wheelchair to a bed, mat table, or any other surface. A transfer moves the center of gravity from one base of support to another, sometimes with a transitional base in the middle. When the center of gravity projection moves smoothly from one base to another with no more than a momentary projection between the old and new bases of support, we can maintain our sense of balance.

As Mary Smith transfers from her wheelchair to the mat table in a stand-pivot movement, the four points at which the wheels contact the floor outline her existing base of support. The mat table becomes her target base. A box drawn around the outer edges of Mary's shoes defines her transitional base of support. Because an OT practitioner supports Mary, his shoes enlarge the transitional base. Mary and her OT practitioner share this base for a short time.

One day Mary almost fell during a transfer because the OT practitioner placed Mary's feet too close to the wheelchair. While pulling Mary forward in her seat to prepare for the transfer, he placed Mary's feet on the ground between the chair's two front casters, nearly tucked under the chair. As soon as Mary stood up, her center of gravity projected to the very front edge of the transitional base (Figure 3-8). Mary felt like she was falling forward; the OT practitioner then sat Mary back down in her chair.

During the next transfer attempt, the OT practitioner overcompensated and placed Mary's feet too far in front of her knees. This transfer required too much forward travel, and Mary felt her gravity projection fall behind the transitional base (Figure 3-9).

Often, OT practitioners in similar situations make a strong, sudden rotation to complete a transfer rather than stop it. This maneuver requires a ballistic-type muscle contraction in the OT practitioner's lower back and generally leads to a low-back injury. Easing a client back into the original position or onto the floor provide better options.

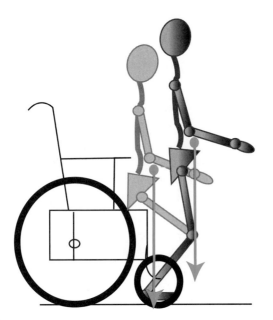

FIGURE **3-8**
Mary's transitional base of support is too close to the wheelchair. Once she stands, she has difficulty preventing her center of gravity from projecting in front of her transitional base of support.

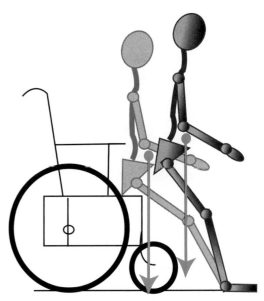

FIGURE **3-9**
Mary's transitional base of support is too far forward. When she moves to stand, she must travel forward more than is possible. Mary finds that with too little momentum, her center of gravity projects behind the transitional base.

The most stable stand-pivot transfer involves consideration of placements at all three bases of support before movement begins. The OT practitioner moves the chair and mat as close together as possible without restricting his own base of support. The client scoots forward in the chair, with her feet directly under her knees. As soon as the client's knees and hips extend into standing, the center of gravity projection automatically moves through the center of the transitional base. With a closely placed chair the client moves easily onto the mat. She can pivot and begin flexing her hips and knees. The center of gravity projects behind her feet, but the mat supplies a final base of support.

Meanwhile, the OT practitioner must ensure his own stability. Reaching out too far in front puts him at a disadvantage and requires him to lean forward, forcing his center of gravity forward near his anterior base of support (Figure 3-10, A).

As the OT practitioner provides more assistance, he gets pulled toward the client. The OT practitioner should anticipate this forward weight shift and adjust his stance before a transfer by moving as close to the client as possible. Instead of leaning forward and down to reach for a transfer belt, the OT practitioner bends his knees and maintains the center of gravity projection through his base of support. He reaches forward with the upper extremities only, to prevent a forward shift in his center of gravity. This keeps the OT practitioner's projection closer to the center of the base of support (Figure 3-10, *B*).

In moderate- to maximum-assist transfers the weight of the client becomes a forward drag that moves the OT practitioner's center of gravity projection to the front edge of his base. This unstable situation puts both the OT practitioner and the client at risk of falling. The OT practitioner anticipates and balances this added weight by synchronizing his posterior weight shift with the amount of assistance he provides. The posterior weight shift gives him a supportive lifting force far superior to his upper-body strength. The net effect maintains the OT practitioner's center of gravity projection through the center of the base and provides assistance using his body weight rather than his upper-body strength (A Closer Look Box 3-5).

WHEELCHAIRS

Wheelchairs have large bases of support, substantial weight, relatively low centers of gravity, and projections of centers of gravity well within the chairs' bases of support. Usually these factors work together to make them stable. There are some conditions in which wheelchairs are less stable. The back of a reclining wheelchair may recline far enough back that it outdistances its rear base of support. An individual with bilateral lower-extremity amputation may feel unstable in a standard wheelchair

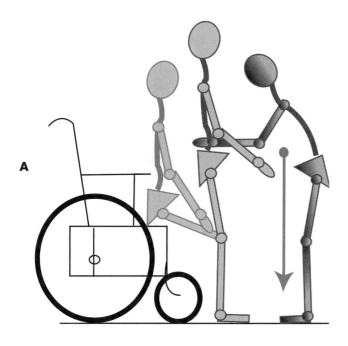

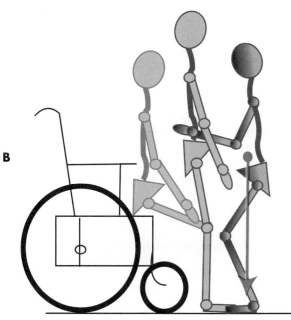

FIGURE 3-10

A, Leaning and reaching forward to assist the client moves the OT practitioner's center of gravity projection too far forward relative to the base of support. **B**, Standing close and bending at the knees keeps the OT practitioner's projection more centralized in the base of support and decreases the risk of falling into the client.

because of the backward shift in his center of gravity projection. Lightweight sport wheelchairs often have built-in rearward centers of gravity projection to ease maneuverability. The sport wheelchair's front wheels pop up easily, making it possible for the user to hop curbs

BOX 3-5

A CLOSER LOOK

Transfers as Therapy

Practitioners often perform transfers hastily. Instead of viewing transfers simply as part of getting the client to the clinic, we need to think of them as opportunities to improve body awareness, strength, balance, impulse control, and sequencing skills. Transfers as therapy involve more than movement from one place to another.

Engage clients in the transfer for full therapeutic value. Talk to clients about the transfer before, during, and after it occurs. Before the transfer, review the steps and reassure clients about safety. Instruct the clients in the importance of wheelchair positioning and proper use of transfer belts.

If possible, engage the help of an aide, who can watch and provide standby assistance. Use clear physical and verbal prompts during the transfer. In stand-pivot and sliding-board transfers, pause for quick assessments when reaching the transitional base of support, and after completing the transfer, assess the full process with the experience still fresh in your mind.

Above all, do not use transfers as opportunities to prove your strength and experience. Taking time to assist clients in transfers may save time later. Poor judgments present unnecessary risks to clients and threaten the trust between the client and the practitioner.

and maneuver stairs. However, these "wheelies" require practice to reduce the risk of backward falls in this unstable position.

Reclining Wheelchairs

A fully reclined wheelchair back results in a redistribution of the wheelchair's mass such that more mass is located farther back in the chair and the new center of gravity projects closer to the rearward border of the base of support. Full recliners have extended frames to accommodate this projection. Semireclining wheelchairs allow some degree of tilt but have shorter wheel bases to improve maneuverability. Because a semirecliner has a shorter base of support than a full recliner, when the center of gravity projection moves backward it comes close to the rear limit of the base of support in the "full" semireclined position (Figure 3-11). As long as the projection stays within the base of support, the semirecliner remains upright. However, in this unstable position even a slight forward force, such as a sudden push by the user, can throw the

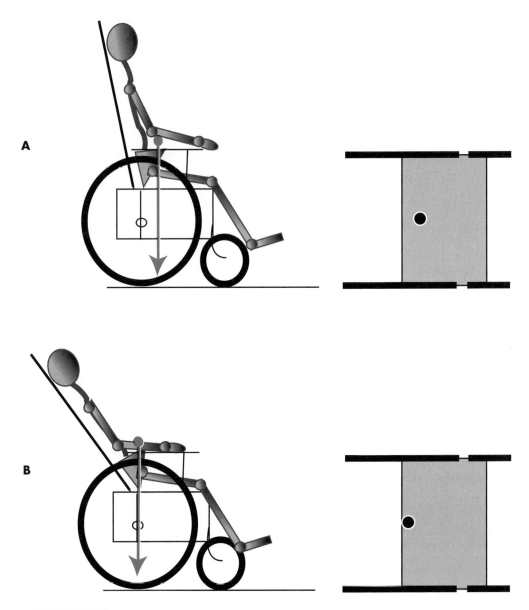

FIGURE **3-11**
A, Side view of a semirecliner and top view of the base of support and projected center of gravity when the chair back is upright. **B**, Same two views when the chair back is fully reclined.

chair off balance enough to cause a backward fall. The forward push moves the wheels, which form the base of support, in front of the center of gravity projection, tipping the chair backward (Figure 3-12). The same quick start creates little risk with an upright chair back because the center of gravity projection lies farther forward.

Wheels

Changing the positions of the front casters and rear wheels changes a wheelchair's stability. The front casters change positions every time the wheelchair reverses direction, which modifies the depth (front-to-rear dimensions) of the chair's base of support. The front casters point toward the rear when the chair stops moving forward and toward the front when it stops backing up (Figure 3-13). As a result a chair moving forward has a shorter base of support than a chair moving backward (Figure 3-14). When the forward-moving user stops the chair and bends forward to pick up an object on the floor, his weight shifts onto the footrests, moving his center of gravity and its projection forward in the base of support. If the user reaches too far forward, the projection pushes in front of the base, causing the chair to fall forward (Figure 3-15).

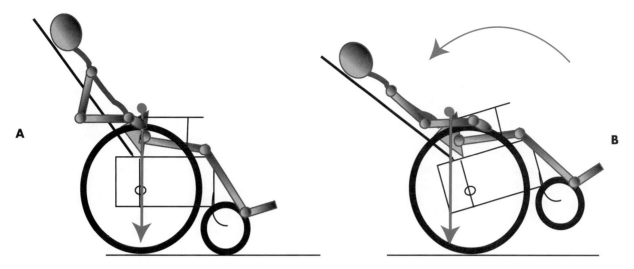

FIGURE **3-12**
A, The reclined position moves the center of gravity projection toward the back of the base of support. **B**, The quick start moves the base of support from under the center of gravity projection, and the chair falls backward.

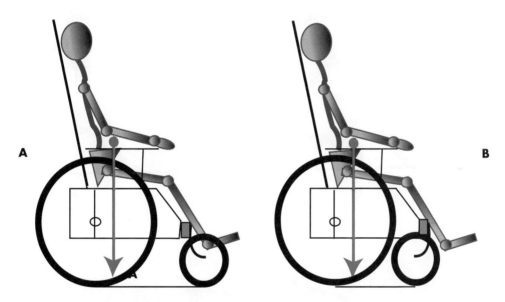

FIGURE **3-13**
The front casters swivel to point to the front when the chair stops backing up **(A)** and to the rear when it stops moving forward **(B)**.

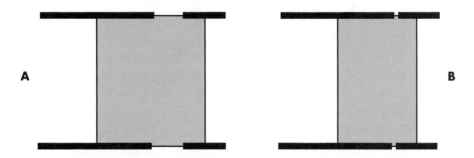

FIGURE **3-14**
Top view of the base of support as affected by the position of the front casters. As the chair backs up, it has a longer base of support **(A)** than when it moves forward **(B)**.

Xavier Morales often wears prostheses to stand for presentations and uses a standard wheelchair at work. When Xavier reaches for his briefcase and other objects on the floor, he pivots to place objects to his side between his casters and wheels and leans to the side rather than forward. If he needs to get something in a corner or tight place, Xavier automatically pushes his chair slightly backward to pivot his casters forward, making a larger base of support. Sometimes he leans forward using the shorter casters-backward base of support to tip his chair onto its footrests and increase his reach, but only when he can use his desk or wall as a brace to regain an upright position.

Xavier can adjust his lightweight wheelchair's base of support easily by moving the wheels forward or backward. Normally the center of gravity projects near the rear edge of his wheelchair base, so moving the wheels forward brings this projection closer to the rear edge. Xavier intentionally adjusts his wheelchair this way so that he can pop up the front casters in a wheelie. Xavier maintains his balance in a wheelie by keeping the center of gravity projection through the axle of the rear wheels. This limits the front-to-back dimension of his base of support to about an inch where his rear wheels touch the ground directly under he axle (Figure 3-16). Balanced on these two rear wheels, Xavier can hop up or down curbs and even some short flights of stairs.

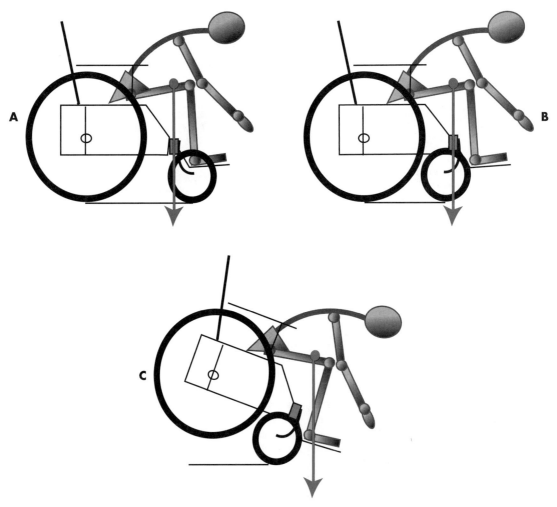

FIGURE 3-15
Forward leaning moves the center of gravity projection forward. **A**, It remains inside the base of support when the casters point forward. **B**, It moves outside the base of support when the casters point to the rear. **C**, This causes the chair to fall forward.

Xavier first learned this technique in the veterans' rehabilitation hospital, where he practiced with mats while OT staff members guided him. He tried for months before he learned the proper control. A slightly too forceful forward push would move the projection of gravity too far behind his base of support, quickly spinning his chair backward on its wheels, accelerating him backward until something hit the ground. When this happened, Xavier's push handles usually hit the ground and his quick reflexes and strong neck flexors saved him from injury. A couple of times Xavier hit his head hard enough to "see stars," but he continued to practice this technique on his own in wheelchair athletics. Eventually wheelies became natural and safe, and their advantage in overcoming architectural barriers made them worth the practice.

Camber, tilting the rear wheels so that the bottoms of the rims are farther apart than the tops, makes maneuvering the chair easier (Figure 3-17). The shoulders push from a more relaxed position (less shoulder abduction and scapular elevation) because the tops of the wheels lie closer to the body than the bottoms. Slight abduction of the arms as the hands follow the rims also makes the forward stroke more natural.

Camber widens the base of support and increases the chair's side-to-side stability. More sideways stability combined with greater maneuverability makes camber an essential feature in all sport wheelchairs. Just as athletic shoes have found their way into the workplace, lightweight sports chairs also have become a preferred choice for active wheelchair users.

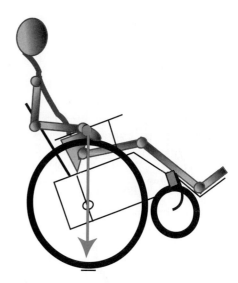

FIGURE **3-16**
Xavier balances his chair in a wheelie.

Instability after Amputation

Xavier Morales' center of gravity shifts substantially when he does not wear his prostheses. Without this weight, contributing their segmental centers of gravity, Xavier loses much of the forward-placed body mass in sitting and his center of gravity projects more toward the rear (Figure 3-18). Like the person in the

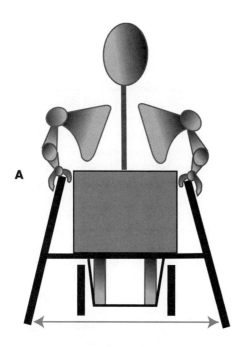

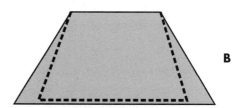

FIGURE **3-17**
Rear-wheel camber **(A)** and its effect on the width of the base of support **(B)**.

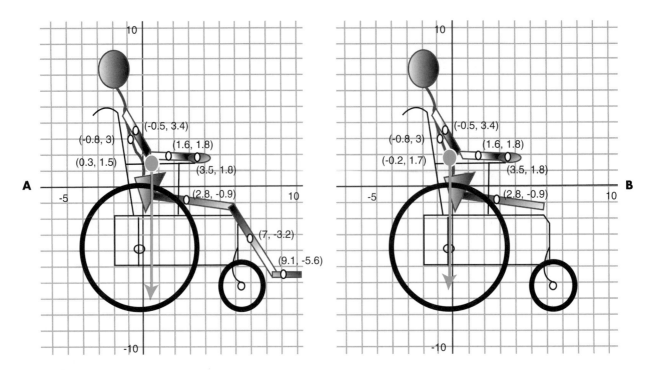

FIGURE **3-18**
A, The segmental centers of gravity are determined using the process described in this chapter. **B**, The center of gravity projection shifts toward the rear when an individual whose lower extremities have been amputated sits in a wheelchair.

semirecliner wheelchair, Xavier has a greater risk of falling backward. In his case the posterior center of gravity projection results from loss of anterior mass, not the chair's reclined position. Quick pushes on his wheels move this projection behind Xavier's base of support, and the front of his chair tips up. Before Xavier entered the rehabilitation hospital he had a standard wheelchair, and its instability made him insecure about moving. Xavier could not adjust his balance in time, and fear of falling kept him rooted in one spot, dependent on others for mobility.

As soon as Xavier got to the rehabilitation hospital, hospital staff placed sandbag weights on his footrests. The added weight anterior to his center of gravity adjusted his center of gravity projection and gave him immediate relief. As a longer-term adaptation, he received a rear-axle extender. This piece of metal tubing bolted onto the original frame to provide a place to attach the rear wheels in a more posterior position. Extending Xavier's base of support caused his center of gravity projection to fall more toward the center. Xavier became more mobile and eventually moved into a lightweight wheelchair to pursue a more active lifestyle.

Summary

Newton envisioned gravitational attraction like the attraction of magnets. Einstein envisioned space as a fabric in which large objects such as planets, stars, and black holes created deep pockets that drew smaller objects such as light rays inward on a curved trajectory. The conceptual models these mathematicians developed have kept physicists employed for centuries!

For our purposes the specific details of the conceptual models seem less relevant. Objects move downward toward the Earth in direct proportion to their mass. Although the force of that attraction depends on mass, the acceleration of all objects remains constant, which means a larger, heavier object falls to the ground just as fast as a smaller, lighter one. However, a heavier object requires more force to push it over an edge than the lighter one does. We use these important concepts to visualize gravity's effect on movement by drawing objects with vectors that demonstrate gravity's ever-present influence. Our understanding of gravity informs our practice allowing us to perform safer, more effective transfers and troubleshoot problems of stability in sitting, standing, and wheelchair use.

Applications

■ APPLICATION 3-1
Creation of a Mobile

Make a mobile from three to five objects in the room. Hang the objects from a clothes hanger. Can you find each object's center of gravity? How do you know when you have each object balanced? Which objects suspend most easily?

■ APPLICATION 3-2
Scale Drawing of Your Lab Partner

On a scale drawing of your lab partner, find each body segment's center of gravity and mark it with a dot.

■ APPLICATION 3-3
Vector Indicating Gravity's Effect on a Laundry Basket

Figure 3-19 shows a laundry basket weighing 10 kg. Show the effect of gravity on the full basket by drawing a vector from its center of gravity. Also, show the effect of gravity on a basket that is half full, or 5 kg.

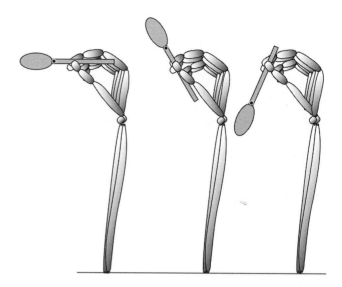

FIGURE **3-20**
This spoon weighs 0.04 kg. Draw a vector representing the force of gravity in each position.

■ APPLICATION 3-4
Force of Gravity Acting on a Spoon

The spoon in Figure 3-20 weighs 0.04 kg. Draw a vector for the force of gravity acting on the spoon in each of the three different positions. Does the center of gravity or its action on the spoon change as the position changes?

■ APPLICATION 3-5
Force of Gravity Acting on Spoons of Different Weights

In Figure 3-21 a spoon with a built-up handle weighs 0.06 kg, and a regular spoon weighs 0.04 kg. Indicate the force of gravity acting on each spoon. Does weight affect each spoon's center of gravity?

See Appendix C for solutions to Applications.

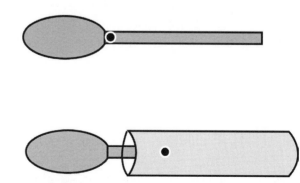

FIGURE **3-21**
The spoon without the adapted handle weighs 0.04 kg, and the spoon with the built-up handle weighs 0.06 kg. Draw a vector representing the force of gravity in each spoon.

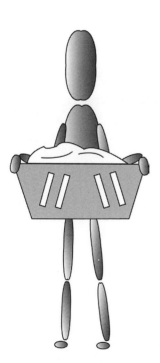

FIGURE **3-19**
This laundry basket weighs 10 kg. Draw the vector representing its weight.

REFERENCES

1. Leveau BF: *Williams and Lissner's biomechanics of human motion*, ed 3, Philadelphia, 1992, WB Saunders.
2. McCance KL, Huether SE: *Pathophysiology: the biologic basis for disease in adults and children*, ed 2, St Louis, 1994, Mosby.
3. Williams PL, Bannister LH: *Gray's anatomy: the anatomical basis of medicine and surgery*, ed 38, New York, 1995, Churchill Livingstone.
4. World Health Organization: International Classification of Function, Disability and Health (ICF). Available from: http://www3.who.int/icf/onlinebrowser/icf.cfm found on 3-1-04 [Cited 03-01-2004].

RELATED READINGS

Fritjof C: *The Tao of physics*, New York, 1994, Bantam.
Krauss LM: *Fear of physics: a guide for the perplexed*, New York, 1993, Basic Books.
Luttgens K, Wells K: *Kinesiology: scientific basis of human motion*, ed 9, Madison, Wis, 1997, Brown & Benchmark.
Nordin M, Frankel VH: *Basic biomechanics of the musculoskeletal system*, Philadelphia, 1989, Lea & Febiger.
Norkin CC, Levangie PK: *Joint structure and function: a comprehensive analysis*, ed 2, Philadelphia, 1992, FA Davis.
Wiktorin CH, Nordin M: *Introduction to problem solving in biomechanics*, Philadelphia, 1986, Lea & Febiger.

LAB BOX

Find applied activities exploring concepts in Chapter 3 in the following laboratory exercises:

Topic	Laboratory
Wheelchair stability	**Lab 2** Stability, Balance, Wheelchairs, Min Assist Transfers
• Wheelies	
• Base of support affected by front caster position	
• Rear wheel camber and stability and mobility	
Amputation and wheelchair stability	**Lab 2** Stability, Balance, Wheelchairs, Min Assist Transfers
Transfers:	**Lab 2** Stability, Balance, Wheelchairs, Min Assist Transfers
• Changing centers of gravity	
• Foot placement and stability	**Lab 4** (max assist)

4 *Linear Force and Motion*

KEY**TERMS**

Law of Inertia
Law of Acceleration
Law of Action-Reaction
Equilibrium
Compressive
Tensile
Elasticity
Shear
Resultant Force
Distensibility
Multijoint Muscle
Active Insufficiency
Passive Insufficiency

F *orces surround us.* Though we cannot see them, we feel their effects as deeply as we sense our own breathing. An apple falls from a tree to the ground. Two automobile bumpers collide. These examples of external linear forces operate in patterns similar to those of the internal forces that exist within our bodies. Both the action of the tiny spindles pulling chromosomes to their respective poles in cell division and the contraction and substantial excursion of the sartorius muscle forcefully flexing the knee follow the same rules as external linear forces. This chapter explores the laws that govern motion caused by linear forces and details the effects of linear forces within the musculoskeletal system.

External Forces

External forces affect the body from the outside. Isaac Newton explained the effects of forces on objects in his three laws of motion. As OT practitioners, we observe Newton's laws at work every day. When we relate what we observe to the underlying principles involved, we can understand our observations more completely.

LAW OF INERTIA

*Bernice Richards has quadriplegia and minimal control of the muscles balancing her trunk. She directs her electric wheelchair through the main thoroughfare of a shopping mall, and a child darts in front of her. As she stops the chair, Bernice demonstrates Newton's first law, the **law of inertia**. The chair quickly decelerates, but Bernice continues moving forward within the chair, stopped only by her chest and pelvic seat belts.*

This isolated event demonstrates a valuable lesson. Bernice, like other individuals with weak trunk muscles, needs seat belts to provide trunk support. Analyzing this event from a physics perspective increases our ability to generalize principles from previous chapters.

All matter has inertia. We see this applied every day—nearly every moment of our lives. A coffee cup placed on a table remains there until picked up for a sip. The table and chairs, in fact all the furniture in the house, remain at rest until acted upon by some outside force (Newton's first law). Moving the cup or the chair requires an outside force greater than the inertia of the cup, the chair, or any other object we plan to move.

Understanding Newton's first law requires nothing more than common sense. *A body at rest remains at rest unless acted on by an outside force, and a body in motion remains so unless acted on by an outside force.* The second part of this law was demonstrated by Bernice's sudden stop. We can appreciate the concept of momentum, but

we know that nothing lasts forever, including motion. We have pushed cars, bikes, and carts that move for a bit and then stop. Therefore despite what Newton says about remaining in motion our experience informs us that an object has a natural tendency to stop.

In truth, objects do not stop because of a natural tendency. Some outside force stops them, a force we cannot see. Friction, for example, stopped Bernice's wheelchair by the drag of the turned-off motor and the resistance of the rubber tires on the floor. The seat belts provided a more obvious source of friction. In other words, an outside force, friction, slowed the chair, but Bernice's body continued moving forward (law of inertia). The force of friction on the chair did not affect Bernice's body. A separate, outside force, provided by the seat belts, stopped her body from continuing forward.

Understanding this event according to Newton's law allows us to extrapolate our understanding and predict the outcomes of different, perhaps less obvious situations.

Because she was a nightclub singer, Bernice was concerned that a chest strap would ruin her sequined tops, but she needed some way to prevent herself from falling forward. Her OT practitioner understood the underlying principle, inertia, and devised an alternative solution for Bernice by focusing on the force of gravity. He tilted her seat and the back of her chair to increase the effect of gravity as it acted to extend Bernice's trunk and hips.

We will examine "tilt-in-space" more closely in a later chapter. For now, realize that a variety of solutions exist to solve the same problem. We can recognize these solutions only when we look past the event and understand the nature of the problem.

LAW OF ACCELERATION

Newton's second law, *force equals mass times acceleration,* often causes undo concern. We imagine that application involves solving algebraic formulas from lengthy word problems requiring complicated diagrams. In reality most students and all OT practitioners apply Newton's second law every day.

Although often stated in its algebraic form ($F = ma$), force equals mass times acceleration simply means that it takes less effort to push a broken-down Volkswagen than a stalled Cadillac. A Volkswagen, which has less mass than a Cadillac, requires less force to move. (Simplify the equation by considering acceleration as movement.) Look at the equation from a different perspective. Consider that if we hold force constant and push the Volkswagen as hard as the Cadillac, the Volkswagen will move farther faster. Paraphrasing Newton, *objects that have more mass require more force to move (accelerate), and if two objects, each with a different mass, are under the influence of one force, the object with the least mass moves first.* We commonly see this application of Newton's **law of acceleration** in various regions of the body.

Eduardo Ybarra severed his radial nerve with a power saw while making his son a rocking horse for Christmas. As a result, Eduardo cannot extend his wrist and fingers. An OT practitioner uses a splint to extend Eduardo's wrist, but unfamiliar with underlying splinting principles, she applied the extension force to the fingers. To her surprise, the splint overextended Eduardo's fingers before fully extending his wrist. She failed to appreciate the effect of his fingers being lighter (having less mass) than his hand.

*The same rule applies to **Tony Adams**, whose scapular stabilizers were paralyzed by a gunshot wound. When Tony contracts his deltoid muscle to abduct the arm at the shoulder, he gets an undesired downward movement of the scapula and cannot raise his injured arm. Like any muscle, when the deltoid shortens, it can move either of its attachments. If the scapular stabilizers are paralyzed, attempts to abduct the arm result in scapular movement because the scapula has less mass than the entire upper extremity* (Figure 4-1).

LAW OF ACTION-REACTION

Most people know Newton's third law, commonly referred to as the **law of action-reaction**, popularized in cartoons as "what goes up, must come down." *If a force acts on an object, that object remains stationary for as long as an equal force acts on the object in the opposite direction.* We usually remain unaware of these opposing forces on stationary objects until one force fails.

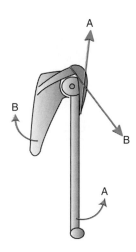

FIGURE **4-1**
A, The deltoid muscle moves its insertion and abducts the humerus with the scapula stabilized. B, The deltoid muscle acts on its origin, the scapula, without scapular stabilization.

Imagine an individual sitting in a chair, listening to a conference speaker. Suddenly, this attentive listener falls to the ground as the chair collapses with a loud bang. What happened? The listener's action (force of body weight downward) did not change, but the chair's reaction (force provided by the legs of the chair upward) decreased when the structure of the chair failed.

The listener's original force, body weight, took over. This downward force was present the entire time but the equal and opposite upward force of the chair's legs held it in balance. No movement occurred until the collapse of the chair. In truth, as long as the two forces remained equal the chair and listener appeared to be bodies at rest. Newton's third law describes this condition of **equilibrium**.

An OT practitioner uses clinical applications of this law to make lateral trunk supports for Bernice Richard's wheelchair. These supports counteract the effect of gravity on her otherwise unsupported trunk. Gravity's downward pull on Bernice's upright vertebral column results in lateral shifts that produce an S curve. Without support, that spinal curve could develop into scoliosis.

Lateral supports on Bernice's wheelchair help prevent formation of the S curve. Gravity pulls downward on the vertebral column, which causes a lateral shift in the vertebral segments. The OT practitioner considers this lateral movement of the vertebrae caused by gravity as the action. He provides the reaction, which counterbalances gravity's effect, through pads attached to the back of the chair's seat directing a medial force. A strong trunk movement from Bernice could cause the support pad to give way. A support pad that pushed medially with too much force could overcorrect Bernice's posture and cause her trunk to develop a curve in the opposite direction.

Unbalanced forces upset equilibrium. We will see that our essential objective in wheelchair seating and positioning depends on understanding and neutralizing the effects of gravity to create a state of equilibrium between its force and the forces provided by critically placed supports.

Force Equilibrium

The carefully placed supports that hold Bernice's trunk erect provide an example of a way to obtain equilibrium. The law of inertia applies: Her body remains at rest. The absence of lateral supports or poorly adjusted supports on Bernice's chair may lead to formation of an S curve, the result of unbalanced forces and a body in motion. Newton's second law (the law of acceleration) helps us understand what happens between periods of equilibrium. Will the lateral support pad apply sufficient force to balance the mass of the vertebral column and the effects of gravity's force on that mass? Will too great a force from the lateral support pads cause the vertebral segments to accelerate in the opposite direction?

Donna Nelson, a food server in a small Italian restaurant, encounters force equilibrium every day. Management wants its food servers to carry dinner orders out to the tables using large trays. Donna knows that to work at this restaurant she must be able to hold extremely heavy trays at shoulder height. Therefore in order for Donna to return to work after hospitalization, her OT practioner must develop a strengthening program that will maintain Donna's ability to carry heavy trays at shoulder height.

Donna encounters linear force equilibrium daily. She may not remember Newton's third law of motion, but her tips depend on her body's ability to respond to the law of action-reaction. Every time she carries her tray, Donna's upper extremities provide a combined upward force equal in magnitude and opposite in direction to the downward-directed weight of the tray. Consider the tray's weight as the action and the upward force of her muscle contractions as the reaction (Figure 4-2).

When Donna carries the tray at shoulder height, she exhibits isometric contractions of her muscles at a number of joints. These contractions bring about equilibrium between the weight of the tray and her effort in the upward (opposite) direction. Gravity pulls the tray downward while contractions in muscles opposing gravity balance its effect, pushing the tray upward (in the opposite direction).

Donna uses a concentric contraction to overcome the external force of the tray's weight when she lifts it over her head to negotiate her way around another server, momentarily moving the tray out of equilibrium. Finally, she yields slightly to the weight of the tray when she lowers it back to shoulder height. Donna uses an eccentric contraction to lower the tray, which changes the system's equilibrium in the direction of the external force (weight of the tray). (In the next chapter, we will see how Donna balances large orders and, more importantly, how she removes items without upsetting this balance.)

Normal Forces

Normal forces are external forces that either push joint surfaces together or pull them apart. In Figure 4-3 Donna leans on a table, pushing her joint surfaces together at the elbow joint. In Figure 4-4 she hangs motionless from an overhead bar, pulling these same joint surfaces apart. In each case the force moves perpendicular to the surface on which it acts.

Anatomical structures alter their shapes in response to these forces. **Compressive** forces push tissues together, causing anatomical structures to become shorter and wider. **Tensile** forces pull tissues apart, causing anatomical structures to become longer and narrower. Anatomical structures usually return to their original shapes once the forces acting on them stop. **Elasticity** describes a structure's ability to return to its original shape. Injury happens when normal forces exceed a tissue's elasticity. For instance, joint sprains occur when forces acting around joints tear ligamentous tissues.

Shear Forces

External forces also can operate parallel to a surface. Raising your arm over your head causes the weight of the humerus to produce a **shear** force on the glenoid fossa. Because these forces operate on the periphery of surfaces, we also call shear forces *tangential* forces. Shear and normal forces of the same magnitude have drastically

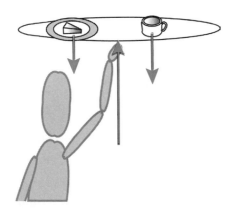

FIGURE **4-2**
Vertical forces upward must equal vertical forces downward for the tray and its contents to remain stable (in equilibrium).

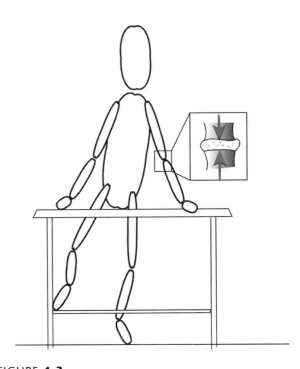

FIGURE **4-3**
When Donna Nelson leans on a table, she causes compressive forces to operate at her elbow with corresponding compressive stress in her joint tissues.

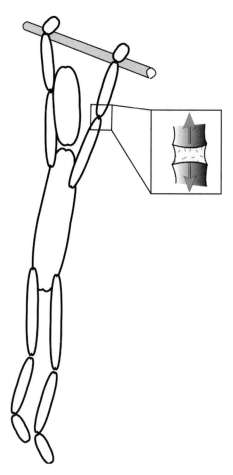

FIGURE **4-4**
When Donna Nelson hangs on a bar, she causes tensile forces to operate at her elbow and shoulder with corresponding tensile stress in her joint tissues.

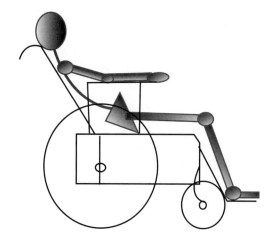

FIGURE **4-5**
Bernice's reclined position, combined with inadequate support, puts her at risk for developing decubiti from shear forces caused by sliding forward.

different effects; shear forces can cause more damage to tissues. For example, Figure 4-5 represents Bernice Richards in a recliner wheelchair. The reclined position, together with inadequate support, causes her to slide down on the seat. This sliding produces a dangerous shear force that acts on the skin of her buttocks. If she resumes this position frequently, Bernice will develop pressure sores, or decubiti, even though the normal force created by her upright weight greatly exceeds the magnitude of the shear force caused during sliding. Therefore the OT practitioner concerned with Bernice's wheelchair positioning focuses first on preventing shear.

Stress

When external forces act on material substances, like a joint capsule, they cause stress within that material. We measure stress as force exerted per unit area of tissue, in newtons/meter^2 (N/m^2, metric measure) or in pounds per square inch (lb/in^2, English measure). When stress within human tissue exceeds the tissue's elasticity, tissue breaks down, causing injury.

Internal Forces

Body tissues generate internal forces. Our experience with internal forces mainly involves those of muscle contractions. Muscle contractions generate linear forces, and we must understand the characteristics of these forces before we consider the anatomical movements they cause. (In Chapter 5, we will learn that the connection of these straight-line forces to articulated skeletal segments results in circular or rotary motion).

FORCE MAGNITUDE AND ORIENTATION

We diagram the forces of muscle contractions as vectors (A Closer Look Box 4-1). We must use correct orientation and direction to understand the function of these forces. In its simplest function, a muscle like the brachialis acts through a straight path, represented with an arrow drawn through the longitudinal aspect of the muscle. Its orientation lies parallel to the direction of muscle fibers.

The number of active muscle fibers determines a muscle force's magnitude. The specific length of the vector, according to a chosen scale, represents magnitude. Graphic units of length equal specific units of force. A force drawn 0.5 inch long represents 50 lb on a scale of 1 inch = 100 lb.

In Figure 4-6 we see Donna Nelson's brachialis muscle pulling at the elbow with a 90-lb force indicated by the vector. The force aligns with her muscle fibers, which operate nearly parallel to the humerus from origin to insertion.

BOX 4-1

A CLOSER LOOK

Using Line Drawings To Organize Problems in Biomechanics

Line drawings accurately represent biomechanics in functional activity and do not require artistic skill. They can communicate information to bioengineers, physicians, orthotists, clients, and others involved in the treatment process. Biomechanics provides a framework for OT practitioners to understand movement and the forces responsible for movement. To organize information into a line drawing, follow these steps:

1. Look at the body parts used in an activity. Observe the activity as a whole to determine where movement takes place. Note all important movements.

2. Identify which specific joints and active muscle groups play major roles in the activity. Some muscles and joints have less importance than others. Joints and muscles that play major roles can change as the movements change.

3. Determine which plane or planes of motion provide the most information about an activity. The individual who makes the drawing determines the plane of view. A drawing of motion in the sagittal plane, for example, using elbow and shoulder flexion to place dishes in an overhead cabinet, requires a view of the client from the side. Frontal plane movement, such as a wave of the hand to greet someone, should depict the client from the front. Identify the plane of motion (where movement occurs) and draw body segments with the surface of the paper serving as that plane. Different phases of an activity may require different views.

4. A line drawing should include the following relevant information:

   a. Movement of skeletal segments—To indicate moving segments use curved arrows drawn from the point at which a segment began moving to its final location in the drawing.

   b. Joints—Use dots to indicate the axis where motion takes place. Each axis for a plane of movement should orient 90 degrees to the plane. Imagine the axis sticking out of the paper like a pin so it appears as a dot on the paper.

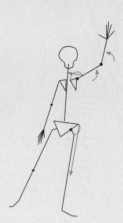

   c. Muscles—Use light lines from the muscle's point of origin to its point of insertion, making sure to draw around any point the muscle circumnavigates. For example, draw the middle deltoid from its insertion on the humerus around the tip of the shoulder to its origin on the acromion, not through the acromion itself.

   d. Objects or tools—Use circles, squares, or other simple geometric shapes that approximate the object's size.

5. Determine where and how gravity acts on the human body, tools, or other objects. Determine the segmental centers of gravity where needed and the center of gravity of the entire body using the methods described in Chapter 3.

6. Determine the forces that help move specific body parts, objects, or tools. Draw these forces as vectors scaled for magnitude, with an arrowhead pointing in the direction of force. Remember, the vector should orient parallel to the muscle fibers in the center of the muscle. Draw the vector straight from the point of a muscle's attachment, even if the muscle fibers curve around some anatomical pulley.

Colored pens or pencils can help differentiate muscles, bones, and forces in a schematic drawing. Use different colors for curved arrows showing movement versus straight arrows indicating forces. Use a goniometer to measure joint angles.

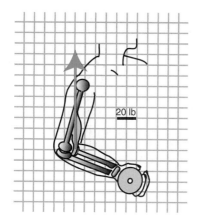

FIGURE **4-6**
A vector drawn to scale indicates a force of 90 lb generated by the brachialis muscle (20 lb = 2 boxes).

In many muscles a tendon transmits force to the skeletal segment. The tendon may travel around various bony protuberances, completely reorienting the direction of the force by the time this force reaches the bony segment serving as its insertion. The force of Iris Clark's flexor hallucis longus (the long flexor of the great toe) lies parallel to her tibia in the leg but parallel to her foot (90 degrees to the leg) at the point of the muscle's insertion (Figure 4-7). The tendon travels around and turns behind the medial malleolus, creating a pulley effect to flex the great toe. (See Chapters 7 and 8 for a discussion of how forces commonly can be redirected around pulleys that are within the hand.)

Some muscles have fibers oriented in different directions. The forces created by these fibers combine to form a **resultant force** that we can determine through careful drawing. For example, the pectoralis major muscle has a fan shape. The active muscle fibers pull in the same plane but in different directions. To determine the resultant force and direction of contraction for the combined fibers of the pectoralis major, use the parallelogram method of graphic representation.

In this method, construct a parallelogram using two representative forces of this muscle as sides. [Figure 4-8 shows the two most contrasting forces in the muscle (the clavicular and inferior sternal fibers) represented as sides of a parallelogram.] A diagonal line down the center of the parallelogram represents the resultant force. This intersects the middle-lying fibers and gives us a general idea of the overall effect caused by simultaneous contraction of all fibers, or maximal effort.

FORCE DIRECTION

Pay attention to the direction of forces. An arrow drawn from a muscle's insertion (distal attachment) toward its origin (proximal attachment) implies the muscle moves the more distal part of the extremity. This happens with a stabilized origin. In Figure 4-6 Donna's brachialis muscle pulls a hand-held weight toward her shoulder, which she stabilizes with scapular muscles. The force of flexion generated by the brachialis and other elbow flexors operates almost parallel to her humerus, directed proximally, pulling the distal insertion toward the proximal origin.

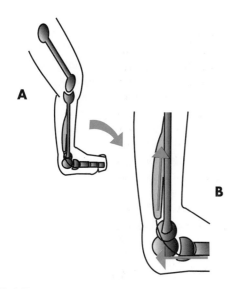

FIGURE **4-7**
A, The lower extremity. **B,** Close-up of the lower leg. The direction of the force as indicated by the placement of the arrowhead changes as the direction of the muscle fibers and tendon travel around bony protuberances.

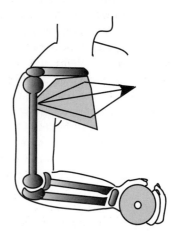

FIGURE **4-8**
The parallelogram method determines the combined effect of muscle fibers in the pectoralis major. The greater resultant force travels in a different direction from the two component forces that represent divergent fibers of the same muscle.

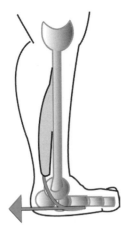

FIGURE **4-9**
The force vector continues in a straight path, although muscle fibers curve around the ankle.

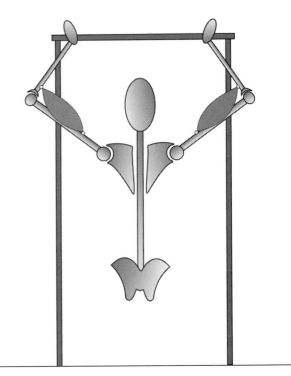

FIGURE **4-10**
When Donna Nelson pulls up on a bar, it stabilizes her wrist and hand, causing the elbow flexors to bring her body closer to the forearm.

To represent the effect of force vectors in a drawing, draw a straight arrow from the moving part along the muscle fiber or tendon. Draw the arrow long enough to represent the magnitude (strength) of the force according to a chosen scale. If the muscle or tendon curves in its path, never follow the turn with the arrow; keep the arrow straight (Figure 4-9).

How we represent the direction of muscle contraction depends on which part—the origin or insertion—moves in a contraction. We generally assume muscles' distal attachments (insertions) move in relation to their proximal attachments (origins), but real life has more variation. Figure 4-10 demonstrates schematically how Donna's elbow flexors pull her body (proximal) toward a bar she holds in her hands (distal). In this case Donna's grip on the bar stabilizes her muscle's insertion, which allows the origin to move distally. The direction of elbow flexor force runs proximal to distal, pulling the origin (humerus) toward the insertion (ulna and radius). Donna performs a push-up in the same way, by contracting her triceps to extend her elbow, moving her body away from her hand. Because the floor stabilizes her hand, Donna's body moves away from it.

Tony Adams, whose gunshot wound paralyzed some of his upward scapular rotators, provides another example of a muscle that moves its origin instead of its insertion. The bullet that barely missed his spinal cord partially damaged the ventral rami of cervical roots 3, 4, and 5, which supply a variety of nerves to scapular muscles. When Tony's deltoid muscle contracts, it moves the unstabilized scapula instead of the upper extremity (via the humerus), resulting in a contraction directed proximal to distal (Figure 4-1).

Muscle Contraction Types

When muscles contract the two ends of the muscle move closer together. Movement occurs when one end, either the proximal or the distal attachment of the muscle, remains stable. This occurs because other muscle contractions prevent either the proximal or the distal end from moving. We have previously considered how scapular stabilizers allow the deltoid to abduct the humerus instead of downwardly rotating the scapula (Figure 4-1). In this case, muscles inserting on the scapula contract to stabilize it while the deltoid, arising from the scapula, contracts to move the humerus.

We represent the force of muscle contraction with an arrow drawn along the lines of the muscle fibers. The arrow begins from its attachment on the moving segment, and points in the direction of the contraction. This indicates which point—the origin or insertion—moves.

Remember that whether the muscle shortens (concentric), stays the same (isometric), or lengthens (eccentric), it always attempts to shorten. Draw the force the same way regardless of the type of contraction. We need to determine which attachment moves, or in the case of isometric contractions, which attachment would move if equilibrium were altered.

Muscle Force

Absolute strength, the maximum amount of force a muscle can exert, depends on the bulk or girth of a muscle's cross section (A Closer Look Box 4-2). Muscle girth depends on the amount of contractile protein packed into a muscle. Muscle length, when one muscle is compared to another, does not determine strength. However, the amount of force one muscle generates when it contracts with maximal effort varies according to its length at the beginning of the contraction.[2] This length determines the state of overlap of the actin and myosin myofilaments. At optimum overlap, the "just-right" length, the muscle generates the maximum amount of force.

Positioning the joint slightly before midrange typically yields this "just-right" muscle length. For example, 70 to 80 degrees of elbow flexion positions the biceps and brachialis at a length associated with maximum strength.

This means there are positions associated with "feeling weaker." A muscle produces less force when it begins a contraction near the end of the joint range because at this short length the myofilaments are bunched together and have poor overlap. Beginning the contraction at the start of the joint range results in similar poor strength due to insufficient overlap.

Excursion

The resting length of muscle fibers determines excursion, the distance a muscle can shorten (A Closer Look Box 4-3). Generally, a muscle can contract to half its

BOX 4-2

A CLOSER LOOK

Determining the Maximum Strength Capability of a Muscle

Common sense tells us that a muscle's size determines its strength. If larger means more bulk and more bulk means a larger cross section, we can express strength clearly. Measurements of bulk determine muscle strength.

Researchers measure the strength of a muscle with special laboratory equipment, dividing the amount of strength (in units of force) by the cross section of the muscle to determine how much force it produces per amount of bulk. Although 10 different muscles of different sizes would produce 10 different force values, dividing each force value by the cross section of the muscle produces approximately the same answer, a constant. The constant commonly used for vertebrate skeletal muscle is approximately 10 kg/cm². *

We use this constant to estimate the maximum force a muscle generates at the beginning of the contraction from its ideal resting length. Use this formula:

$$F = k \times cs$$

F is muscle strength, k is the constant (10 kg/cm²), and cs is the muscle's cross section measured at a place in the belly of the muscle where a cut intersects all the fibers at 90 degrees to the length of the fiber. For example, if a pronator teres has a cross section of 3 cm², its force capability at optimum length would be 3 cm² × 10 kg/cm² = 30 kg. In comparison, a brachialis with a cross section of 6 cm² could produce 60 kg of force.

BOX 4-3

A CLOSER LOOK

Determining Muscle Excursion

As OT practitioners, we rarely need to determine active excursion, the distance through which a muscle contracts. However, when we measure active and passive range of motion, we indirectly measure active and passive excursion. Joints move because the agonist has sufficient active excursion to pull the joint through a range of motion. On the other side of the joint, the antagonist must simultaneously have adequate passive excursion (**distensibility**) to allow joint movement.

Approximate values for muscle excursion give us a deeper understanding of common range of motion measurements. Although experimental findings vary, average excursion equals 50% of a muscle's longest length.[5] Measure the longest length of a muscle when the joints it crosses have moved fully in the antagonistic position. While not exact, positioning the muscle at its longest length and measuring this length based on knowledge of the muscle's attachments provide an approximate but reliable calculation. For the brachioradialis, measure the longest length from just above the lateral epicondyle to the distal tip of the radius in a position of full elbow extension and forearm pronation.

When Eduardo Ybarra holds his upper extremity in full shoulder and elbow flexion, the long head of his triceps from the infraglenoid tubercle to the olecranon measures 35 cm. Based on the 50% estimate, we know that the maximum excursion of his triceps equals approximately 17.5 cm.

*Different authors have reported the strength capability per cross section for human skeletal muscle.[1,3,4] The range of reported results is from 3.6 to 10 kg/cm².

length, but some muscles do vary. Consider muscle *fiber* length, not overall muscle length, to determine muscle excursion. Fusiform muscles like the biceps have fibers running the length of the muscle. If an individual's biceps muscle measures 15 cm from tendon of origin to insertion, so do its muscle fibers. In pennate muscles, tendons run almost the full length of the muscle resulting in shorter muscle fibers. The tendon of the long thumb flexor may measure 20 cm from attachment to attachment; however, it has muscle fiber lengths only 4 cm long because they bridge from bone to tendon (Figure 4-11).

Each joint movement we observe requires some muscle fiber shortening. The more a joint moves, the greater the amount of shortening, or muscle excursion, it needs. A **multijoint muscle** produces movement at more than one joint. It cannot move all these joints simultaneously through complete range of motion because it would have to shorten more than possible (excursion requirement). If stabilization does not occur at one of the joints crossed by a multijoint muscle, the muscle shortens through its full excursion but the range of motion in the various joints remains incomplete. When a muscle's full excursion cannot complete range of motion at all joints, we call it **active insufficiency**.

Because of the injury to his radial nerve, Eduardo Ybarra finds that he can no longer pick up a hammer. His OT practitioner

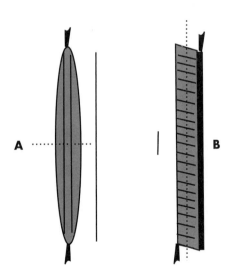

FIGURE 4-11
Comparison of fusiform **(A)** and pennate **(B)** fiber lengths. The *multiple solid lines* within each muscle indicate actual fiber lengths. A *solid line* to the right of **A** and to the left of **B** represents the different lengths of individual muscle fibers. These two muscles measure the same general gross length between attachments. *Dotted lines* indicate the different orientations necessary to measure a cross section, or where a cut will intersect all the fibers.

says that active insufficiency in his flexor digitorum profundus means he lacks the shortening ability to move all its joints simultaneously. She explains that this multijoint muscle crosses the wrist, metacarpophalangeal, and both interphalangeal joints. When Eduardo tries to flex his fingers and close his hand around the handle of a hammer, his fingers cannot form a grasp forceful or complete enough to pick it up. The flexor digitorum profundus contracts, but Eduardo no longer has active wrist extensors to prevent the wrist from flexing. As a result, the flexor digitorum profundus acts unopposed across all of its joints simultaneously. It cannot flex the metacarpophalangeal and interphalangeal joints through full range because it "spends" some of its excursion flexing the wrist as well. The OT practitioner makes a splint to stabilize Eduardo's wrist. Once his wrist no longer flexes Eduardo has sufficient excursion to bring his metacarpophalangeal and interphalangeal joints through enough range to grip the handle.*

Insufficiency in an *antagonist* muscle also can cause incomplete movement or render the muscle(s) on the other side of the joint immobile. For any movement to occur, antagonist muscles located on the opposite side of the joint must allow agonist muscles to concentrically contract. For example, while the long finger flexor contracts, the long finger extensor stretches passively in the distal direction across the flexing joints. The extensor must have enough length to allow full proximal excursion of the flexor yielding full joint flexion.

Directly after his injury, emergency room staff placed Eduardo's left forearm in a cast that held his fingers in slight flexion, his wrist in about 15 degrees of extension, and his elbow in about 90 degrees of flexion. Eduardo's surgeon wanted to ensure that his radial nerve had sufficient time to heal. During that 5-week period, Eduardo used his hand very little. The cast prevented Eduardo from stretching his wrist and finger extensors and led to shortening of the extensor digitorum tendons.

When the hand clinic staff removed Eduardo's cast they found his laceration had healed but radial nerve function had not returned. His grasp efforts produced unwanted wrist flexion along with incomplete finger flexion. To make matters worse, Eduardo's shortened finger extensors limited finger flexion for grasp even sooner than normal in the flexion range because of passive insufficiency of the extensor digitorum muscle.

Passive insufficiency restricts motion in the opposite direction because muscles antagonistic to the desired motion cannot stretch adequately to permit full movement in the desired direction. Active insufficiency involves

---

*To understand active insufficiency imagine trying to push the clutch pedal fully down in a car where the seat slips backward due to a broken latch. The seat moves back before the clutch goes all the way to the floor. Knee and hip extension, or excursion, can push the clutch fully down only if the seat stays in position. The lock on the seat acts like muscles stabilizing the wrist in extension.

insufficient shortening ability (active excursion) in the desired direction, and passive insufficiency involves insufficient passive stretch (passive excursion) in the opposite direction. Both result in incomplete movement of some or all of the joints crossed by the muscles involved.*

MULTIPLE FORCES

Suppose two or more forces act on a body simultaneously. For example, when we considered the various fibers of the pectoralis major, we saw that the forces they produce combine to determine how they act together. This combination of forces, called resultant force, depends on the various directions and amounts of forces involved to determine its magnitude.

Forces Along the Same Line

Forces acting along the same line of application each originate from a single point. That point of application always lies in a straight line with the force represented by the vector.

Force Combination

When forces have the same point of origin and the same direction, we add them.

In a hospital-based clinic OT practitioners use a variety of force combinations in treatment. Spiros Prasso exercises his elbow flexors as part of a regular strength-building circuit in a work-oriented treatment program (Figure 4-12). He uses a 5-kg wrist weight. With a bucket of sand weighing 5 kg attached to the wrist weight, the resultant force equals the sum of both forces. If we draw these vectors to a scale of 1 kg = 0.5 cm, the resultant force will measure 5 cm:

$$5 \text{ kg} + 5 \text{ kg} = 10 \text{ kg}$$

When forces have the same point of application but opposite directions, we subtract them.

In Figure 4-13 Henry Isaacs plays a board game requiring elbow and shoulder flexion to reach and position markers. An overhead pulley system provides the assistance Henry needs to lift his forearm and a cast weighing 6 kg. The 5-kg weight on the pulley helps elevate the upper extremity. To determine the amount of assistance, subtract the 5-kg upward force from the 6-kg downward force of the cast:

$$6 \text{ kg} - 5 \text{ kg} = 1 \text{ kg}$$

---

*Tight jeans or too many layers of clothing can restrict movement in the same way a shortened muscle causes passive insufficiency. As muscles move the joints, the movement meets the resistance of cloth that cannot stretch any further. The cloth rather than muscle length restricts full movement. Movement beyond this point would cause cloth to tear.

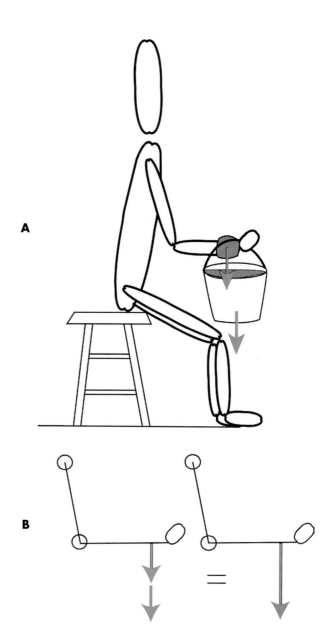

FIGURE **4-12**
A, A 5-kg bucket of sand added to a 5-kg wrist weight increases the amount of weight Spiros Prasso lifts. **B,** The 5-kg force of the bucket added to the 5-kg force of the wrist weight increases the force Spiros needs to lift to 10 kg.

The balance of 1 kg moves in a downward direction; therefore Henry lifts with only 1 kg of additional force instead of 6 kg to move a game marker. The overhead pulley helps maximize Henry's available muscle strength.

Multiple Force Combination

Concurrent forces may act on the same point but come from different directions. We use two methods to find the resultant force of concurrent forces—the parallelogram and the polygon methods. We used the parallelogram

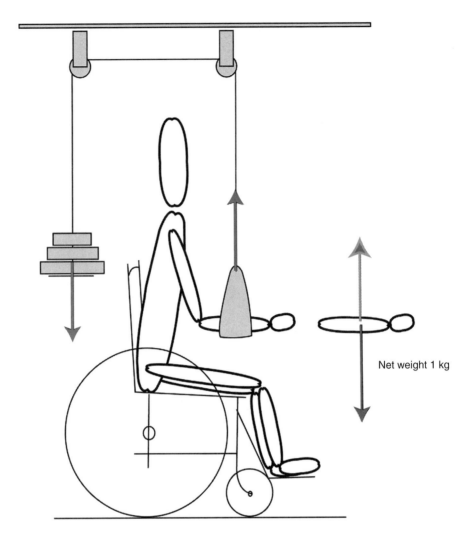

FIGURE **4-13**
The 5-kg weight applied through an overhead pulley offsets the weight of a 6-kg cast on
Henry Isaac's forearm.

method earlier to determine the resultant force of different forces active within the belly of the pectoralis major muscle.

The OT practitioner visiting a metal shop uses this method to answer questions from the staff about worker safety. As part of their daily routine George O'Hara and Raul Estrada must move a 1 m × 1 m × 1.5 m cart filled with metal parts (Figure 4-14). George often complains that Raul does not help him, and sometimes the two fight. The OT practitioner uses a bathroom scale to determine that Raul and George each push with a force of 12.5 kg. The parallelogram method shows us how much force one worker would need to move the cart.

The OT practitioner draws vectors representing the two workers' efforts: Raul pushes 12.5 kg upward and George the same amount on another side of the box (pushing to the right in the figure). She draws these vectors accurately and to scale; then she draws two more sides of the same length parallel to each of the first two to form a parallelogram. Once she has completed the parallelogram, a diagonal line, drawn in the direction the box will move, represents the magnitude of force necessary to move it. By measuring the length of this diagonal vector, the OT practitioner finds the resultant force magnitude, or the amount of force required for one worker to push the cart. The determination helps George and Raul realize they both contribute equally to the task and that having to do it alone would be much more difficult!

Although the measurement of the vector provides a numerical answer sufficient for this work situation, drawing and measuring errors could make this unsuitable for a situation requiring a more accurate solution to safety

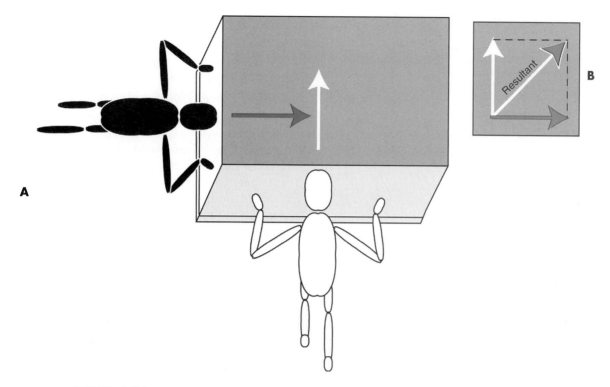

FIGURE **4-14**
A, Raul and George each push a cart using 12.5 kg of force exerted in different directions.
B, The force diagram indicates that one person pushing the same cart must use 17.7 kg of force.

questions. Because these vectors intersect at 90 degrees, the Pythagorean theorem* would give a more accurate absolute value:

$$a^2 + b^2 = c^2$$
$$12.5^2 + 12.5^2 = c^2$$
$$156.25 + 156.25 = 312.50$$
$$c^2 = 312.50$$
$$c = 17.7 \text{ kg}$$

When more than two forces act on an object, use the polygon method to determine the combined effect. Draw arrows representing the forces sequentially, with the base or beginning of one to the tip of the preceding one. Scale the arrow lengths in proportion to the force magnitudes. Orient the arrows in the original direction of the forces.

---

*The Pythagorean theorem states that in a right triangle (a triangle with one angle equal to 90 degrees) the square of the hypotenuse equals the sum of the squares of the two sides. If we know the length of two sides, we can use algebra to determine the exact length of a triangle's hypotenuse.

Fred Jackson underwent surgery to replace a deteriorated metacarpophalangeal joint. As part of his postsurgical therapy program, he needs to wear a splint that provides rubber-band traction to the metacarpophalangeal joint in the direction of extension and radial deviation. An OT practitioner at a hand clinic uses the polygon method to determine the effect of two or more forces on a digit in Fred's splint. The resultant force combines these two separately directed forces (Figure 4-15).

Diagramming the separate forces makes it easier to understand what a splint does. The forces produced by two rubber bands occur simultaneously, pulling the proximal phalanx along a diagonal resultant force that moves radially as it extends. Recognizing that two separate, simultaneous forces combine to form the resultant force allows us to make corrections in the final position. For example, tightening the radial pull yields stronger, more radially-directed extension.

Some practitioners apply dynamic force using one rubber band angled to follow the path of the resultant force. Whether one or two forces are used, being able to understand the combined effect of two forces or conceive of the resultant force as two components helps us visualize how to adjust the force to obtain the desired result. The OT practitioner who does not understand

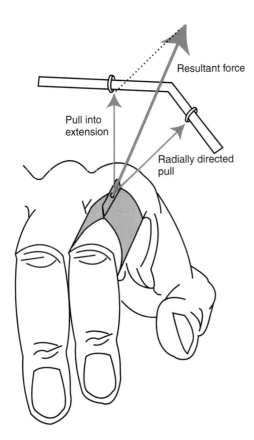

FIGURE 4-15
In this splint the forces from two rubber bands combine to determine a resultant force. An *arrow* directed from the finger cuff toward the point of attachment represents the force of each rubber band.

this process sees the finger moving in an undesirable way, and attempts to correct the force through trial and error, a time-consuming and often frustrating endeavor.

Summary

The topics in this chapter all point to the need for us, as OT practitioners, to understand the physics underlying our observations of functional activity. Failing to understand, we may turn to other sources for ideas, often matching our observations to a list of problems and solutions suggested by a particular protocol. This "cookbook" approach limits therapy to (1) finding a problem on a list, (2) using others' solutions, or (3) settling for a solution that does not exactly match the unique aspects of an individual's life.

Each observation represents a separate situation, and a few fundamental laws explain many different problems. As we develop a greater sense of how these laws interconnect, our understanding of what we observe deepens and our solutions become more effective.

Applications

■ **APPLICATION 4-1**
Adding Forces and Establishing Equilibrium
Donna Nelson carries a tray weighing 0.35 kg. It contains a soft drink weighing 0.5 kg and a sandwich weighing 0.3 kg. How much downward force must Donna match to hold the tray at shoulder height? Draw a graphic representation of this force, indicating the direction and magnitude of the force. Include arrows representing the force of gravity acting on the tray, soft drink, and sandwich.

■ **APPLICATION 4-2**
Adding Forces
Spiros Prasso, advancing in his work treatment program, wears a 6-kg wrist weight and picks up a 7-kg bucket of sand. What downward force must Spiros overcome to lift both the wrist weight and the bucket of sand?

■ **APPLICATION 4-3**
Finding the Resultant Force
Henry Isaacs plays checkers using the overhead pulley. He still wears the 6-kg cast, but only needs a 4-kg weight on the end of the pulley. How much downward force from the weight of his cast must Henry overcome to lift his arm?

■ **APPLICATION 4-4**
Combining Forces
George and Raul must move another 1 m × 1 m × 1.5 m cart filled with metal parts. It takes 35 kg of force to move the cart this time. George can only push with a force of 22.5 kg. How much harder must Raul push to make the cart move?

■ **APPLICATION 4-5**
Determining Force Capability
Measure the girth of your lab partner's biceps and estimate the amount of force this muscle can generate. Use the formula from A Closer Look Box 4-2.

■ **APPLICATION 4-6**
Determining Excursion
Measure the long head of your partner's triceps at its longest length and estimate its maximum excursion.

■ **APPLICATION 4-7**
Drawing Vectors Indicating Contractions
Look at the three drawings in Figure 4-16 and draw a vector representing contraction of the brachialis in each condition.

See Appendix C for solutions to Applications.

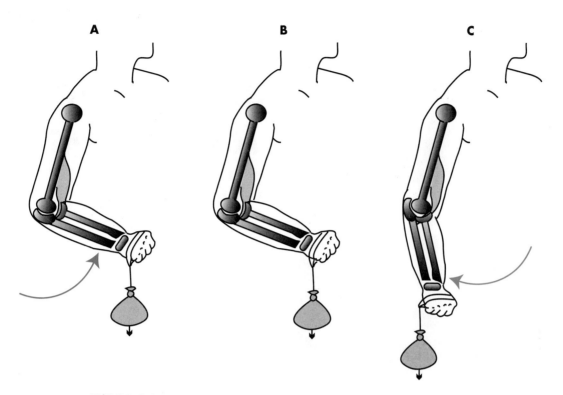

FIGURE **4-16**
Three contraction types: concentric **(A)**, isometric **(B)**, and eccentric **(C)**.

REFERENCES

1. Fick R: *Anatomie und Mechanik der Gelenke: Teil III spezielle Gelenk und Muskelmechanik,* Jena, 1911, Fisher.
2. Gordon AM and others: Variation in isometric tension with sarcomere length in vertebrate muscle fibers, *J Physiol* 184:170-192, 1966.
3. Haxton HA: Absolute muscle force in the ankle flexors of man, *J Physiol* 103:267-273, 1944.
4. Von Recklinghausen N: *Gliedermechanik und Lahmungsprothesen,* Berlin, 1920, J Springer.
5. Weber EF: *Ueber die Langeverhaltnisse der Muskeln im allgemeinen,* Leipzig, Germany, 1851, Verh Kgl Sach Ges d Wiss.

RELATED READINGS

Luttgens K, Hamilton N: *Kinesiology: scientific basis of human motion,* ed 9, Madison, Wis, 1997, Brown & Benchmark.
Nordin M, Frankel VH: *Basic biomechanics of the musculoskeletal system,* ed 2, Philadelphia, 1989, Lea & Febiger.
Wiktorin CH, Nordin M: *Introduction to problem solving in biomechanics,* Philadelphia, 1986, Lea & Febiger.

LAB BOX

Find applied activities exploring concepts in Chapter 4 in the following laboratory exercises:

Topic	*Laboratory*
Muscle excursion	**Lab 4** Accessory Joint Motions/Muscle Excursion/ Active & Passive Insufficiency/Max Assist Transfers
External and internal forces	**Lab 5** Torque and Equilibrium Conditions
Types of muscle contraction	Biomechanical Analysis Lab

5

Rotary Force, Torque, and Motion

ike linear forces and motion, we experience **rotary motion** every day without ever having to think about how it affects us. Examples of rotary motion are everywhere. They include swinging doors, turning doorknobs, and rolling wheelchair wheels. All these objects demonstrate motion around a central point. We see the rotary nature of most skeletal movements when we look for an axis of movement.

For example, the brachialis attaches proximally to the humerus and distally to the ulna. With the humerus stabilized the brachialis contracts concentrically, moving the ulna the only way it will move—around an arc centered in the side-to-side axis of the elbow joint. The brachialis exhibits shortening (excursion) proportional to the amount of movement of the insertion in its arc. This movement, flexion, occurs because the brachialis lies anterior to the flexion/extension axis; we say it has an anterior relationship (Figure 5-1). The rotary motion of elbow flexion results from the linear force created by contraction of the brachialis.

In Chapter 4 we discussed Newton's second law: greater force will have a greater effect on the movement of an object. In this chapter we see that force alone does not determine rotary motion. Another condition, the distance of force from a joint axis, can minimize or enhance the effect of force.

Rotary Motion

Rotary motion differs from linear motion because rotary motion occurs in a circular pattern. Rotary motion of a skeletal segment occurs when the force of a muscle contraction is applied to one segment attached to another segment via a joint. The joint stabilizes the segment at one end, stopping that end from moving while the muscle force moves the other end.

We all recognize that linear movement allows us to go somewhere. Objects in rotary motion travel distances but never get from one place to another except in the path of a circle. Musculoskeletal segments move only in circular paths, but combinations of rotary movements at different joints take us from place to place on linear paths.

The rotary movements of the hands of a clock bring those hands to the same places again and again. Traveling through one circle after another, they measure the passage of time, a linear concept. A clock demonstrates

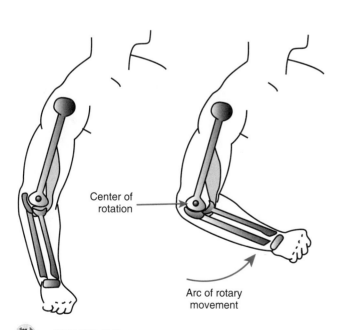

FIGURE **5-1**
The brachialis flexes the forearm at the elbow with a side-to-side axis as its center of rotation. The forearm bones comprise the rotationally moving segment.

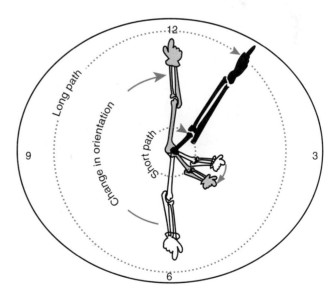

FIGURE **5-2**
The hands of this clock demonstrate the fundamental characteristics of rotary motion. They move in a circular path around a central point and change orientation as they move. The elbow point on the second hand moves at a slower speed than the wrist, which lies farther from the center and moves through a greater circumference in the same amount of time.

the fundamental characteristics of rotary motion (Figure 5-2). The clock's hands move in a circle around a central point. They change orientation, pointing up, right, down, then left. If we tracked different points on the second hand, we would notice these points appear to move at different speeds. In a drawing, the circumference of the circle traced by a point close to the center measures less distance than that of a point on the end of the second hand. Because both points complete one revolution in 1 minute and the end point travels a greater distance in that time, the end point travels faster than the point closer to the center.

As we observe the movement of the second hand, three clear differences between rotary and linear motion emerge (Figure 5-3):

1. Rotary motion occurs in a circular path around a central point, the **center of rotation.** Linear motion occurs along a linear path, starting in one place and ending in a different place.
2. Objects that rotate change orientation during movement. Objects in linear motion remain in their original orientation throughout.
3. Two points in a segment moving around an axis move at different speeds, the point farther from

the center of rotation moves faster than the other. Two points in a segment moving in a line from one place to another move at the same speed. Otherwise, the segment would rotate or break apart.

Tendency to Rotate

In rotary motion, both the force and the point of action of the force on the object are important. Opening and closing a door requires a certain amount of force. However, we must also realize that the point of application affects the amount of force needed.

Crystal Turner, a 4-year-old with Down syndrome, tries to open a heavy glass door for her OT practitioner. Because she cannot reach the handle, Crystal pushes the glass toward the center of the door's width. When the door does not give way, she automatically moves her hand toward the door's swinging edge. Using the same amount of force, Crystal succeeds.

We experience a similar event when we try to open a door with a lock release on a bar handle that spans the width of the door (commonly found in public places). As we try to open the door, we find it easier to place our hand on the far end of the bar, away from the hinge.

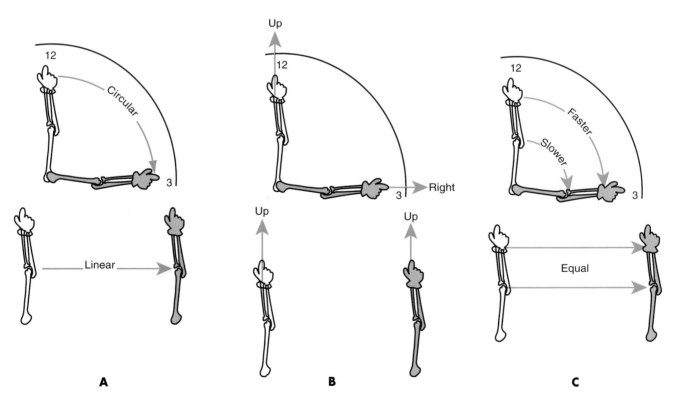

A   **B**   **C**

FIGURE **5-3**
Rotary motion has three unique characteristics: movement in a circular path **(A)**, orientation change **(B)**, and movement that occurs at different speeds depending on distance from the center of rotation **(C)**.

Attempts to open the door by pushing closer to the hinge edge usually fail.

The tendency of a force to cause rotation relates to the spot where force acts. Crystal and her brother experience this fundamental truth of mechanical physics on a playground seesaw. Crystal's older and heavier brother can sit at the bottom and keep her at the top. The seesaw remains stationary until Crystal's brother slides toward the center, closer to the pivot point.

A mechanical engineer may say that the brother's weight (force of gravity) must pull down closer to the pivot in order to give Crystal's weight the **mechanical advantage.** We call this mechanical advantage **leverage.** We lose leverage by applying a force close to a pivot and gain leverage by applying the same force farther away. Thus a lighter weight with enough leverage operates as effectively as a heavier weight. The weight is a force creating a **tendency to rotate** when applied to a segment at some distance from the pivot. Rotation depends as much on where a force acts—its distance from the pivot—as it does on the amount of force exerted.

Torque describes the effectiveness of a force to cause rotation. Torque means tendency to rotate and depends on the amount of force applied and the distance between the force and its pivot, or **axis,** the center of rotation. The formula to determine the value of torque (how much tendency toward rotation exists) is torque (T) equals force (F) times **moment arm** (MA), the distance from the force to the axis (Figure 5-4):

$$T = F \times MA$$

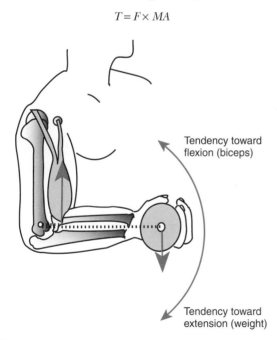

Tendency toward flexion (biceps)

Tendency toward extension (weight)

FIGURE **5-4**

The force of contraction in the biceps and its distance from the axis create a tendency toward elbow flexion. The weight of an object held in the hand and its distance from the axis at the elbow create a tendency toward elbow extension.

The **point of application** (the exact place on the lever or bony segment where force acts) determines a moment arm. On a skeletal segment we find the point of application is synonymous with the muscle's attachment. This attachment and the direction of the force created by muscle contraction determine its moment arm.

Equilibrium of Torques

As we know from studying inertia and linear force, an object at rest remains at rest unless some external force moves it. At rest, all forces associated with an object stay in equilibrium; gravity pulls downward and the reaction of the surface pushes upward. Linear movement occurs along a surface when an external force pushes or pulls in a direction with enough force to overcome the resistance of friction. We say the disturbing force has upset equilibrium. Rotary motion also involves overcoming resistance to upset the existing balance or equilibrium. However, rotary equilibrium involves more than a balance of forces. Whether an object rotates depends on upsetting the balance of tendencies to rotate in one direction versus the other.

Achieving elbow flexion involves upsetting the equilibrium of tendencies toward extension. As the biceps contracts concentrically its tendency toward elbow flexion overcomes a hand weight's tendency toward extension. A heavier weight placed in the hand in a position of mid-elbow flexion might result in an eccentric contraction as the biceps struggled unsuccessfully to create a tendency toward flexion great enough to unbalance the weight's tendency toward extension.

To balance a weight held in the hand at a certain position of elbow flexion, the biceps creates a flexion tendency with an isometric contraction that matches the weight's extension tendency. Because the balance describes equal tendencies for rotation into flexion and extension, equilibrium of rotary tendencies, or **equilibrium of torques,** exists.

We constantly confront equilibrium of torques. *Donna Nelson* provides a clear example as she carries a tray of food. In Chapter 4 we considered her use of linear equilibrium (up and down forces) to hold the tray. Donna must simultaneously create an equilibrium of torques as she prevents the tray from tipping while she removes food items. Donna positions items on the tray based on their relative weights. Heavier food items go near the center, where her hand elevates the tray. She places lighter items closer to the edge.

Figure 5-5 shows Donna's tray in rotary equilibrium. For the purpose of our discussion, assume the tray rotates clockwise or counterclockwise in the plane of the page. Donna's hand provides an axis of rotation, and items on the tray to the right and left of her hand exert

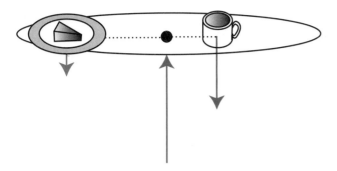

FIGURE **5-5**
Donna's tray rests in rotary equilibrium. The force vectors, drawn to scale, indicate greater force for the full mug of coffee. Notice also the greater distance, or moment arm, between the axis and the dessert. This longer moment arm gives the lighter weight dessert an advantage equal to the heavier coffee mug.

opposite tendencies toward rotation because of their weight and distance from her hand. Serving the coffee mug removes its tendency to rotate the tray clockwise. In the cup's absence the plate of cheesecake produces a tendency toward counterclockwise rotation. Donna must balance the weight of the cheesecake side of the tray before she removes the coffee cup. She does this by moving the plate toward the center of her tray or moving her hand (pivot) closer to the plate.

Lever Systems

Because torque involves both force and moment arm (distance of the muscle force from the joint axis), we cannot use a 4.45-kg muscle contraction force to counteract 4.45 kg of resistance unless both forces act at identical moment arms. In rotary motion we consider forces *and* moment arms; the amount of muscle force required depends on the muscle's moment arm and the moment arm of its resistance. The arrangements of the two moment arms on a lever with respect to each other and the axis of motion vary. The following three variations represent three classes of levers (Table 5-1).

EVERYDAY LEVERS

We use lever systems every day to make our lives easier. Without these adaptive devices, we could not perform many common functions. A lever allows us to use a handle to extend the moment arm, which changes the mechanical advantage of the forces we exert to overcome resistance.

On the seesaw Crystal and her brother experience a first-class lever; one where the mechanical advantage of

effort more or less balances the mechanical advantage of resistance on the opposite side of the axis. Doorknobs, steering wheels, and circular faucet valves all involve exerting forces in opposite directions on opposite sides of a central axis.

Placing a lever extension on circular doorknobs or faucets turns them into second-class levers, a popular adaptive device. Second-class levers lend a mechanical advantage to the force of effort. The amount of force necessary to operate a second-class lever decreases in proportion to the length of the handle. Most bottle openers work as second-class levers (Figure 5-6) as do wheelbarrows (Figure 5-7).

The helpfulness of second-class levers rests in their inherent mechanical advantage. A second-class lever allows the force of effort to operate on a longer moment arm than the resistance force. We choose a wrench with a longer handle to loosen a stubborn nut because this arrangement extends the exertion force moment arm. The hand must travel a greater distance as it applies force to the handle, but the reduced effort required usually outweighs this one disadvantage. Once the nut loosens, we usually grab the handle closer to the nut because we no longer need so much leverage. The inconvenience of moving the handle through all that distance points to a property of rotary motion: a circular path has greater distance farther from its center of rotation.

Third-class levers, which favor the mechanical advantage of resistance, lack the popularity of second-class levers, except for one infamous example from history. Medieval warriors who wanted to hurl objects toward castle walls as fast and as high as possible designed the catapult. Because plenty of warriors existed to provide the effort, flinging objects over great distance with as much force as possible became their primary concern. A third-class lever provided the speed and distance the warriors needed (Figure 5-8). Again, this points out a characteristic of rotary motion: faster movement results farther from the axis of motion. (See Figure 5-2 where the wrist point of the clock's second hand moves faster than the elbow.)

MUSCULOSKELETAL LEVERS

In the body, most musculoskeletal lever systems act as third-class levers (Table 5-1), giving the mechanical advantage not to the muscle trying to lift the load but to the load itself. Most muscle insertions lie close to the joint axis, resulting in short muscle moment arms. Because they operate with short moment arms, muscles must typically generate greater forces than the resistance loads they encounter. Weights held in the hand have the mechanical advantage of being an arm's length from the joint axis. Why would the body evolve to require more

TABLE 5-1 *Classification of Levers*				
We classify levers according to the placement of the axis, resistance force, and machine (muscle) force used to move the resistance.				
	LOCATION OF AXIS	LENGTHS OF *MAs*	DIRECTION OF FORCES*	DIRECTION OF MOTION
First Class	Between the two forces	Resistance force *MA* equal, or one greater than the other	Same	Opposite
Second Class	On one end	Resistance force *MA* always less	Opposite	Same
Third Class	On one end	Resistance force *MA* always greater	Opposite	Same

MA, Moment arm.
*Forces in equilibrium

effort from muscles? Short moment arms for muscles move the ends of the extremities (hands and feet) through greater distances at high speeds, which favors locomotion and tool use.

We often consider third-class levers as examples of poor mechanical advantage to avoid in tools and adaptive devices. But most bone–joint chains, or kinematic chains, work as third-class levers because third-class levers provide advantages in amount and speed of movement. In our bodies, musculoskeletal segments move in rotary motion around joint axes. In this way, distal parts of extremities travel greater distances at faster speeds than proximal body parts. If the body's lever systems were configured as second-class levers, we would have great ability to lift heavy loads but little ability to move them through great distances at fast speeds. Third-class levers provide the only way to position an object at the end of a lever to deliver speed and distance.

Another advantage of the third-class lever lies in the nature of muscle contraction. Muscles can shorten only

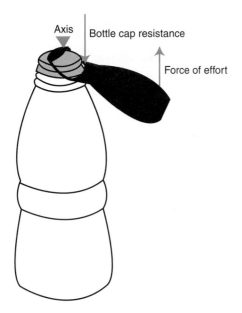

FIGURE 5-6
A bottle opener works as a second-class lever.

a limited distance; they have limited excursion capabilities. If muscles operated within second-class lever systems, muscle moment arms would exceed those of the resistance being moved. As in the case of the wrench handle, the longer muscle moment arm (handle) would

have to travel greater distance. Moving a muscle attachment through a great distance requires greater amounts of muscle excursion than skeletal muscles have available.

Imagine the hand extending from mid-forearm and the brachialis inserting on the distal radius [a second-class lever (Table 5-1)]. The brachialis would have a mechanical advantage, a longer lever arm, compared with the resistance (Figure 5-9). However, because the distal end of the radius lies farther from the axis (elbow joint), it moves through a greater distance at greater speed than the hand. The brachialis attached to this more distal insertion would have to contract through twice the distance the hand would move. It also would have to contract faster, because regardless of its speed, the hand would move at half that speed. We already have seen that muscles have the ability to contract only a limited amount of distance. In addition, the force of contraction suffers if the muscle contracts too fast (A Closer Look Box 5-1).

The third-class lever makes more sense in muscle movement. The muscle operating at a short moment arm can contract slowly and through much less excursion to move the hand faster in a greater arc of motion. Muscles must shorten one-fourth or less the length of distance the hand travels. However, a muscle must generate enough force to make up for its short moment arm (poor mechanical advantage). We increase muscle strength far more easily than muscle excursion.

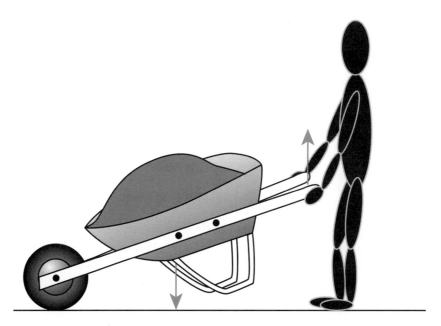

FIGURE 5-7
This wheelbarrow has handles 1.5 m long from axis to hand placement. The hands on the handles apply an upward force, making the handle distance the moment arm for a force exerted by the body. The load (135 kg) projects downward and closer to the axis. The exertion force operates at a longer moment arm.

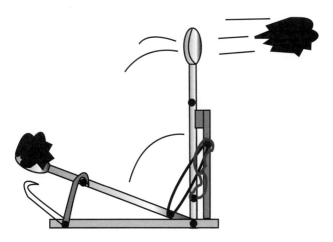

FIGURE **5-8**
The catapult works as a third-class lever.

External and Internal Torques

Two kinds of torque—internal and external—operate on the human body. Forces operating outside the body produce **external torque.** The external torques produced by various food items are Donna's main considerations in balancing her food tray.

A Hand in a Different Place
Switching the hand's location from the end to the middle of the forearm poses a number of problems. A few we have not yet considered follow:

1. Functional reach would greatly decrease.

2. Clothing would require a different design.

3. Eating would require more effort and planning. You would have to position your drink at arm's length because your distal forearm would reach beyond the far side of the plate every time your hand scooped food on the near side.

4. Shaking hands would pose a threat. It would require great care not to poke your acquaintance in the nose with your distal forearm.

5. Decreased typing speed would require you to learn touch typing. (But with practice, you could possibly use your distal forearms to turn the pages of the book from which you are typing.)

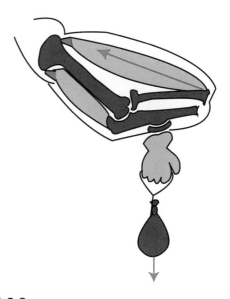

FIGURE **5-9**
If the upper extremity operated as a second-class lever with a moment arm for resistance less than that for muscle force, several problems would result.

Muscles acting on their attachments to bony segments produce **internal torque.** We think of these bony segments as a system of levers. Internal forces of muscle contraction and external forces of the loads we lift create tendencies to rotate in opposite directions of each other at the same joint.

Although Donna may not concentrate on internal torque, it plays just as important a role in the tray's balance as its external counterpart. Once Donna positions items on her tray to equalize their clockwise and counterclockwise tendencies, her shoulder reacts to the external torque of the full tray. The tray exerts an external tendency toward shoulder adduction. Donna's shoulder abductors create an equal internal tendency toward abduction. When the two tendencies balance, she successfully holds up the tray.

We must be careful and notice the words used in the previous statement. Donna supports the tray when the adduction and abduction *tendencies* equalize, in spite of the fact that the forces contributing to these equalized tendencies have very different values. We might ask how tendencies in opposite directions can equalize with disparate forces at work.

To move a load in rotary motion, we must consider both a force and its moment arm. The shoulder abductors create a tendency of rotary motion toward abduction at the shoulder; the weight of the tray creates a tendency toward adduction at the same joint. According to Figure 5-10, these forces operate at very different moment arms. The shoulder abductors attach close to

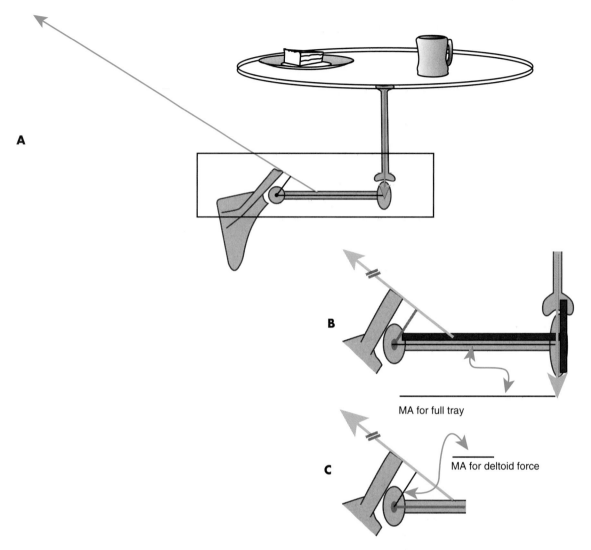

FIGURE **5-10**
A, Equilibrium of abduction/adduction torque at the shoulder. Notice the greater deltoid force needed to compensate for its short moment arm (*MA*). **B**, The T square placed to assist in drawing a tray force moment arm. **C**, The deltoid force (only partly shown in this enlargement) has a poorer mechanical advantage—a shorter moment arm or shorter lever.

the joint and have a short moment arm while the weight of the tray pulls down through the forearm, with a moment arm the length of the humerus. As a third-class lever, the tray has the mechanical advantage—a longer moment arm. Whatever the tray weighs, the shoulder abductors must generate a much greater force to create a tendency toward abduction equal to the adduction tendency created by the tray.

Differentiating between equal tendencies and force magnitude is important. When forces operate on different moment arms, disparate magnitudes of opposing forces allow these forces to generate equal and opposite

tendencies to rotate. We determine the actual value of opposing forces and the torque they generate with a simple formula.

TORQUE VALUE

To determine specific tendencies toward rotary motion, identify and draw the forces and moment arms involved in each tendency. When Donna holds up her tray, shoulder adduction and abduction produce opposing tendencies. We note the humerus, the shoulder joint, and the front-to-back rotational axis for abduction/adduction. The weight of the food tray produces a force for shoulder adduction counteracted by contraction of the deltoid muscle producing a force for shoulder abduction. (Other shoulder abductors also work, but for simplicity we will consider only the deltoid.) We represent the forces of both adduction and abduction as vectors.

Let us consider how we diagram the deltoid force and its moment arm. If we visualize abduction and adduction as a balance between two sets of factors (two force–moment arm sets creating opposite tendencies), we can determine how much force the deltoid muscle must exert to balance the tray. We know the weight of the tray and, using a drawing, can measure the moment arms. To complete the drawing, we must determine deltoid force.

The tray's force (i.e., weight) is 10 pounds. Measure the moment arm by measuring the distance from the tray's force vector (projected from its center of gravity) to the axis of movement. Use a homemade T square made from two cardboard strips attached to each other at 90-degree angles (Figure 5-11). Place the short arm of the T square on the force vector (originating where Donna balances the tray with her hand) and slide the T square along the vector in the direction of the elbow. Stop when the long arm of the T square intercepts the axis of the shoulder joint and draw a line connecting the axis to the force vector. This perpendicular distance is the moment arm of the resistance force. (Figure 5-10 shows this placement. Figure 5-12 shows a similar example that identifies the moment arm for the biceps with the forearm body segment.)

Draw a vector originating from the deltoid's insertion along its fibers to indicate the direction deltoid muscle fibers contract. (Do not draw an arrowhead because we do not yet know the magnitude of this force.) Use the

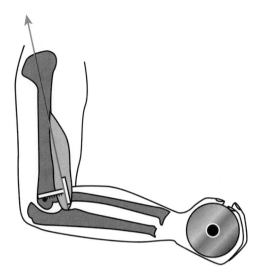

FIGURE **5-12**
Using the T square to determine the distance from force to axis.

sliding T square to measure the distance from the muscle force to the axis and draw this line, the moment arm for deltoid force.

The weight of the food tray and its contents project straight downward from the tray's center of gravity. The weight of the tray times its moment arm (the distance from a vector representing the tray's weight to the axis in the shoulder joint) creates a tendency toward adduction. Because Donna carries the 10-lb tray of food about 10 inches from her shoulder joint, the torque or tendency involved toward shoulder adduction equals the product of the 10-lb tray and the 10-inch moment arm. In other words, multiply force by moment arm to yield a shoulder adduction tendency equal to 100 inch-lb.

Because Donna can elevate and hold the tray up successfully, we know she balances the 100 inch-lb adduction tendency by the abduction effort of her deltoid. But take note! This 100 inch-lb tendency toward abduction (by the deltoid) involves a different combination of force and moment arm because the deltoid inserts so close to the shoulder axis of abduction/adduction. To generate the 100 inch-lb abduction tendency to balance the food tray, the deltoid must produce a 33.3-lb force.

Why must the deltoid create a 33.3-lb force to balance a 10-lb food tray? The food tray weight (force) lies farther (10 inches) from the shoulder joint axis, and therefore has greater leverage than the deltoid. The deltoid pulls with greater force closer to the axis to compensate for its inferior lever (3 inches). Figure 5-10 indicates the different amounts of force with different length vectors.

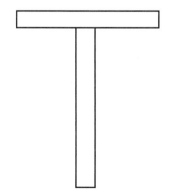

FIGURE **5-11**
A T square helps identify the true (perpendicular) distance from force to axis.

Once we have diagramed both moment arms, we can measure their lengths and calculate the force of the deltoid.

When Donna holds her food tray, the equation looks like this, with the answer rounded down to one decimal place:

Shoulder adduction tendency = Shoulder abduction tendency

$$10 \text{ lb} \times 10 \text{ inches} = \underline{\quad} \text{ lb} \times 3 \text{ inches}$$

$$100 \text{ inch-lb} - \underline{\quad} \text{ lb} \times 3 \text{ inches}$$

$$\frac{100 \text{ inch-lb}}{3 \text{ inches}} = 33.3 \text{ lb}$$

The deltoid needs a 33.3-lb force to balance the tray. Now that we know the magnitude of the deltoid force, we can go back to the line drawn from the deltoid insertion. Measuring the distance along this vector according to the scale used to draw the tray's force vector, place the arrow indicating the deltoid force vector roughly 3 times the length of the vector for the tray's weight.

CHANGING FACTORS DURING CONSTANT TORQUE

We have thought about, measured, determined, and drawn the values of factors (force magnitude and moment arm) that produce a tendency toward rotary motion (torque). These factors often change during movement involving submaximal efforts, even though the amount of torque this combination generates remains the same. When effort increases to a level of maximal strength, torque no longer remains constant but changes depending on joint position.

Torque during maximal effort changes as the magnitude of force and moment arms change. We notice that we may not feel torque as strongly in one joint position as in another. This puzzles us because movement does not change the cross section of a muscle, and cross section determines strength. However, movement does change the length of the muscle, and the length of a muscle at the start of its contraction can affect the amount of force a muscle can generate. Movement also often results in changes to the length of a moment arm. The combination of these changes, including muscle length and moment arm, produces different torques at different joint positions.

We can actually feel these changes of moment arm in the biceps tendon anterior to the elbow. With the forearm supinated and the elbow flexed to 90 degrees, find the moment arm by placing your thumb on the medial epicondyle of the humerus, the approximate location of a side-to-side axis, and your index finger on the biceps tendon. Slowly extend the forearm. The distance between the thumb and finger decreases, providing a good approximation of the changing moment arm length for the biceps.

We use a goniometer and force gauge (dynamometer) to perform a technical but simple measurement of the effect of changes in force magnitude (muscle contraction) and moment arm. Measure the strength of a series of isometric efforts at different joint positions. Each contraction begins at a different point in the range, and we meet maximal effort by matching resistance so that no movement occurs during the contraction. Figure 5-13 shows a maximum isometric torque curve used to plot the results of this measurement.

Isometric torque curves provide values to illustrate the concept that positioning affects the available amount of maximal strength.

For example, Jason Black has an annual school goal to eat independently, but he cannot completely lift a utensil to his mouth. Jason performs best with the table height adjusted so that he starts bringing his hand to his mouth at 90 degrees of elbow flexion. Jason makes a good start away from the plate but as he brings his hand toward his mouth he loses strength and the spoon never quite gets there as long as he sits erect with proper vertebral extension. He begins the motion at the strongest point in the torque-curve range. However, continued flexion brings his elbow to a position that produces less torque. (The changing moment arm and muscle length are shown in Figure 5-14.)

Jason's OT practitioner wonders what causes this problem; too short a moment arm or too short a muscle? In elbow flexion, both occur at joint positions beyond 90 degrees of flexion. Perhaps if Jason had better synergistic function from select shoulder muscles, less biceps muscle shortening would occur and improved muscle length could compensate for the shorter moment

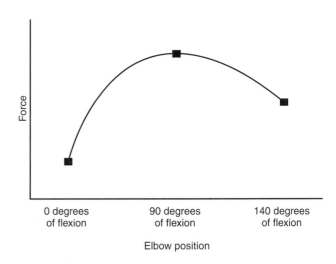

FIGURE **5-13**

Torque generated by contraction of the elbow flexors shown at different places in the elbow-flexion arc.

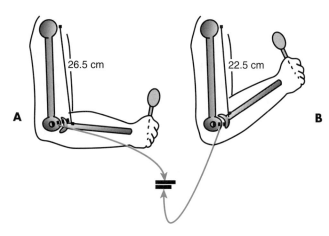

FIGURE 5-14
Changes in length of both Jason's muscle and its moment arm affect Jason's internal torque. **A,** He begins the movement with his elbow flexed to 90 degrees. **B,** He reaches an elbow position that shortens the moment arm and muscle, resulting in loss of strength.

arm, permitting torque to remain more constant. The OT practitioner resolves to facilitate a different movement pattern to test this theory. More shoulder extension will provide better biceps length by preventing the biceps from shortening at the elbow and the shoulder.

Summary

We usually associate force with movement and thus more force with faster movement or greater strength. Rotary movement expands our thinking and helps us realize that the amount of force only partially affects movement. Placement of force with respect to the axis of motion also plays a key role. Together, magnitude and placement result in a tendency to set bony segments and external objects into circular motion. (The tendencies of different muscles to cause circular motion and affect activity will be further discussed in Chapters 6 through 9.)

Applications

■ APPLICATION 5-1
Effort Needed to Open and Close a Valve
Find a sink on which lever faucet handles have replaced round handles. With the faucet securely off, try to turn on the water using one finger placed at the end of the handle. Close the valve and try again, placing your finger closer to the screw connecting the handle to the valve. Can you feel a difference in how easily the valve opens? Identify the axis of rotation and the moment arm.

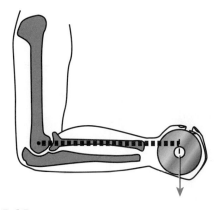

FIGURE 5-15
External torque provides the tendency of a weight to produce elbow extension.

■ APPLICATION 5-2
External Torque Produced by a Barbell
In Chapter 4, we considered some activities in *Spiros Prasso's* work treatment program. Continuing to build his upper-extremity strength, Spiros lifts a 5-kg barbell from a seated position (Figure 5-15). His forearm measures 35 cm from the elbow-joint axis to the palmar crease where the barbell rests. How much external torque does the barbell produce with the elbow flexed to 30, 60, 90, and 120 degrees? Does the external torque remain the same throughout the range of motion? If not, how does it change and why?

■ APPLICATION 5-3
Force Produced by the Biceps
In Figure 5-16, Spiros supports the same 5-kg barbell from a seated position. Let us identify the only functioning elbow flexor as the biceps brachii. It inserts 8.5 cm

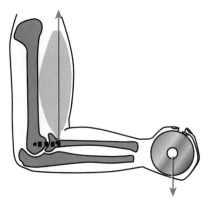

FIGURE 5-16
Internal torque provides the tendency of the biceps to produce elbow flexion.

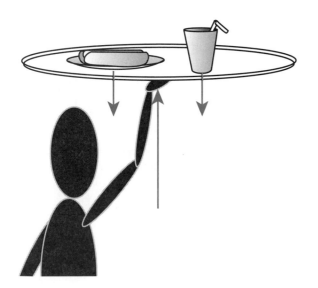

FIGURE **5-17**
Donna's tray holds two food items, a sandwich and a drink, each weighing different amounts. To balance her tray of food with one hand under the tray's center, a torque produced by the drink must equal a torque produced by the sandwich. Different weights can produce equal torques by adjusting each item's moment arm. This skill alone should earn Donna a 20% tip!

from the elbow's side-to-side axis for flexion. The torque produced by the biceps matches the amount of torque at each joint position in the previous application because the biceps supports the barbell. The moment arms for the biceps at the different joint positions are as follows: 6 cm at 30 degrees, 8 cm at 60 degrees, 8.5 cm at 90 degrees, and 6 cm at 120 degrees of flexion. How much force does the biceps produce at 30, 60, 90, and 120 degrees of flexion to support the barbell in an isometric contraction? Does the amount of biceps force remain the same in each contraction? If not, how does it change and why?

■ APPLICATION **5-4**
Balance Needed to Hold a Tray of Food

In Figure 5-17, Donna carefully places each item a certain distance from the center of her tray. If she positions a 0.5-lb sandwich 6 inches from the center of the tray, how far from the center of the tray must she place a soft drink weighing 1 lb?

See Appendix C for solutions to Applications.

RELATED READINGS

Hall SJ: *Basic biomechanics*, ed 4, New York, 2002, McGraw-Hill.

Luttgens K, Hamilton N: *Kinesiology: scientific basis of human motion*, ed 10, New York, 2001, McGraw-Hill.

Nordin M, Frankel VH: *Basic biomechanics of the musculoskeletal system*, ed 3, Philadelphia, 2001, Lippincott Williams & Wilkins.

Wiktorin CH, Nordin M: *Introduction to problem solving in biomechanics*, Philadelphia, 1986, Lea & Febiger.

LAB BOX

Find applied activities exploring concepts in Chapter 5 in the following laboratory exercises:

Topic	*Laboratory*
Rotary motion, axis of movement, moment arm, musculoskeletal levers, changing factors during constant torque, equilibrium of torques, external torque & internal torque	**Lab 5** Torque and Equilibrium Conditions
Rotary motion, axis of movement, moment arm, internal torque	**Labs 7 & 8** Shoulder Complex: Scapular Movement, Differential Functions of Scapular and Glenohumeral Muscles, Differential Functions of Supraspinatus and Deltoid in GH Abduction
Rotary motion, planes, axis of motion, internal and external torques	**Lab 3** Overview of ROM & MMT Motion CD

Basic Concepts Applied to Musculoskeletal Regions

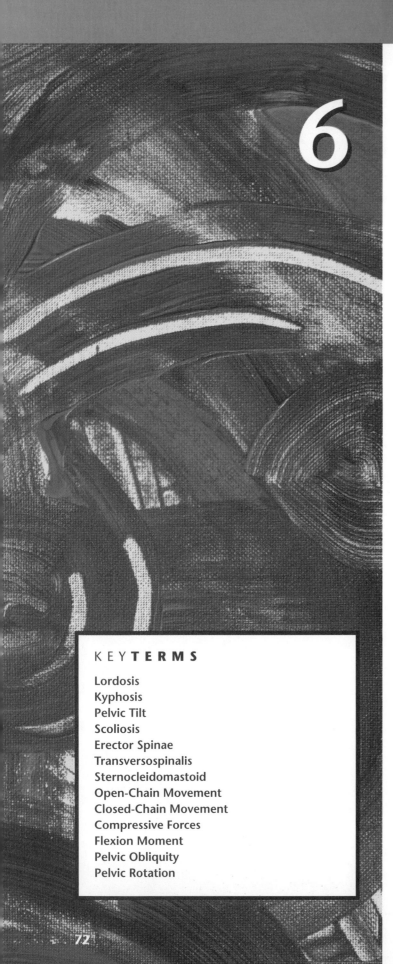

6

The Head and Torso

K E Y **T E R M S**

Lordosis
Kyphosis
Pelvic Tilt
Scoliosis
Erector Spinae
Transversospinalis
Sternocleidomastoid
Open-Chain Movement
Closed-Chain Movement
Compressive Forces
Flexion Moment
Pelvic Obliquity
Pelvic Rotation

The skull, spine, rib cage, and pelvis, by virtue of their strong structure, protect delicate life-supporting organs. Skin, tendons, ligaments, cartilage, and fascia supply additional protection. The torso provides a stable base for the attachment of the extremities and adds to their movement capabilities.

Although the fragile structures enclosed have their greatest security when we assume a fetal position, daily survival depends on our ability to move the bony structures of the head and torso frequently in a variety of amazing ways. Some of these movements reposition the trunk; more often the head, vertebrae, and pelvis accompany upper- and lower-extremity movement.

Background

Twenty-three bones comprise the skull. These connect primarily by fibrous, suture-type joints. A synovial joint called the *temporomandibular joint* joins the jaw to the skull. The combination of this joint and the head's muscle mass allows us to perform the essential activities of eating and communication. Numerous small muscles controlling eye movement, eyelid blinking, facial expression, and attenuation of the hearing mechanism make subtle but important contributions to our ability to interact with the environment.[1]

All the vertebral bodies, except for the first two, attach via *symphyses*, cartilaginous joints containing intervertebral disks. These disks, made up of cartilaginous tissue, attach to the vertebral bodies at their top and bottom edges. A jellylike substance known as the *nucleus pulposus* makes up each disk's center. The structure of the vertebrae and the intervening disks form a strong, flexible column capable of absorbing a great deal of shock without crushing the spinal nerves that exit through foramina between adjacent vertebral segments. Additional intervertebral articulations function more for movement than for shock absorption. These small synovial facet joints allow the vertebral arches (spinous and transverse processes) to move—one on the other—in small amounts. The combined articulations allow one vertebra to move on the other in three planes, although the amount of movement per plane differs from one region to the next.

The cervical vertebrae and disks often are involved in disease and injury. Various tests exist to assess the degree of this involvement (A Closer Look Box 6-1).

Three vertebral curves occur in the sagittal plane. These structural curves occur independently of muscle function, but change shape in response to muscle

contractions. The seven cervical vertebrae form an anterior convex curve (Figure 6-1).

The 12 units of the thoracic spine form a posterior convex curve (Figure 6-2). The thoracic vertebrae stand out because each body has articulating surfaces directed laterally to receive the ribs. Each rib connects with its matching surfaces. All but the first, tenth, eleventh, and twelfth ribs also connect to adjacent vertebrae, thus spanning the disk between. These nonaxial costal articulations permit only slight gliding motion. This added stability in the thoracic spine means that disks of the thoracic spine experience less frequent herniations than those of the lumbar or cervical spine.

The rib cage protects the heart and lungs with a bony enclosure that limits movement of the thoracic spine in both flexion and extension. Seven pairs of true ribs attach directly to the sternum and five pairs of false ribs attach indirectly through cartilage.

The low back has five lumbar vertebrae forming an anterior convex curve like that in the cervical region. The lumbar curve develops its shape as a child learns to stand upright, sit, and walk. It serves to keep the head's

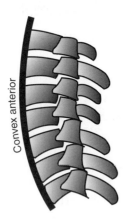

FIGURE **6-1**
Like other curves, the cervical curve has a variety of names. The clearest language consistently names only the orientation of the convexity, as shown here.

center of gravity in line with the pelvis. The lumbar region bears the brunt of poor lifting practices that result in many disk injuries.

The lumbar region joins the five sacral vertebrae, fused together into the *sacrum*, at the lumbosacral joint. The sacrum also articulates with the ilia of the pelvis at the sacroiliac joint. This connection intimately relates pelvic position to vertebral curves. Likewise, shortening of hip and knee muscles that attach to the pelvis directly affects pelvic position and vertebral posture.

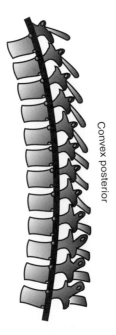

FIGURE **6-2**
The thoracic curve orients in reverse of the cervical and lumbar curves.

PATHOLOGICAL CURVES

The normal curves just described can change for several reasons, including poor posture and abnormal pelvic position. The cervical and lumbar curves may increase (**lordosis**), flatten, or even reverse. (Figure 6-3 shows the normal lumbar curve, which is convex anteriorly *[A]*, and a flattened lumbar curve *[B]*.) The thoracic curve typically increases (**kyphosis**) as upright posture declines. Because the thoracic region links to those regions above and below it, kyphotic posture may occur in association with cervical lordosis, to maintain visual gaze, and flattened or reversed lumbar curve, a rounding of the lower back.

Lordosis of the lumbar curve, commonly called "sway back," occurs with an exaggerated anterior **pelvic tilt.** Likewise, a flattened or reversed lumbar curve occurs with a posterior pelvic tilt. Sometimes the pelvic position develops in response to a change in the lumbar curve. Because of their intimate connection, change in one affects change in the other.

Lumbar Curve
Without regular stretching, hip flexors and extensors may assume shorter resting lengths (contracture). We often notice shortened hamstrings (hip extensors)

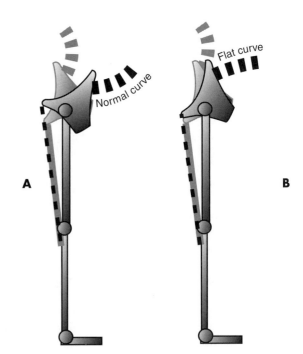

FIGURE **6-3**
A, Normal-length hamstrings allow full flexion of the trunk and pelvis. **B**, Short hamstrings become stretched early as the trunk and pelvis flex onto the thigh. Once the hamstrings reach the limits of stretchability, they prevent further movement of the pelvis. Continued efforts to bend must all occur in the vertebral column through a reversal of the lumbar curve.

when attempting to touch our toes while keeping our knees extended. First the torso flexes onto the lower extremities at the hip. Then, as hip flexion reaches its extreme, the back begins to flex and round out, accommodating the shortened hamstrings (passive insufficiency). We usually feel tightness in the posterior thighs as the stretched hip extensors pull inferiorly on the ischial tuberosity (origin), limiting further hip flexion by stopping pelvic motion (Figure 6-3, *B*).

Extremely short hamstrings can exert this same pull on the pelvis with even less hip flexion, in activities like walking or sitting in a chair. Short hip extensors cause the pelvis to assume a posterior tilt that pulls the lower lumbar vertebrae along with it, reducing, flattening, or even reversing the lumbar curve (Figure 6-4).

Scoliosis

The curves previously described occur in the sagittal plane, visible only from a side view. Even though they may become exaggerated in pathological conditions, we consider these sagittal-plane curves as essentially normal.

Scoliosis describes a curve in the frontal plane, visible from an anterior view. Scoliosis always describes a pathological condition. Extreme cases involve two or more curves in opposite directions that give the appearance of an "S". Scoliosis has a unique orientation in the frontal plane as well as accompanying rotation of vertebral bodies in the horizontal plane.

When scoliosis occurs in the thoracic region, the ribs that attach to vertebrae move along with the vertebrae in a horizontal plane. Because the ribs attach to the vertebral bodies and each body rotates, each pair of ribs turns like a steering wheel (Figure 6-5). This motion forms a raised area, or hump, posteriorly as the posterior aspect of the moving ribs pushes on superficial soft tissue. The posterior ridge occurs on the side of the convexity of the scoliotic curve; therefore a convex scoliosis on the right side produces a hump on the right side of

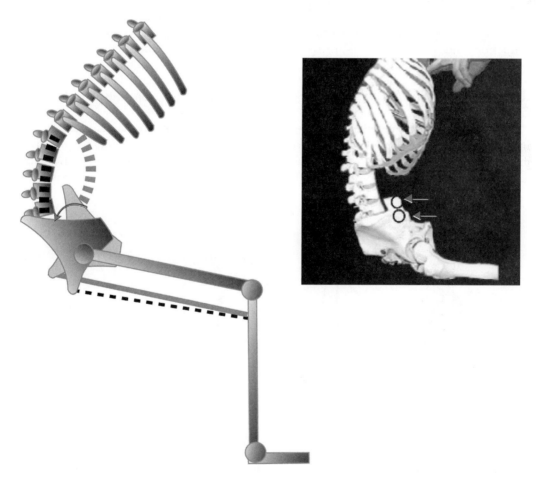

FIGURE **6-4**
Posterior pelvic tilt and a resting posture of reversed lumbar curve secondary to short hamstring length. Note that the description of pelvic position corresponds to the direction of movement at the anterior superior iliac spine.

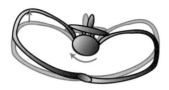

FIGURE **6-5**
In a view from above, a vertebra turns with the rib pair attached to it.

the back. (Figure 6-6 summarizes and compares these three pathological curves with normal alignment.)

Torso Movements

The deep muscles of the back attach to the skull, vertebrae, ribs, and pelvis. These deep muscles maintain the strength and integrity of the spinal column and allow for postural control and movement. Movements of the vertebral column occur in all three planes of motion: extension and forward flexion in the sagittal plane, lateral flexion to either side in the frontal plane, and rotation to either side in the horizontal plane (Figure 6-7).

BILATERAL AND UNILATERAL CONTRACTIONS

The head must have a wide range of motion to position sensory organs such as the eyes, ears, nose, and mouth for optimal gathering of information. For this reason the cervical vertebrae form the most mobile section of the spine and allow movement in all three planes.

The first cervical vertebra, or *atlas*, has a ringlike structure that attaches to the skull via bilateral synovial joints. These joints primarily allow flexion and extension of the skull on the neck.

The second cervical vertebra, or *axis*, has a toothlike protuberance, the dens (odontoid process), onto which the atlas fits and rotates. The head rotates on the neck at this joint, but the entire cervical region rotates as the head shakes "no" or turns to allow the eyes to track a moving object. (Watch a crowd of spectators at a tennis match to see the cervical region operating at its best!)

Muscle contractions in three major groups of muscles produce cervical, thoracic, and lumbar movements in all directions. The erector spinae and transversospinalis produce cervical, thoracic, and lumbar motion, while four pairs of abdominal flexors control only thoracic and lumbar movement.

The first two groups occur segmentally. They originate deep in the back on lower segments and insert into higher segments. These muscles, paired right and left, derive their names from their respective spinal segments of insertion. For example, the longissimus thoracis and longissimus cervicis make up two sections of the erector spinae group. As a rule, more superficially placed fibers span a number of vertebrae and deeper fibers span fewer segments.

Erector Spinae
Because our interest inclines toward structural relationships leading to movement, rather than the specific names of anatomical connections, we differentiate the

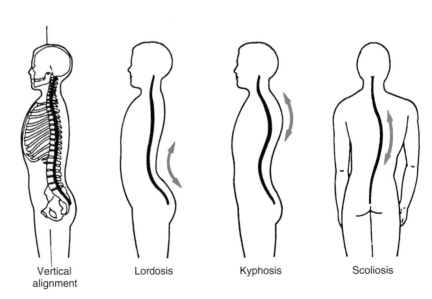

Vertical alignment   Lordosis   Kyphosis   Scoliosis

FIGURE **6-6**
Normal alignment versus three pathological curves. (Modified from Hall SJ: *Basic biomechanics,* ed 4, New York, 2002, McGraw-Hill.)

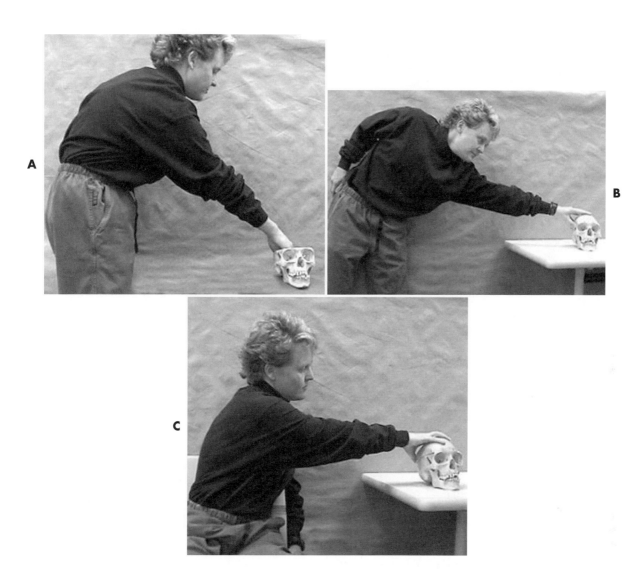

FIGURE **6-7**
The three pure movements of the vertebral column: **A**, forward flexion; **B**, lateral flexion—
to the left; and **C**, rotation—anterior to the left.

two groups of deep back muscles by the directions of their fibers. The **erector spinae** muscles mostly run parallel to the vertebral column and consist of three major divisions: the spinalis, running spine to spine; the longissimus, running largely from transverse process to transverse process; and the most laterally placed iliocostalis, running from rib to rib.

Based on our fundamental knowledge of muscle action on joints, we know that a muscle force pulling through the axis of motion produces no tendency for rotation and no movement. We say no "moment" occurs for the movement because although force exists, it lacks a moment arm and therefore has no tendency to rotate (torque). A contraction force pulling at some distance from the axis produces torque so movement occurs when the muscle contracts.

All three divisions of the erector spinae lie posterior to the side-to-side axes for flexion and extension so they extend the vertebral column. Except for the spinalis division, erector spinae muscles also lie to the left and right of the front-to-back axes for lateral flexion and move the trunk side-to-side in the frontal plane. (Figure 6-8).

Notice that although these relationships exist the erector spinae have very short moment arms. Short moment arms put spinal muscles at a mechanical disadvantage, a prime factor in back injury (disk herniation and rupture). Lifting from a bent-over position instead of using hip and knee extension puts most of the work on these mechanically disadvantaged spinal muscles. If the back extensors attached to a long handle, such as the backwards rib shown in Figure 6-9, they would have longer

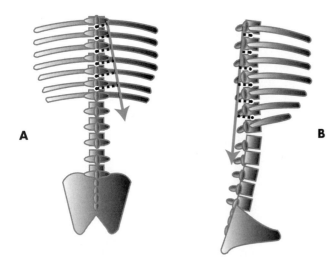

FIGURE **6-8**
The relationship of the erector spinae muscles to the **A,** front-to-back and **B,** side-to-side axes. Notice that a moment arm drawn from force to axis quantifies the distance from the axis at which the force pulls. Different views (posterior for lateral flexion and side for extension) show movement in different planes.

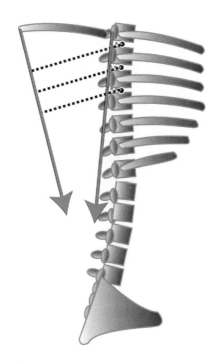

FIGURE **6-9**
Extra help for the back extensors—mechanically wonderful—but a functional disaster for daily living.

moment arms at each side-to-side axis. However, imagine the difficulty in wearing a shirt or a slip-over sweater!

Since one muscle group produces both trunk extension and lateral flexion, how can one movement occur independently from the other two? Consider what happens when parts of a muscle act in isolation from the rest. Contraction of the left erector spinae laterally flexes the column to the left (the same side); contraction of the right erector spinae laterally flexes the column to the right. These statements describe unilateral contractions and actions are based on left and right relationships to the front-to-back axes. A bilateral contraction of the erector spinae (left and right sides) cancels the lateral flexion effects (equilibrium of tendencies in opposite directions) and produces extension. Every vertebral muscle has the potential for action at multiple axes, requiring us to differentiate between unilateral and bilateral functions for each muscle group.

Transversospinalis

The **transversospinalis** group is primarily responsible for rotation of the vertebral column. This group, segmented and paired like the erector spinae group, contains fibers running diagonally rather than parallel to the column. Generally, as concentric contractions occur, the group's laterally placed origins (transverse processes) pull their more superiormedial attachments on spinous processes laterally. These contractions serve mainly to rotate the vertebrae. For example, the left transversospinalis rotates the trunk so that the front turns to face right (Figure 6-10).

Sternocleidomastoid

The head and cervical region most often move together, sometimes independent of but often in conjunction with the entire vertebral column. The **sternocleidomastoid,** the most prominent of the anterior neck muscles attaching to the head, functions across all cervical axes and the

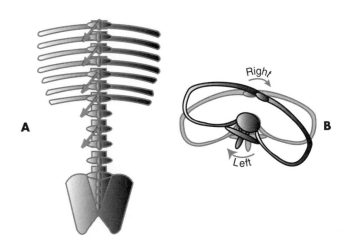

FIGURE **6-10**
A, The transversospinalis group rotates the vertebrae by pulling the medial insertion (spinous process) toward the lateral origin (transverse process). **B,** One point of confusion in the terminology occurs when the trunk "turns right" (anterior facing right) and the spinous process "moves left" (posterior facing left).

atlanto-occipital joint. Each side of this paired muscle originates from the sternum and proximal clavicle anteriorly and inserts posteriorly on the mastoid process of the skull. Many misunderstand the sternocleidomastoid as a simple head flexor. The muscle actually provides different functions at different levels of the head and neck. As always, attention to the relationship of muscle fibers to the axis of movement goes a long way toward explaining the variety of functions available (Figure 6-11).

To fully understand the sternocleidomastoid we need to look at the head and neck as separate units. The head may move independently of the neck or the head and neck may move as a unit in relation to the trunk. At its insertion on the mastoid process, the sternocleidomastoid lies posterior and inferior to side-to-side axes of the sagittal plane. From the cervical segments lying anterior to the muscle, the sternocleidomastoid extends the head in relation to the neck. Near its origin on the sternum, the force of contraction runs anterior to the side-to-side axis at the base of the neck, so from there the sternocleidomastoid flexes the head and neck as a unit in relation to the trunk. All these functions involve bilateral contractions of the sternocleidomastoid and synergistic function of other muscles.

Considering the movements possible at the numerous axes, bilateral contraction of the sternocleidomastoid muscle alone results in extension of the head, hyperextension approaching virtual collapse of the cervical region, and flexion of the head and neck onto the trunk (Figure 6-12). Production of the movements we associate

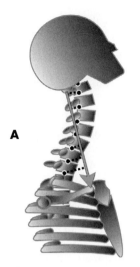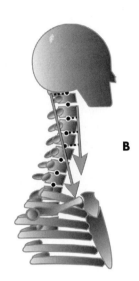

FIGURE 6-12
A, Appearance of the head and neck when the sternocleidomastoid acts alone. **B,** The same muscle acts in conjunction with a deep cervical flexor, the longus colli, to prevent hyperextension of cervical vertebrae.

with the sternocleidomastoid actually involves reliance on the synergistic function of a deep cervical flexor.

"Why can't Jason Black chew with his mouth closed?" asks one of the teaching assistants during lunch one day. The occupational therapy practitioner draws a picture to show what happens when Jason's sternocleidomastoid muscles contract without proper synergistic coordination from his other neck muscles. She points out Jason's lack of chin tuck and inability to elongate his neck. The OT practitioner has the teaching assistant attempt similar positioning while chewing a piece of cracker. "Now I see why he does better when repositioned," says the assistant.

Normally the sternocleidomastoid contracts with a deep cervical flexor, the longus colli, preventing hyperextension in the cervical vertebrae. These two muscles, together with vertebral extensors, help individuals gaze forward, elongate the neck, and tuck the chin. Specifically, the sternocleidomastoid partially extends the head on the neck while the longus colli prevents cervical hyperextension. The highest segments of the erector spinae group partially extend the head and neck in relation to the trunk.

Flexor (Abdominal)
The four paired abdominal muscles help the trunk flex and rotate. They also protect the internal contents of the abdominal and pelvic cavities.

The rectus abdominis flexes the trunk as contraction pulls its superior attachment on the sternum inferiorly toward its attachment on the pelvis. Overstretching the rectus abdominis, from excessive weight gain or pregnancy, creates less upward force on the pubic symphysis, which can cause anterior pelvic tilt and lumbar lordosis.

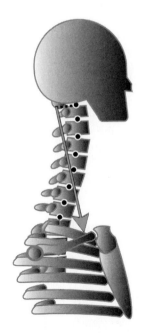

FIGURE 6-11
The sternocleidomastoid muscle in relation to various head and neck side-to-side axes.

The fibers of the external abdominis oblique follow an angle similar to that seen when the fingers are placed in front trouser pockets. Each side of the external abdominis oblique attaches inferiorly and medially to the pelvis and usually pulls the superior lateral insertion diagonally in a unilateral contraction. For example, the right external oblique rotates the trunk, turning the front leftward. Like the transversospinalis, the external abdominis oblique rotates the trunk to the opposite side of the muscle's location. Some lateral flexion to the same side also occurs because of the muscle's lateral relationship to the front-to-back axis of the frontal plane. Finally, this paired muscle has an anterior relationship to the side-to-side axis of the sagittal plane; a bilateral contraction cancels all rotational and lateral flexion and flexes the trunk forward.

One layer deeper, the fibers of the internal abdominis oblique run opposite those of the external oblique. Unilateral contraction of the internal oblique pulls the medial, superior attachment on the lower ribs diagonally downward toward the more lateral attachment on the pelvis, rotating the trunk to the same side. In other words, the right internal oblique rotates the trunk anterior to the right with some lateral flexion to the same side. Bilateral contraction flexes the trunk.

The transversus abdominis inhabits the innermost layer, and its fibers run horizontally. This layer primarily supports the internal organs; it also helps the trunk laterally flex and rotate.

Posteriorly, two major muscles—the quadratus lumborum and the iliopsoas—protect the abdominal contents. The quadratus lies next to the spine from the lower ribs to the iliac crest of the pelvis. Its fibers run mostly vertically, laterally flexing the vertebral column to the same side in a unilateral contraction. Working on its inferior attachment, the quadratus lumborum raises the pelvis on one side with a unilateral contraction or raises the entire pelvis with bilateral contractions.

Two muscles comprise the iliopsoas—the psoas major, originating on the lumbar spine, and the iliacus, originating on the pelvis. These two muscles join in a tendon that attaches to the lesser trochanter of the femur. The iliopsoas flexes the thighs at the hips. With the insertion at the femur stabilized, the iliopsoas acts on its more proximal attachment and pulls the pelvis forward into flexion over the thigh. The iliopsoas, through its effect on anterior pelvic tilt, contributes to the normal lumbar curve.

OPEN- AND CLOSED-CHAIN MOVEMENTS

The upper extremity consists of a chain of segments connected at joints. When the free distal end of the extremity moves, we call it an **open-chain movement**.

Open-chain movements involve stabilization of the muscle origin, concentric contraction, and movement of the muscle insertion. This combination yields motion of the distal end of the extremity. Many functional movements involving lifting of objects or movement of the hands in various personal hygiene and home-management tasks use open-chain movements.

The phrase *open-chain* helps differentiate specific movements. Muscles shorten but cannot control whether the proximal or distal attachments move. With the proximal attachment (origin) stabilized, a concentric contraction moves the distal segment in relation to more proximal segments and the trunk. For example, the forearm flexes onto the arm through open-chain elbow flexion, whereas the entire upper extremity flexes in relation to the trunk through open-chain shoulder flexion.

Closed-chain movements do not follow this scheme. In a push-up or pull-up, the hand, as distal end of the chain, remains stable and the trunk moves in relation to the hand for closed-chain elbow flexion. In a sit-up, the trunk flexes over the hip onto the thigh for closed-chain hip flexion. A deep-knee bend brings the anterior leg to the dorsum of the foot in closed-chain dorsiflexion. In each case the insertion remains stable and the origin moves. (Review Figure 4-10 to see closed-chain elbow flexion and shoulder extension.)

The status of the distal end of the chain distinguishes closed versus open-chain movements. In open-chain movements, muscles contract across joints to move a segment's distal end in space. The same muscles contract across the same joints to produce closed-chain movements when distal ends remain stationary. The stabilization of the distal end occurs either by holding onto a stationary object, in the case of the upper extremity, or by bearing the weight of the body.

The trunk produces many closed-chain types of shoulder and hip movements. Lifting a suitcase involves open-chain shoulder extension and elbow flexion resulting in upward movement of the hand. Chin-ups involve the same shoulder extension and elbow flexion in a closed-chain. The hand remains stable by holding the bar. It cannot move downward to the body, so the body moves up to the hand. Kicking the foot up in front of the body involves open-chain hip flexion (the foot moves), whereas bending the trunk forward at the hips to touch the toes involves closed-chain hip flexion (trunk moves, Figure 6-13). Walking produces the most commonly experienced closed-chain movements. After the foot is planted, the trunk moves over it in closed-chain hip extension. This alternates with open-chain hip flexion as the lower extremity swings forward to take another step.

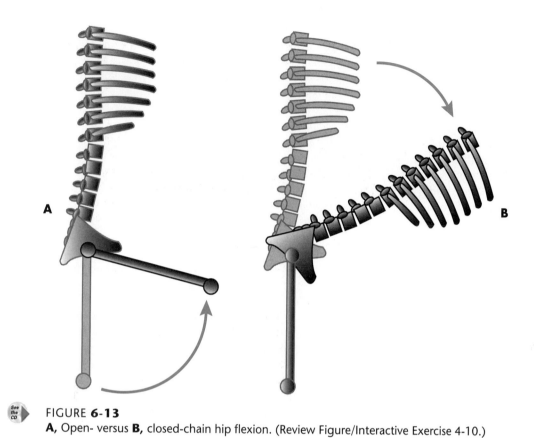

FIGURE **6-13**
A, Open- versus **B,** closed-chain hip flexion. (Review Figure/Interactive Exercise 4-10.)

TRUNK POSITIONING

Effective use of the extremities requires a stable base. In many cases this base (the trunk) not only provides stability but also contributes to movement. In forward reach the trunk remains upright. As the body reaches farther forward, vertebral flexion accompanies scapular protraction, shoulder flexion, and elbow extension. In side reach the trunk flexes laterally. Reaching across the chest with the right arm to grab an object on the left involves trunk rotation. Upright posture and the three major vertebral movements accompany a multitude of upper-extremity movements.

Stabilization
Any examination of trunk movements associated with extremity functions leads to a focus on the scapula and pelvis. Movements of the arm at the shoulder and of the thigh at the hip involve activation of muscles inserting on the humerus and femur, respectively. Movements of insertions (open-chain motions) require stabilization of origins; this stabilization involves activation of muscles originating in the trunk and inserting on the scapula or pelvis.

While lying in a supine position to perform straight-leg raises, the abdominals tighten. Why do the abdominals contract when the hips simply flex to raise the lower extremities slightly into the air? Remember, muscles shorten and move that attachment connected to the lightest segment—the segment that moves most easily. Hip flexors originating from the pelvis and crossing the hip to insert on the femur can tilt the pelvis forward more easily than they can raise the entire lower extremity against the pull of gravity. Without the pelvis (origin) stabilized, the hip flexors would tilt the pelvis and have little contractility left to flex the hip and raise the lower extremity (Figure 6-14).

Thus the rectus abdominis guarantees a stable pelvis by pulling upward on its attachment to the pubic

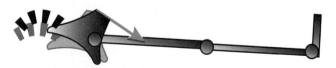

FIGURE **6-14**
Movement of the pelvis with unstabilized hip flexor origins.

symphysis as the hip flexors contract. Because the hip flexors cannot move their origins, they shorten and move their insertions, achieving the desired leg raise by flexing the hip. We observe open-chain hip flexion.

The OT practitioner evaluating Tony Adams holds out a large beach ball. Tony reaches for it with both hands but has two different movement patterns. On the left side his shoulder abducts and his elbow extends, placing his hand on the ball. On the right side Tony's elbow is slower to move away from the trunk—the shoulder does not achieve the same amount of abduction as on the left. His elbow partially extends, and he manages to place his right hand on the ball with a small trunk rotation to the left side. A stray bullet has permanently altered Tony's ability to abduct his right shoulder.

Both glenohumeral abductors originate largely from the scapula and insert onto the humerus. As they shorten, Tony's unstabilized scapula, weighing less than his upper extremity, moves first. In Tony's case the right abductors waste excursion rotating the scapula downward instead of fully abducting the arm (Figure 6-15 and Figure 4-1). In the normal pattern, contraction of Tony's left upward scapular rotators stabilizes the scapula against this downward pull, preventing movement of the origin of the arm abductors. These scapular muscles originating on the trunk and inserting onto the left scapula perform upward rotation, contributing to full shoulder abduction. On the right side Tony's external abdominis compensates for his shortened reach with trunk rotation. Similar stabilizing and mobilizing trunk muscles play an essential role in all extremity movements.

FORCES ACTING ON THE HEAD AND TORSO

Clinical observation of the head and vertebral column involves the realization that we live, play, and work under gravity's constant influence. Muscle contractions that maintain upright posture inevitably cause **compressive forces** to act on the vertebral bodies and disks. We must account for these forces in activity analysis.

Neck

The department head of an occupational therapy educational program contracts with the Assistive Technology Resource Center (ATRC) on campus after several OT students complain of neck pain and upper-back tightness associated with time spent completing assignments on departmental laptop computers in their new wireless biomechanics laboratory. All students use identical equipment and spend approximately 3 hours at their computers. The most seriously affected student, Olivia Xiong generally sits with her head flexed to 30 degrees. She stands about 2 meters (m) tall and weighs 65 kilograms (kg). Nancy Grant, another student, has fewer problems and is observed sittting

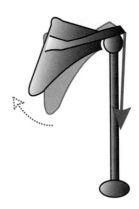

FIGURE **6-15**
Tony's scapula downwardly rotates when his shoulder abductors act on their origins because of his paralyzed upward scapular rotators. (Review Figure/Interactive Exercise 4-1.)

with her head erect. Nancy stands about 1.6 m tall and weighs 60 kg. The OT practitioners from ATRC estimate that the students' heads each weigh about 5 kg (see Appendix B, Table B-1). Figure 6-16 shows these students at their laptops.

The OT practitioners want to know the force, or load, on each operator's intervertebral disks and the force of contraction in the head extensors, and how these values change with different head positions. First, they determine the force of muscle contraction in the spinal extensors because contraction of these muscles to extend the cervical region produces substantial compression (linear force) and extension (rotary force).

Although the cervical region contains a number of side-to-side axes, the OT practitioners focus on the axis of motion at cervical vertebra 5 (C5), about 3 centimeters (cm) above the palpable spine of C7. The head's center of gravity lies between the temples where they come closest to the temporomandibular joint. With the head erect, the distance from the axis of motion to the center of gravity in the head equals about 2 cm. With the head flexed, this same distance measures about 6 cm. The distance of the erector spinae to the axis of motion equals about 4 cm with the head erect or flexed to 30 degrees.

In Figure 6-17 a diagram of Nancy's head shows the opposing forces and their moment arms. Forces play in opposite directions, which normally causes tendencies toward rotation in opposite directions. Because little or no movement occurs, equilibrium exists. The torques (tendencies) in opposite directions remain equal; thus torque of flexion, caused by head weight, equals torque of extension, caused by muscle contraction in the head extensors. The sum of all torques (T) equals zero ($T = 0$).

Calculate the force of the erector spinae muscles by using the formula for equilibrium of torques, which considers the force (F) and moment arms (MA) in opposite directions. Engineers and physicists set this up first with a summary statement indicating torques (tendencies

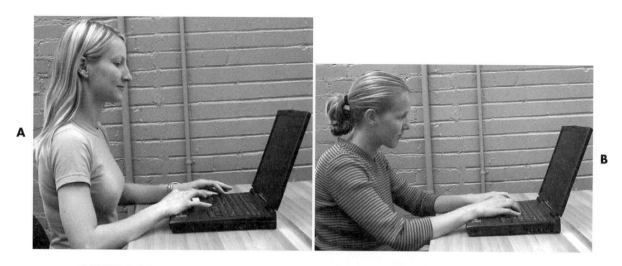

FIGURE **6-16**
A, Nancy, an occupational therapy student, sits with her head erect. **B**, Olivia, a fellow student, sits with her head held in a slight amount of flexion (30-degree angle from vertical).

to rotate) in the two opposite directions are equal ($\Sigma T = 0$). Correct procedure specifies conversion of mass units to force units: all kilogram measures convert to newtons by multiplying the mass amount by the acceleration of gravity. We will use this method to solve the first problem but take a shortcut in later calculations.

$$\Sigma T = 0$$

$$\text{Torque}_{\text{extensors}} = \text{Torque}_{\text{gravity}}$$

$$F_{\text{extensors}} \times MA_{\text{extensors}} = F_{\text{gravity}} \times MA_{\text{gravity}}$$

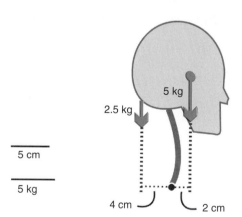

FIGURE **6-17**
To maintain the head in erect posture, the erector spinae muscles must exert 2.5 kg of force. This causes a reaction force of 7.5 kg upward on the C5 disk, determined by adding the two forces (head weight and muscle force) directed downward.

In this equation, $F_{\text{extensors}}$ and F_{gravity} represent the forces created by the erector spinae and gravity, respectively. Moment arms (distance or force from the axis) for the extensors and gravity become $MA_{\text{extensors}}$ and MA_{gravity}. Remember to convert centimeters to meters and kilograms to newtons (N): 5 kg ×10 kg-m/sec² = 50 N (head weight represented as a force). Now we have the torque equation and can solve for the force of the extensors:

$$F_{\text{extensors}} \times 0.04 \text{ m} = 50 \text{ N} \times 0.02 \text{ m}$$

$$F_{\text{extensors}} = 1 \text{ Nm}/0.04 \text{ m}$$

$$F_{\text{extensors}} = 25 \text{ N}$$

Disk compression involves a linear force in which both gravity and the erector spinae muscles pull downward, so the reaction force on the disk must be an equal upward force. Forces up equal forces down, or the sum of all forces equals zero ($\Sigma F = 0$). Converting kilograms to newtons, calculate the reaction force on the C5 disk by using the formula for equilibrium of forces.

$$\Sigma F = 0$$

$$F_{\text{reaction}} = 25 \text{ N} + 50 \text{ N}$$

$$F_{\text{reaction}} = 75 \text{ N}$$

The abbreviated method would look similar to the calculations most likely used in practice settings. Start by equating the tendency in one direction with the tendency in the opposite direction. Then move directly to solving for the muscle force and omit conversion of kilograms to newtons. Although formally incorrect in terms of units, the relative values of force tendency remain essentially correct.

$$F_{extensors} \times 4 \text{ cm} = 5 \text{ kg} \times 2 \text{ cm}$$

$$F_{extensors} = 10 \text{ kg cm}/4 \text{ cm}$$

$$F_{extensors} = 2.5 \text{ kg}$$

The relative values of extensor and flexor force have the greatest importance in this type of real world problem. To balance Nancy's 5 kg of erect head weight, her extensors generate half as much force (2.5 kg). Why? Because Nancy's extensors work at a longer moment arm than the weight of her head. The location of the center of gravity in Nancy's head and the attachment of her extensor muscles determine the moment arms. The head's center of gravity projects closer to the axis at C5 (2 cm) than does the line of force of her extensors (4 cm). We will see this relationship over and over: because the extensor force has a moment arm twice that of the head weight, the extensor force generates the same amount of **tendency** as the head weight with half the force— a convenient arrangement to conserve energy with correct posture!

When Olivia holds her head flexed to 30 degrees, the compressive forces are amplified because the increased torque produced by gravity acts on the head and causes a stronger contraction in the erector spinae to maintain neck extension. This deserves some thought; why does gravity have a greater effect when the head is held in a flexed position?

Consider an extension ladder: holding the ladder vertical takes less effort than picking up the ladder from the ground. The ladder weighs the same in the vertical position, but in this position gravity pulls though the legs. Because the ladder rests on an axis where the legs meet the ground, gravity's force pulls through the axis, creating no tendency to fall. If the ladder leans, gravity begins to project away from the axis, creating a moment arm and thus creating a tendency to fall. This tendency increases in proportion to the amount the ladder leans (Figure 6-18).

Likewise Olivia's 30 degrees of neck flexion creates a longer moment arm than in the case of Nancy's erect posture. Calculate the force of Olivia's erector spinae:

$$F_{extensors} \times 4 \text{ cm} = 5 \text{ kg} \times 6 \text{ cm}$$

$$F_{extensors} = 30 \text{ kg cm}/4 \text{ cm}$$

$$F_{extensors} = 7.5 \text{ kg}$$

Although not all the head's weight in this position compresses her spine, the reaction force is greater at 30-degrees flexion than in the upright position. More than half the weight of Olivia's head compresses her

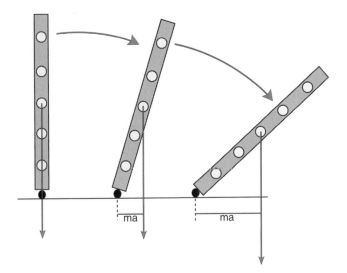

FIGURE **6-18**
The extension ladder's weight creates no tendency toward falling in the upright position. Tendency to fall begins as the ladder leans. The tendency increases the more the ladder leans because the projection of gravity moves farther away from the axis, creating a longer and longer moment arm.

spine, and the contraction force of her head and neck extensors more than doubles (see Figure 6-19).

Thus the longer Olivia maintains her head in a flexed position, the greater the effect of gravity and more erector spinae strength will be required to balance her head. This in turn causes greater compression of the cervical spine. The OT practitioners from ATRC must make a number of determinations to draw this scenario. In establishing a class of lever, the practitioner determines relationships between the forces of effort and resistance to the axis of motion. In this case the axis of motion lies between the two forces, creating a first-class lever. Spinal muscles must exert greater effort when Olivia's head moves from alignment with the spinal axis of motion. This effort increases in direct proportion to the distance of the head's center of gravity from the spinal axis of motion. The effort force increases quickly with a minimal increase in head flexion.

Nancy requires minimal effort to keep her head erect, but Olivia, who holds her head flexed to 30 degrees, needs three times as much effort. This produces about 50% more compressive force on her corresponding disk. Olivia pulls her head erect frequently while working on the laptop and experiences muscle fatigue and soreness. Placing the laptop and its screen higher encourages an erect rather than flexed posture and relieves some muscle fatigue. The OT practitioners from ATRC recommend that Olivia, Nancy, and the other students properly position their monitors and take frequent breaks, slowly stretching their neck muscles to relieve the forces of neck flexion and extension.

OT practitioners know the importance of posture when considering fatigue and discomfort in activity.

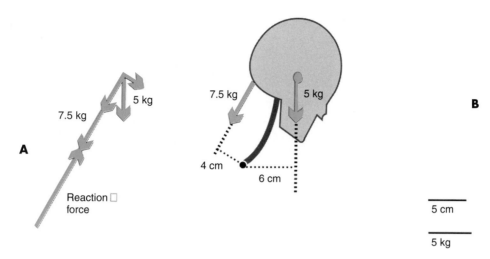

FIGURE **6-19**

To maintain the head at a 30-degree angle, the erector spinae muscles must exert a force of 7.5 kg **(A)**. The reaction force increases accordingly. With the head at 30 degrees, most of the weight exerts a compression effect on the vertebral column, and the compression from the erector spinae contraction increases compared to the erect position. The reaction force (at least 7.5 kg) exerted toward the head equals the sum of the two forces directed toward the shoulders (7.5 kg plus a portion of the head's weight). As before, these two forces consist of the muscle contraction force and the portion of the head weight directed into the cervical disk **(B)**.

Poor head alignment yields greater difficulty, resulting in accelerated fatigue.

Figure 6-20 shows Jason Black, a student with cerebral palsy, trying to eat his lunch in the school cafeteria. He has difficulty lifting the utensil to his mouth. To compensate for his upper-extremity difficulties, Jason flexes his head forward to meet the spoon. This solves one problem but creates another. The greater degree of flexion requires more effort to support his head than Jason would need with better posture. Poorly coordinated bilateral activation of his sternocleidomastoids increases his difficulties with chewing and swallowing. The added fatigue and discomfort he experiences cause him to stop eating before he has satisfied his hunger.

Erector Spinae

Spiros Prasso's job requires he lift 25- and 46-cm boxes to shoulder height. All boxes weigh 18 kg. While his upper extremities lift the boxes, Spiros' erector spinae maintain back extension. The OT practitioner working with Spiros must determine the force his erector spinae muscles need to lift each box and the reaction force (load) on the L5 disk in each case. How can the OT practitioner adapt the work environment when the loads on the disk exceed recommended levels?

The OT practitioner visiting Spiros' job site uses the following information to determine the forces involved:

The force of Spiros' erector spinae group operates an estimated 5 cm from the axis of motion at his L5 disk.

Spiros weighs 70 kg, so the OT practitioner estimates his upper-body weight at about 40 kg.

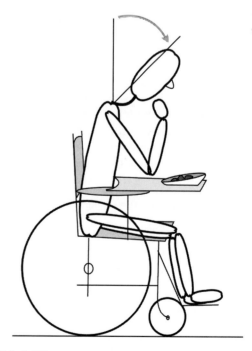

FIGURE **6-20**

Eating with his head angled forward, Jason requires more endurance than his neck muscles can sustain.

Spiros holds the 25-cm box with its center of gravity 20 cm from his axis of motion.

Spiros holds the 46-cm box with its center of gravity 40 cm from his axis of motion.

The weight of Spiros' upper trunk falls dorsal to the axis of motion and contributes to extension; however, its negligible moment arm means it lacks sufficient force to consider in this problem.

Figure 6-21 shows a diagram of the relevant forces and moment arms. Using the formula for equilibrium of torques, calculate the tendency toward extension created by Spiros' erector spinae muscles. The weight of the box (18 kg) creates a tendency toward flexion; the erector spinae force creates the tendency toward extension.

$$(F_{extensors} \times MA_{extensors}) = (F_{box} \times MA_{box})$$

$$(F_{extensors} \times 5\ cm) = (18\ kg \times 20\ cm)$$

$$(F_{extensors} \times 5\ cm) = 360\ kg\ cm$$

$$F_{extensors} = 360\ kg\ cm/5\ cm$$

$$F_{extensors} = 72\ kg$$

Remember our answer falls short of absolute value as we did not account for the weight of the trunk and its extension effect. Still, we can appreciate from our solution that the back extensors must generate a force many times that of the box weight to support the spine in extension.

Calculate the reaction force on the L5 disk based on the force equilibrium condition $\Sigma F = 0$. The weights of the box and body and the contraction force of the erector spinae muscle all pull downward. The reaction force through the disk must push upward with equal force:

$$F_{reaction} = 18\ kg + 40\ kg + 72\ kg$$

$$F_{reaction} = 130\ kg$$

Figure 6-22 shows the forces and moment arms involved in lifting the larger box. Use the same calculation as before to determine the muscle force, substituting the greater distance of the box away from the body:

$$(F_{extensors} \times 5\ cm) = (18\ kg \times 40\ cm)$$

$$(F_{extensors} \times 5\ cm) = 720\ kg\ cm$$

$$F_{extensors} = 720\ kg\ cm/5\ cm$$

$$F_{extensors} = 144\ kg$$

Calculate the reaction force:

$$F_{reaction} = 18\ kg + 40\ kg + 144\ kg$$

$$F_{reaction} = 202\ kg$$

As the size of the box increases, its center of gravity moves farther from the axis of motion in the L5 disk and

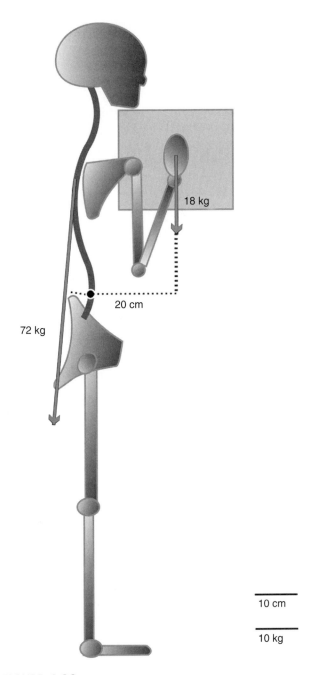

18 kg

72 kg

20 cm

10 cm

10 kg

FIGURE 6-21
Spiros' erector spinae muscles exert an approximate force of 72 kg to hold 18 kg in a 25-cm box 20 cm from the axis of motion at his L5 disk. Carrying the box in this position causes an upward reaction force of about 130 kg on his L5 disk.

the box's moment arm for flexion increases. The longer moment arm means the weight creates a greater tendency toward vertebral flexion, or a greater **flexion moment.** To balance this tendency, Spiros uses twice as much force to lift the larger box, even though it weighs the same as the smaller box. The larger box creates a larger disk load. Using the smallest possible box reduces the magnitude of the moment arm of the box, decreasing

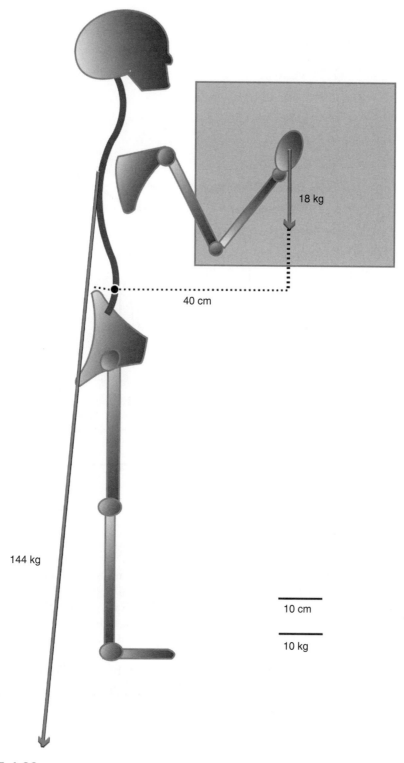

18 kg

40 cm

144 kg

10 cm

10 kg

FIGURE **6-22**
Spiros' erector spinae muscles exert a force of about 144 kg to hold 18 kg in a 46-cm box 40 cm from the axis of motion at his L5 disk. Carrying the box in this position causes an approximate upward reaction force of 202 kg on his L5 disk.

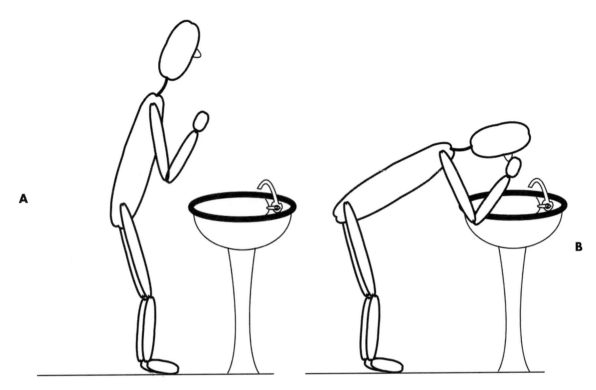

FIGURE **6-23**
A, When Nancy stands at the sink, the L5 vertebra forms a 30-degree angle to the floor. Her elbows project 20 cm from the axis of motion at her L5 disk. **B**, When she bends over the sink, the L5 vertebra forms a 70-degree angle to the floor. Her elbows project 52 cm from the axis of motion at her L5 disk.

the amount of effort required to lift it, and thus decreasing the disk load.

As Spiros' muscles become fatigued, he compensates by using rapid, jerking motions to shift the load's center of gravity as close to his axis of motion as possible. He arches his back, shifting his body's center of gravity farther back to lengthen his upper trunk's moment arm. The OT practitioner notes that this works because it intensifies the effect of his body weight as an extensor. However, she reminds Spiros that hyperextension increases the load on the smaller facet joints of his vertebrae and creates stress on ligaments along the anterior vertebral bodies. Because no safe way exists to compensate for the large flexion moment the boxes create, the OT practitioner encourages Spiros' employer to use the smallest boxes possible and package each load so its center of gravity remains close to the body at all times.

L5 Disk*

The Assistive Technology Resource Center in the OT program where Olivia and Nancy attend university presents a program on preventing computing-related injury with improved body

*See Appendix C for graphic and mathematical solutions to this problem.

mechanics. During the program, Nancy explains that she often notices back pain when she prepares for bed. Figure 6-23 shows how she leans over a sink to perform personal-hygiene activities. To demonstrate why back pain occurs, an OT practitioner uses a diagram with both arms held in a bilaterally symmetrical posture.

When Nancy stands, the center of gravity for her head and trunk falls 17 cm from the axis of motion in the L5 disk and the center of gravity for her arms falls 20 cm from the L5 disk. When Nancy bends, the center of gravity for her head and trunk falls 31 cm from the L5 disk and the center of gravity for her arms falls 52 cm away from the L5 disk. Nancy weighs 60 kg.

The erector spinae force needed to counteract the force of gravity lies 5 cm from the axis of motion in the L5 disk. Remember that a force pulling directly through an axis (zero moment arm) creates no moment, or has no tendency toward extension; thus the force created by contraction produces a linear motion. An extension force acting at a small moment arm creates some extension tendency, but most force moves the segment along a line into the next connecting segment. The erector spinae have a short moment arm, and their linear movement causes the vertebral bodies to move closer and compress the intervertebral disks.

How much force do the erector spinae need to counteract the weight of Nancy's head, trunk, and arms when she stands erect versus when she bends? How much compressive force operates on the L5 disk in each position? How can the OT practitioner adapt this activity to reduce the effort needed by her erector spinae and the load imposed on her L5 disk?

The OT practitioner notes that the weights of Nancy's head, trunk, and arms fall anterior to her axis of motion. In this relationship these segments produce a flexion tendency at the axis. (See Appendix B, Table B-1 for the proportions of body weight of each segment.)

Figures 6-24 and 6-25 show forces and moment arms. Calculate the force of the erector spinae based on the formula for equilibrium of torques ($\sum T = 0$). Nancy's head and trunk together weigh 34 kg and exert force 17 cm from her axis of motion. Her arms weigh 6 kg and have a moment arm of 20 cm. Calculate the force generated by the erector spinae muscles when she stands upright at the sink:

$$(F_{extensors} \times 5 \text{ cm}) = (34 \text{ kg} \times 17 \text{ cm}) + (6 \text{ kg} \times 20 \text{ cm})$$

$$(F_{extensors} \times 5 \text{ cm}) = 578 \text{ kg cm} + 120 \text{ kg cm}$$

$$F_{extensors} = 698 \text{ kg cm}/5 \text{ cm}$$

$$F_{extensors} = 139.6 \text{ kg}$$

When Nancy leans over the sink, her erector spinae must support the increased effect of gravity on her trunk—recall the ladder lesson. Notice how everything changes as the moment arms increase:

$$(F_{extensors} \times 5 \text{ cm}) = (34 \text{ kg} \times 31 \text{ cm}) + (6 \text{ kg} \times 52 \text{ cm})$$

$$(F_{extensors} \times .5 \text{ cm}) = 1054 \text{ kg cm} + 312 \text{ kg cm}$$

$$F_{extensors} = 1366 \text{ kg cm}/5 \text{ cm}$$

$$F_{extensors} = 273.2 \text{ kg}$$

The direct compressive force on the disk caused by the weight of Nancy's body actually diminishes when she bends rather than when she stands, but the erector spinae work twice as hard when Nancy bends over the sink as they do when she stands next to it due to gravity's greater moment arm in bending. Remember that the small moment arm for the back extensors results in more linear (compressive) force than extension force as the back extensors contract to balance the flexion moment. In fact, most compressive forces on the disk result from activation of the erector spinae.

Bending also introduces shear force into the equation. Shear force runs parallel to the surface on which

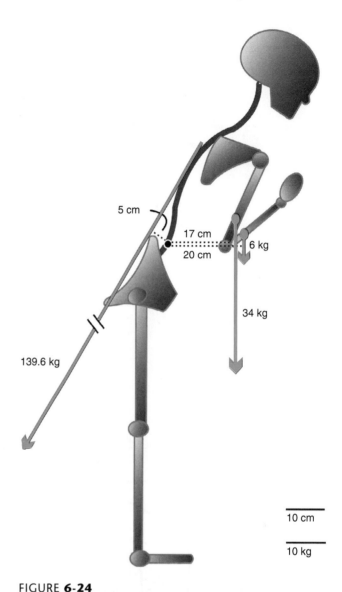

FIGURE 6-24
To maintain standing posture at the sink Nancy's erector spinae muscles exert 139.6 kg of force. This posture causes 174.2 kg of compressive force and 20 kg of shear force on her L5 disk (see Appendix C).

another force acts. In this case the amount of shear is small—about 13%—and negligible compared with the large amount of compressive force acting on the disk (see Appendix C).

Most sinks stand so low that individuals must bend to perform daily tasks like washing the face or brushing the teeth. The OT practitioner shows Nancy how to reduce the stressful forces on her low back by supporting some of her body's weight on one arm (Figure 6-26) and by bending her knees and lowering the body to get her face closer to the sink, requiring less lumbar flexion (Figure 6-27). When Nancy's hip joints move to bend her body, she holds her low back in extension, so her lumbar disks experience less anterior pressure.

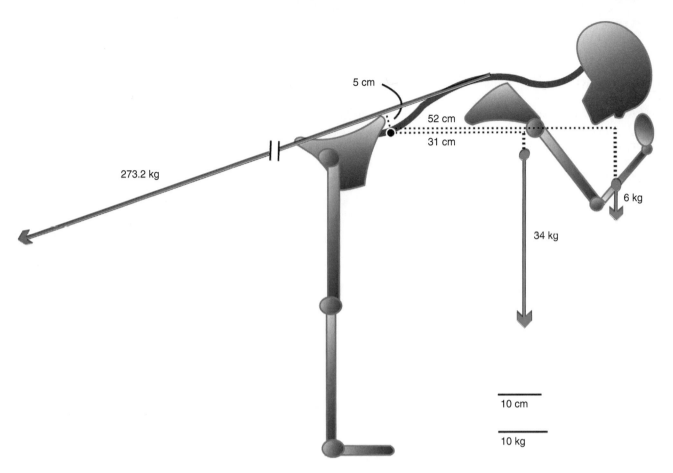

5 cm

52 cm

31 cm

273.2 kg

6 kg

34 kg

10 cm

10 kg

FIGURE **6-25**
To maintain a bending posture at the sink Nancy's erector spinae muscles must exert 273.2 kg of force. This posture causes 286.9 kg of compressive force and 37.6 kg of shear force on her L5 disk (see Appendix C).

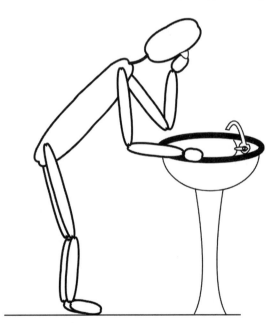

FIGURE **6-26**
Nancy uses less back-extensor force by supporting her body weight with one arm on the countertop. Her upper-extremity muscles share the weight of her upper trunk, generating less compressive force. As Nancy raises the washcloth to her face, her need to flex decreases.

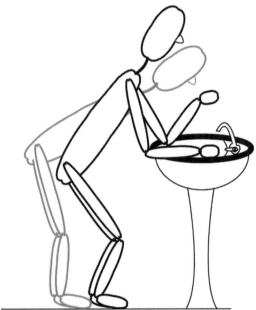

FIGURE **6-27**
Bending at the knees allows a woman to lower her face to the sink without bending her back. The weight of the upper trunk works at a smaller moment arm, and the back extensors produce a smaller contraction force. She keeps the lower portion of her back straight, thus decreasing the forces acting on her lower back as she bends over the sink.

SEATING AND POSITIONING

Muscle weakness or imbalances clearly demonstrate the drastic effect of gravity on the vertebral column. When we look at an unsupported column, we see how the different vertebral muscles manage the column against the predominant influence of gravity.

Stabilization Principles

The pelvis forms a foundation for stabilization. All the straps and pads in the world do very little to support a weak vertebral column without stabilizing the pelvis first. Most of the work areas in the laptop lab where Nancy and Olivia attend university have ergonomically designed desks and chairs. However, as Nancy becomes fatigued and slouches to view her screen, her pelvis slips forward and ruins the vertebral alignment her chair should support.

The pelvis helps the body maintain a normal lumbar curve. We learned how anterior pelvic tilt affects the normal lumbar curve and how posterior tilt accompanies reversed lumbar curve. Positioning the pelvis in a slight anterior tilt allows weight to bear on the ischial tuberosities (as it should) and allows the body to maintain a normal lumbar curve (convex anteriorly) if the lumbar spine remains mobile (A Closer Look Box 6-2). A lumbar pad or cushion placed at the position of normal lumbar curve assists in providing anterior pelvic tilt by reducing lumbar repositioning. Placement too high or too low may put pressure on the thoracic or sacral vertebrae, respectively. Because both these regions normally protrude posteriorly, an improperly placed lumbar roll serves only to push the individual forward from the chair.

At Jason Black's school the OT practitioner struggles to help him achieve a better seating position. First she puts a small roll behind his lumbar spine. Instead of creating an anterior pelvic tilt, the foam roll pushes Jason further forward in the seat.

Overtight hamstrings frustrate attempts at repositioning by prestabilizing the pelvis. The OT practitioner experiences this problem as she attempts to reposition Jason with an anterior pelvic tilt. His short hamstrings stretch to their maximum length early in this manipulation as attempting anterior tilt moves his ischial tuberosities (hamstring origin) backward from the hamstring insertions just below his knees. Tightness in the hamstrings prevents pelvic movement unless the knees are free to flex—an impossibility with Jason's feet strapped into the footrests. Because his standard footrests hold the lower legs at 80-degrees flexion instead of allowing 90 degrees or more, the hamstrings experience constant stretch, pulling his ischial tuberosities forward into posterior pelvic tilt (see A Closer Look Box 6-2).

Freeing his feet of the footrests, the OT practitioner again attempts anterior pelvic tilt. Achieving the desired pelvic position, she secures a 45-degree seat belt but notices Jason's knees have flexed past 90 degrees with his heels now under the chair seat.

Evaluations

The OT practitioner who works with Jason knows that the first step toward improving his positioning involves evaluation. To begin, she determines the mobility of his spine. Some individuals maintain postures so long that they become fixed and require accommodation rather than correction with external supports. Jason has a fixed reversed lumbar curve (convex posteriorly). A lumbar pad puts undue pressure on the posterior spinous processes, and simply pushes Jason from the seat instead of reestablishing lumbar lordosis. Tightly securing his pelvis with a 45-degree belt risks skin breakdown. Without a tightly secured pelvis, the lumbar pad simply pushes Jason from the seat instead of reestablishing lumbar lordosis.

The OT practitioner then determines whether Jason's hamstrings have enough length to position his pelvis in anterior tilt. She compares passive range of motion of hip flexion with his knees extended versus flexed. The larger the discrepancies in the amount of hip flexion, the more his hamstrings limit movement. Jason's shortened hamstrings prevent him from achieving 90 degrees of left hip flexion, even with his knee flexed.

Armed with this information, the OT practitioner begins to develop a seating system that will allow Jason hip flexion at 90 degrees by permitting greater than 90 degrees of knee flexion.

When she tries to reposition his legs to place them into the footrests, he whimpers in discomfort. School staff complain that Jason usually slouches against his seat back whenever they place his feet in the footrests. The OT practitioner also notes that Jason's left knee seems more flexed than the other. When she takes Jason out of the wheelchair and uses a goniometer to measure hip flexion, she finds that his left hip stops at about 85 degrees of flexion even with his knee at 90 degrees of flexion to provide hamstring slack.

Transferring him back to the wheelchair, the OT practitioner notices that Jason's left posterior thigh drags on the front seat edge to a greater degree than his right thigh when she attempts to create a more optimal sitting posture by anchoring his pelvis farther back in the chair. As she pushes him toward the back of the chair, his right hip flexes 90 degrees. Because Jason's left hip cannot flex to 90 degrees, his left pelvis moves upward as his posterior thigh drags on the seat edge. The OT practitioner makes a note about Jason's "pelvic obliquity" to remind herself that his left iliac crest rests higher than his right (Figure 6-28).

The OT practitioner knows that asymmetrical hamstring length and limited hip flexion range often results in another type of pelvic repositioning. Because Jason cannot achieve hip flexion of 90 degrees on his left side, he will probably also shift his pelvis anteriorly. She observes this pelvic rotation by looking at Jason from above and noting that his hips no longer lie in the same frontal plane (Figure 6-29).

Seating must address any pelvic positions that occur because of muscle shortness across the hips. Without accommodating the pelvis all other support attempts remain futile. An asymmetrical seat depth or seat height can often provide a desirable adaptation to the sitting

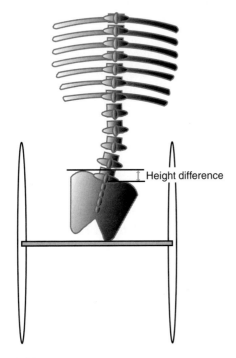

FIGURE 6-28
Jason's asymmetrically short hamstrings cause pelvic obliquity when he attempts to sit.

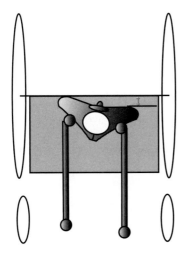

FIGURE 6-29
Jason's pelvic rotation from a top, or superior, view.

surface. A 45-degree seat belt can secure the pelvis, but as Jason reminded us, both hips must be capable of 90 degrees of flexion.

Alignment in superior regions follows pelvic stabilization. Lateral supports medially direct forces in the thoracic region. These lateral supports counter lateral forces of the vertebral segments caused by gravity's downward pull on the column. Straps hold the trunk to the seat back so that lateral supports can apply pressure to the intended regions. In addition, anterior-posterior and lateral supports provide the stabilization required for good head control.

Other vertebral and pelvic issues deal less with orthopedics and more with neurology. For example, a wedge cushion encourages greater than 90 degrees of hip flexion, which can reduce extensor spasms and improve overall sitting posture. A wedge cushion may provide an ideal solution to a seating problem because it addresses the problem with a minimal amount of support.

Sometimes increased support proves itself unnecessary as well as harmful.

Jason's OT practitioner has concerns about the head supports that hold his head against the headrest. He seems most uncomfortable with the unnecessary pressure on his forehead exerted by the anterior support surfaces. She hopes to collaborate with practitioners at the wheelchair clinic to use a wheelchair with a tilt-in-space design that angles Jason backward so his

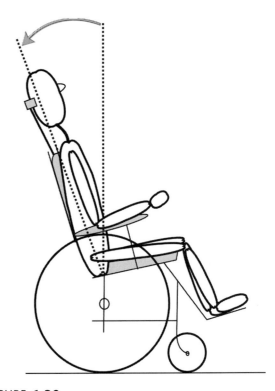

FIGURE 6-30
Jason's tilt-in-space chair. Notice the angle of tilt away from vertical.

head's center of gravity falls just behind his pelvis (Figure 6-30). A small rear support could then provide adequate stabilization. Jason could use his neck flexors to raise his head upright and then relax into neck extension supported by his chair. From this position he also could view his surroundings without becoming unduly fatigued.

OT practitioners must approach external supports in positioning differently than they do when attempting to change alignment and muscle length with orthotics. Good positioning accommodates fixed positions and prevents problems in one area, like the pelvis, from negatively affecting vertebral alignment in other regions. Positioning support should prevent further degradation of alignment. Since external support replaces and does not strengthen muscles, OT practitioners should add extra support only after determining that an individual cannot maintain good sitting posture independently. A deeper understanding of positioning usually requires advanced study and extensive clinical practice.

Common Restraint Systems

Upholstered reclining chairs have a long history in nursing homes. They operate as beltless restraints by increasing gravity's moment arm. Caretakers recline the chair until gravity's moment arm for extension exceeds the ability of the body's trunk flexors to produce enough flexion for the individual to rise from the seat.

Seat belts with buckles or Velcro placed out of reach often are used to restrain active individuals. Usually applied as waist straps, these seat belts feel quite uncomfortable, and this discomfort often causes the individual to attempt to remove the belt. Waist straps that attach to the wheelchair back have no real effect on positioning. The waist strap contacts the soft abdomen. Tightening the belt produces severe discomfort and can even affect breathing. The belt must stay loose to remain tolerable, and the pelvis usually tilts posteriorly and slides forward. This action results from the downward pull of gravity and increases when an individual uses a lower extremity to propel the wheelchair, as commonly occurs with one lower extremity after a stroke.

Nursing staff at Maple Grove Skilled Care Facility request that the OT department outfit Quentin Keller with a lap tray to help improve his positioning. They complain that without a tray the retired farmer always tries to unbuckle his seat belt or slide under it. To make matters worse, Quentin has seriously abraded the skin on his sacrum from shear force by sliding down in his chair, placing him at risk for developing a pressure sore. The nurses hope the lap tray will satisfy regulations about restraints and put to rest their worries that Quentin will fall. Leaning on a tray, they think, might remove some pressure from his sacrum.

The OT practitioner finds Quentin in an old wheelchair dragging himself down the hall with his right leg. She notices that he assumes a posterior tilt when pulling himself down the hall and he has developed a kyphotic thoracic curve. She brings Quentin into the OT clinic for measurements and, by the end of the week, outfits him with a more effective 45-degree seat belt (Figure 6-31 A, B).

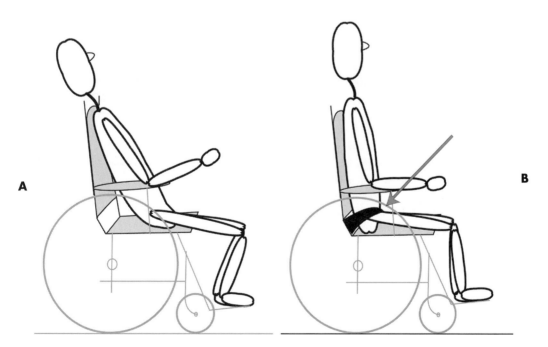

A   **B**

FIGURE **6-31**
Quentin's position **A**, with a waist belt, then with **B**, the 45-degree belt.

The angled belt attaches at the junction of the seat and the back to form a 45-degree angle with the sitting surface. It anchors Quentin's pelvis deep into the corner of the chair and allows him to assume a stable sitting position. He experiences no discomfort, so he does not try to remove it. Because the belt anchors him more securely in the chair, Quentin propels himself more easily. It also facilitates healing the abrasions on his sacrum. The OT practitioner explains to staff that the lap tray would only compound Quentin's problems by stabilizing his trunk at an even higher position that encourages slouching, posterior pelvic tilt, and a forward pelvic slide for escape.

The waist belt and lap tray each fail to do what the 45-degree belt does best—anchor Quentin's pelvis into the corner of the chair. Because the 45-degree belt sits lower than the waist belt and lap tray, it does not compress abdominal and pelvic organs. Tightening it enough to give effective support rarely affects comfort. It puts gentle but firm pressure on the pelvis, preventing a forward slide. An effective and comfortable belt reverses Quentin's original motivation to remove the belt, and with a clasp placed at hand's reach the belt no longer qualifies as a restraint.

Comfortable, and displaying good posture, Quentin frequently returns to the OT clinic, mysteriously appearing just as a fresh batch of cookies comes out of the oven. With a 45-degree belt securing his pelvis, he happily uses a removable lap tray to hold seedling trays during gardening activities.

A wedge cushion also can anchor an individual without using a belt. A wedge places the hips in more than 90 degrees of flexion and produces a similar effect to sitting on a soft sofa. On sofas and overstuffed chairs the hips flex beyond 90 degrees. From this position, the hip and knee extensors, both necessary for standing, operate at weak positions in their range, making them less effective. (Remember isometric torque curves?) The wedge, although effective, produces increased hip flexion and raises the feet. The wedge cushion requires elevating the footrests to support the weight of the lower leg. Without this adjustment, added pressure on the posterior thighs can cause a skin pressure problem.

Bernice Richards, who works as a singer in a cocktail lounge, uses an electric wheelchair. She has the typical trunk instability that accompanies C5 quadriplegia. Like most people with quadriplegia, Bernice uses a chest belt to restrain her body's forward momentum in case her wheelchair made a sudden stop. Now that she has returned to singing she resents the way the belt obscures her sequined tops.

Bernice and her OT practitioner discuss various options. A wedge cushion would increase hip flexion, but would not change the alignment of the trunk—a chest strap still would be needed.

Instead, they decide to use the tilt-in-space feature of her power chair to tilt her chair backward a few degrees. The angle of the chair seat and back places Bernice's upper body center of gravity behind the hip axis for flexion and extension. In this position her upper body produces a tendency toward closed-chain hip extension. This counteracts the forward momentum toward closed-chain hip flexion she experiences when her chair stops suddenly, and it decreases the need for a chest restraint during her singing engagements (Figure 6-32).

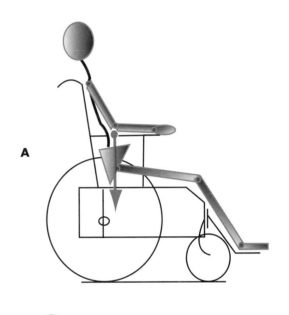

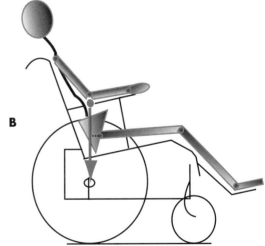

FIGURE **6-32**
Slight backward tilting of Bernice's chair promotes a tendency toward closed-chain hip extension, counteracting the effect of momentum when her chair stops suddenly.

Summary

The bony and soft-tissue structures of the head, neck, and trunk provide a stable but flexible shell to protect vital organs, a stable base for movement of the extremities, and a mobile base from which to extend the upper extremities. Because of its design, the back operates at a disadvantage when lifting the trunk from a forward-flexed position. The vertebral extensors, with their short moment arms, produce more compression than extension force. Maintaining upright posture requires little extensor force and causes minimal compression of the intervertebral disks. In contrast, lifting with the back uses a great deal of extensor force and introduces enough compression to damage disks.

Biomechanics can explain and provide solutions for many common problems associated with body positioning. Basic principles in this chapter serve as a foundation for two of the most common problems an OT practitioner encounters:

1. Providing external support from the pelvis upward along the vertebral column when internal stability fails because of muscle weakness; focusing on the pelvis to identify improper tilt, rotation, and obliquity because of muscle tightness
2. Assessing positioning from the perspective of effectiveness and comfort to avoid misuse of positioning devices that unnecessarily restrain or cause injury to the wearer

Applications

■ APPLICATION 6-1
Upper-Extremity Reach

Identify how the trunk participates in the following reach patterns. Determine the active groups of trunk muscles in each case:

1. Reach forward with both hands as far as you can without flexing the hips past 90 degrees.
2. Reach to one side or the other as far as you can. (Shoulder abduction should be about 90 degrees.)
3. Reach straight up as far as you can.
4. Reach as far as you can to the left side by bringing your right arm in front of your shoulders.

■ APPLICATION 6-2
Open- and Closed-Chain Hip Movements

Sit with your legs crossed in front of you and hips flexed to at least 90 degrees. Compare this with long sitting. (To achieve long sitting, lie in a supine position and sit up so that your hips are flexed to 90 degrees and your knees fully extended with your feet in front.) Is long sitting a different feeling? Compare hip flexion movements for crossed-legged sitting with long sitting. What happens in long sitting when you reach forward to touch your toes?

■ APPLICATION 6-3
Stance

Dr. Paul Zimmerman, a dermatologist with a busy private practice, needs help adapting his office environment to minimize his back pain. He feels most uncomfortable bending over his examination table. Dr. Zimmerman has begun doing some office-based surgery and must hold this position for an hour or more during some procedures. Placing one foot on a step stool relieves the doctor's back pain and makes it possible for him to complete surgical procedures with minimal discomfort. Why?

See Appendix C for solutions to Applications.

REFERENCE

1. Williams PL, Bannister LH: *Gray's anatomy: the anatomical basis of medicine and surgery*, ed 38, New York, 1995, Churchill Livingstone.

RELATED READINGS

Hall SJ: *Basic biomechanics*, ed 2, New York, 1995, McGraw-Hill.

Jacobs J, Bettencourt CM: *Ergonomics for therapists*, Newton, Mass, 1995, Butterworth-Heinemann.

Luttgens K, Hamilton N: *Kinesiology: scientific basis of human motion*, ed 9, New York, 2000, McGraw-Hill.

Magee DJ: *Orthopedic physical assessment*, ed 3, Philadelphia, 1997, WB Saunders.

Moore KL: *Clinically oriented anatomy*, Philadelphia, 1992, Williams & Wilkins.

LAB BOX

Find applied activities exploring concepts in Chapter 6 in the following laboratory exercises:

Topic	*Laboratory*
Vertebral curves, muscular control of the trunk, vertebral motion associated with upper extremity use in reach, vertebral movements and positions, special focus on vertebral rotation	**Lab 6** Head, Neck, and Trunk: Curves, Movements, Measurements, Muscles
Pelvis and vertebral column in positioning in a wheelchair, effect of hamstring length on pelvis and lumbar spine	**Lab 13** Positioning in a wheelchair

7

The Proximal Upper Extremity

K E Y **T E R M S**

Glenohumeral Joint
Scapulothoracic Joint
Sternoclavicular Joint
Scapulohumeral Rhythm
Rotator Cuff
Scaption
Subluxation
Joint Force

Individuals adapt to their environments using tools. Most of us associate tool use with hand use. This chapter focuses on reaching, the important proximal counterpart of tool use. Any meaningful manipulation of materials by the fingers and thumbs depends on arm movement, positioning, and stabilization.

Shoulder motions position the hand an arm's length from the body in a 360-degree arc. With the elbow extended, we touch, adjust, hold, and manipulate objects at the edge of that arc. We extend the shoulder and flex the elbow to reach within the extremes of the arc. Each joint in the upper extremity (UE) has a designated amount of freedom to move. Various combinations of shoulder and elbow movements place the hand at multiple points in space.

The Shoulder Complex

Steindler[6] describes our ability to place the hand in a variety of places as a joint chain displaying degrees of freedom. Each joint contributes to the freedom of the chain based on the number of axes around which movement occurs and the amplitude of movement allowed at the joint. Considering these parameters, the shoulder complex contributes significantly to the freedom of the UE.

We often refer to shoulder movement as if it occurs in a single joint. Early lessons in anatomy highlight the shoulder's classification as a ball-and-socket joint that moves in three planes. This emphasis on glenohumeral (GH) articulation downplays the importance of other joints in the shoulder complex. Acting alone, the **glenohumeral joint,** even in its 3 degrees of freedom, does not allow the hand to reach above the head or in any extreme of forward or backward reach. Clavicular and scapular components of the shoulder prove critical. The shoulder's unmatched mobility makes it challenging to treat because of its corresponding unmatched instability in the presence of trauma.

ARTICULATIONS

We often think of the UE beginning at the GH joint in spite of the fact that its proximal articulations play an equally important role. Freedom of movement in proximal joints allows greater UE movement. Therefore, restrictions proximally reduce distal freedom. For example, if the sternoclavicular joint restricts clavicular movement, scapular movement decreases. In this way, proximal restrictions limit upper-extremity movement and functional use.

The upper extremity's bony attachment to the axial skeleton occurs solely at the **sternoclavicular joint,** a small, freely movable synovial joint. The clavicle projects laterally and articulates with the lateral aspect of the

spine of the scapula, forming the acromioclavicular (AC) joint, the joint involved in the clinical entity "shoulder separation." While not a true synovial joint because of the absence of a capsule, the acromioclavicular ligament surrounds the joint and supports it along with other ligaments at points along the clavicle's length. Further support of the AC joint comes via attachments of the deltoid muscle both proximal and distal to the joint.

The relationships among the sternum, clavicle, and scapula allows free motion of the scapula contributing significantly to upper-extremity movement and function. Its articulation with the thorax (**scapulothoracic joint**) allows movement of the scapula in six directions: elevation and depression; protraction and retraction; and upward and downward rotation (Figure 7-1).

Upper-extremity reach patterns depend on a variety of scapular movements. Forward reach includes scapular protraction as well as elbow extension and shoulder flexion. Placing the hand high above the head requires upward scapular rotation along with full elbow extension and shoulder flexion. Reaching the hand behind the back requires just the opposite—downward scapular

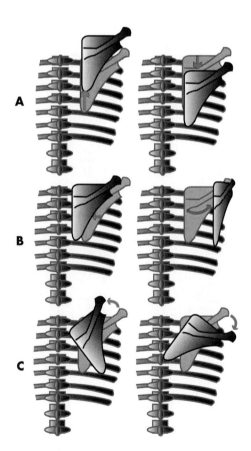

 FIGURE **7-1**
The various movements of the scapula include **(A)** elevation and depression, **(B)** retraction and protraction, and **(C)** upward and downward rotation.

TABLE 7-1

Associated Clavicular, Scapular, and Upper Extremity Motions

CLAVICULAR MOTION	SCAPULAR MOTION	TYPICAL UPPER EXTREMITY MOTION
Motion in frontal plane	Elevation	"I don't know" gesture
	Depression	Transfers; reaching down to pick up a suitcase
	Upward rotation	Reaching high above the head
	Downward rotation	Reaching behind the back
Motion in horizontal plane	Protraction	Reaching forward
	Retraction	Reaching backward with both hands

rotation, full glenohumeral internal rotation and extension, and elbow flexion (Table 7-1).

While the GH joint does not provide all of the UE motions, it still has an amazing repertoire for movement. By itself, it provides UE movement in the three major planes as well as everything in between! Around a dynamic longitudinal axis the humeral head exhibits rolling and gliding/sliding from point to point across the glenoid to position the arm optimally for function. These small-amplitude movements occur during GH flexion/extension, abduction/adduction, and rotation. They result in free placement of the hand at nearly any position we desire. For a more in-depth look at the glenohumeral joint, check out A Closer Look Box 7-1.

MUSCLES AFFECTING THE SCAPULA

Kinesiology involves determining which muscles do what and why. Reviewing anatomy to locate muscle attachments and innervations may help reduce confusion over which muscles move the scapula and which move the humerus at the glenohumeral joint. Instead of memorizing or rememorizing functions, try to develop a three-dimensional image of the entire shoulder region complete with muscles in relation to the joint axes.

The upper trapezius and levator scapulae, originating on the spine and running downward to insert onto the scapula, elevate the scapula, shortening to pull their insertions up toward their origins. Scapular depression occurs mainly through gravity's pull. Scapular depression against resistance, common when walking with crutches or a walker, occurs through concentric contractions of the lower trapezius, latissimus dorsi, and pectoralis major muscles. All of these originate below and reach up to pull the scapula or humerus downward.

These same muscles function to produce closed-chain scapular depression when the hands push down on a surface. This occurs in transfers when the scapular depressors raise the trunk instead of depressing the scapula.

BOX 7-1

A **CLOSER** LOOK

The Capsule, the Glenoid, and the Glenohumeral Ligaments

The glenoid labrum consists of fibrous cartilage that deepens the glenoid by 75% in the vertical plane (superior and inferior) and 57% in the transverse (anterior and posterior) position.

The labrum's wedge shape changes with dynamic shoulder motion, and can even extend to detachment of the inner edge.

Glenohumeral stability decreases 20% without the labrum.

The labrum has a vacuum effect on the head of the humerus, acting more as a suction cup than a physical block to humeral head translation/dislocation.

The synovial sheath surrounding the shoulder capsule originates at the glenoid labrum and inserts onto the anatomical neck of the humerus. An inherently lax structure, the capsule allows 1/2 inch of distraction of the humeral head anteriorly and posteriorly with the shoulder in a relaxed position. Three thickenings or folds of the capsule comprise the glenohumeral ligaments, which along with tendons serve as anterior and posterior reinforcements:

The superior glenohumeral ligament resists inferior translation of the humeral head.

The middle glenohumeral ligament, absent in approximately 30% of the population, limits external rotation and contributes to anterior stability of the shoulder at 45 degrees of abduction.

The inferior glenohumeral ligament (IGHL) posterior band stabilizes the capsule inferiorly and posteriorly, while the anterior band stabilizes anteriorly. Stretch in both ligaments occurs in the externally rotated and abducted position (ERA). Internal rotation is in part stabilized by the posterior band of the IGHL.

Latissimus and pectoralis major move the scapula through their strong attachments to the humerus. Crutch-walking and walker-use serve as other examples of closed-chain scapular depression.

Although they originate in very different places, imagine the upper and lower trapezius together with the lower fibers of the serratus anterior moving toward their origins to clarify how they produce upward scapular rotation. They pull the scapula like three hands on three different points of a steering wheel. A hand on the right pulls down, another on the bottom pulls left, and a hand on the left pushes up, turning the wheel right, or clockwise. The lower trapezius inserts near the root of the scapular spine and pulls down, the lower serratus pulls the inferior angle lateral, and the upper trapezius pulls the acromion up (Figure 7-2 and A Closer Look Box 7-2).

Downward scapular rotation, like scapular depression, occurs most often through gravity's pull. When performed against the resistance, other rhomboids (major and minor) rotate the scapula as in downward pulling downward on a cord to lift a window shade. We achieve full downward rotation when the pectoralis minor tips the top of the scapular forward and downward as we reach behind our backs to touch between our scapulae. The pectoralis minor also contributes to a "winging out" of the scapula when poor stability of the scapula at its medial border allows this muscle to tug on the coracoid process during inhalation (A Closer Look Box 7-3).

The scapula follows the mediolateral contours of the thorax in protraction and retraction (A Closer Look Box 7-2). The insertion of the serratus anterior enables the scapula's costal surface to remain fully adjacent to the convexity of the thorax throughout the arc of movement. The serratus arises from the ribs around the midaxillary line and courses between scapula and thorax to attach to the vertebral border of the scapula. Attachment to the lateral border of the scapula would result in protraction

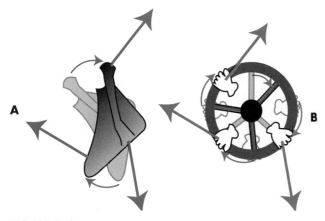

FIGURE **7-2**
(A) The scapula and upward rotation compared with **(B)** the turning of a steering wheel.

Scapular Movement
The terminology for scapular rotation differs depending on the part of the scapula the eye follows. Because the glenoid articulates with the humerus and in a sense points the way for the hand, references to scapular movement refer to glenoid movement. When the glenoid faces upward to allow positioning of the hand above the head, we call it upward scapular rotation. During this movement, the inferior angle moves laterally. The term lateral scapular rotation originates from this perspective. Although technically correct, the description does not depict the direction of distal upper-extremity movement.

The same is true for scapular protraction and retraction versus scapular abduction and adduction. In protraction the glenoid moves around the side of the thorax to face forward, holding the hand in front of the trunk. The vertebral border of the scapula moves from the midline. Emphasis on the movement of the vertebral border leads to a view of protraction as scapular abduction. The opposite movement, retraction, adducts the vertebral border back toward the midline.

accompanied by a rocking motion known as "winging," in which the vertebral border would protrude posteriorly (Figure 7-3, *A*). Coursing under the scapula and inserting onto the vertebral border allows the serratus to push the scapula forward while pulling the vertebral border closer to the ribs instead of pulling the scapula's anterior edge. No scapular winging occurs as long as the serratus anterior remains intact (Figure 7-3, *B*).

Retraction, the opposite of protraction, occurs through a certain amount of recoil in the tissues that stretch during protraction. Because protraction and retraction both occur in the transverse plane, gravity affects neither motion. When retraction occurs against resistance or requires more force than recoil produces, as in pulling an object closer with both hands, the middle fibers of the trapezius create the pure motion or combine with the rhomboids for stronger retraction with downward rotation.

MUSCLES AFFECTING THE HUMERUS

As we learn more about kinesiology, we realize that understanding a muscle's relationship to the axis or axes

A **CLOSER** LOOK

Breathing with the Pectoralis Minor

A relatively small and seemingly insignificant muscle, the pectoralis minor "hides" from attention under the much more appreciated pectoralis major. But an unbalanced pectoralis minor can play an important role in poor posture, shoulder impingement, and even nerve compression of the brachial plexus!

The pectoralis minor attaches proximally to the third, fourth, and fifth ribs and distally to the coracoid process of the scapula. Acting distally, it pulls on the coracoid, tipping the top of the scapula downward when the hand moves behind the back. Place your hand on someone else's scapula. As your subject reaches behind to touch your hand notice how the inferior angle of their scapula protrudes. Acting proximally, when sufficiently stabilized by scapular adductors, the pectoralis minor pulls on the ribs, forcing inhalation.

The pectoralis minor is an important contributor toward widening the lower thorax for "bucket handle breathing." This often desirable mechanism occurs due to repeated elevation–eversion on the lateral aspect of the rib cage. The widening stretches the diaphragm and leads to increased force for inspiration. The pectoralis minor's role in inspiration goes awry when weak scapular adductors (middle trapezius and rhomboids) fail to stabilize the scapula. In this case the pectoralis minor attempts to raise the ribs but produces unwanted scapular motion. Over time repeated winging-out of the scapula contributes to a kyphotic posture.

"Upper-chest" breathers demonstrate the failed function of the pectoralis minor. Upon inspiration, the sternocleidomastoid (SCM) and the scalenes (lateral neck muscles attaching to the upper ribs) begin to compensate for an overall lack of efficiency in "bucket handle breathing." The scalenes and SCM tighten from overuse placing undo tension on the brachial plexus and neurovascular bundle of the neck with every breath. Chronic "upper chest" breathers may develop thoracic outlet syndrome and an overall posture of upper body tension that contributes to impingment syndrome in the shoulders. Smokers, who commonly demonstrate these problems, often inhale using the upper chest.

Interestingly, a number of Eastern disciplines, such as yoga, kung fu, karate, tai chi chuan, and qi-gong, incorporate abdominal breathing into practices that focus on the unity of body, mind, and spirit. These practices combine proper breathing techniques with dynamic standing and sitting postures as well as moving and sitting meditation. Students of kinesiology can use their knowledge of anatomy and movement to bring a special "mindfulness" to any of these practices.

it crosses has more value than simply remembering muscle functions. A review of anatomy refreshes our minds about where muscles attach and their spatial relationships to other structures. Knowing a muscle's location often tells us what tasks it performs in functional activity.

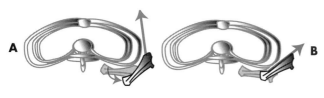

FIGURE **7-3**

A, Scapular protraction and winging would occur if the serratus anterior inserted on the scapula's lateral border. **B**, Its actual insertion on the vertebral border holds the scapula close to the thoracic wall during protraction.

The paired movements of glenohumeral (GH) abduction and adduction occur around a front-to-back axis. All muscles situated lateral or superior to this axis abduct the joint. Imagine a string tied to the insertion and pulled toward the origin parallel to the muscle fibers. As long as the string maintains its same relationship to the axis, it produces the same movement as the muscle. Imagine pulling the string toward a different origin on the opposite side of the axis to produce the opposite motion (Figure 7-4). To assist your imagination try representing a muscle's actions as a relatively simple drawing (A Closer Look Box 7-4).

The middle deltoid and supraspinatus abduct the humerus at the GH joint due to their lateral and superior relationships to the front-to-back abduction axis. The long head of the biceps shares this lateral relationship to the abduction axis only when positioned in UE external rotation (Figure 7-5). On the opposite side of the axis, the pectoralis major (sternal fibers), teres major,

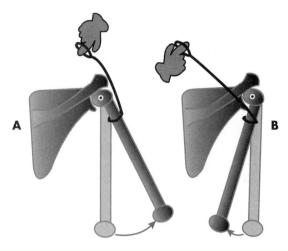

FIGURE **7-4**
A, Pulling a string tied to the deltoid's insertion produces abduction as long as it maintains a lateral relationship to the shoulder axis. **B**, Pulling the string toward a different origin medial to the axis results in adduction.

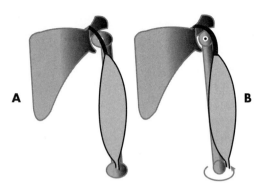

FIGURE **7-5**
A, The humerus rests in a neutral position. **B**, The biceps long head acts as a glenohumeral abductor after externally rotating the humerus.

BOX 7-4

A **CLOSER** LOOK

Drawing Muscle Function: A Review
A drawing of muscle function should include a label identifying the composer's viewpoint. Always conceptualize the motion you draw occurring in a plane along the surface of the paper. Imagine looking down the axis of motion; therefore for flexion you would look down the side-to-side axis. The axis dictates what view you draw: side-to-side, side view; front-to-back, front (or back) view; and up-to-down, horizontal view (from the top). Remember that the axis of motion always sticks into the plane with a 90-degree orientation, so it appears as a dot on the page located in the center of the convex segment of the joint. For glenohumeral flexion, draw a side view and draw the side-to-side axis as a dot in the center of the humeral head.

Draw muscle force as a vector. In a typical open-chain motion in which the insertion moves, place your pencil on the muscle's insertion point and draw a straight line following the direction of muscle fibers toward the origin. If the fibers go around a bony protuberance, do not follow the fibers but continue to draw the arrow straight, as if it were the tangent of a circle. Remember to make a scale and draw the arrow long enough to indicate the strength of the contraction. The arrowhead indicates the direction of the contraction and thus the movement.

---

and latissimus dorsi adduct the humerus (against resistance) due to their inferior relationships to the axis. (Remember that gravity acts as the most constant GH adductor.)

As in abduction and adduction, muscles producing GH flexion, extension, and internal and external rotation function according to their relationships with the axes of these movements. The pectoralis major, coracobrachialis, biceps long head, and anterior deltoid flex because they pull forward on their insertions anterior to the side-to-side axis. The latissimus dorsi, teres major, and posterior deltoid extend because they pull posteriorly with posterior and inferior relationships to the axis. The pectoralis major, teres major, latissimus dorsi, anterior deltoid, and subscapularis all act as internal rotators because they share a medial pull and an anterior relationship to the up-to-down axis for humeral rotation. On the opposite, posterior side of the axis, the infraspinatus, teres minor, and posterior deltoid externally rotate the humerus. Because the supraspinatus pulls through the up-to-down axis and lies neither anterior nor posterior to it, the supraspinatus cannot rotate, regardless of its anatomical designation as part of the *rotator* cuff muscle group.

MOVEMENTS

Scaption
Scaption, a term used widely in the rehabilitation setting, refers to movement of the upper extremity in the plane of the scapula. The scapular plane projects 30 to 45 degrees anterior to the coronal plane. Scaption occurs specifically during elevation of the hand through shoulder abduction by blending movements in the sagittal (flexion) and frontal planes (abduction) to achieve a combination of the two in the scapular plane (Closer Look Box 7-5).

BOX 7-5

A **CLOSER** LOOK

Scaption

The term scaption describes upper-extremity movement in the plane of the scapula, 30 to 45 degrees anterior to the frontal plane. Rehabilitation practitioners emphasize scaption in UE rehabilitation because of the following characteristics: The scapular plane improves the length–tension relationship in the various glenohumeral muscles and provides a more favorable plane of motion if stretching has occurred in the glenohumeral joint capsule. Movement in the frontal plane stretches the anterior pectoralis group and glenohumeral capsule, creating unnecessary tension. Sagittal-plane motion of the glenohumeral joint places the posterior capsule and musculature of the retractors (rhomboids and middle trapezius) in tension.

Specifically:

Scaption achieves a length–tension balance in the anterior and posterior musculature and glenohumeral joint capsule that leads to greater relative stability. Sound shoulder rehabilitation protocols rely on this stability, especially after shoulder surgeries involving tightening procedures to correct shoulder instability.

Scaption combined with a palm-up position of the upper extremity (external shoulder rotation) during shoulder abduction reduces the chance of shoulder impingement during shoulder abduction.

Closed-Chain Scapular Depression

Closed-chain movements involve limiting movement at the distal part of a moving chain through stabilization. In Chapter 4 we used a pull-up to demonstrate how shortening of the shoulder and elbow muscles usually used to move the upper extremity results in trunk movement when the hand grasps an immovable bar. Elbow flexors shorten, flexing the humerus onto the forearm at the elbow; and shoulder muscles bring the trunk closer to the humerus. The trunk rises toward the bar, creating closed-chain elbow flexion and shoulder extension (Figure 4-10).

Closed-chain scapular depression occurs when elevating the trunk for transfer from a wheelchair onto a table or mat. In open-chain depression, the scapula moves downward in relation to the trunk because scapular depressors like the latissimus dorsi and sternal pectoralis major originate lower on the trunk than their insertions on the humerus. With the hand free in space, concentric contractions cause the humerus to move downward. Because the humerus attaches to the scapula at the glenohumeral joint, the scapula moves downward (depression) in relation to the trunk. Closed-chain movement occurs when the hand stabilizes through elbow extension pushing the hand down onto the mat. The depressors shorten, moving the trunk upward toward the scapula (Figure 7-6). Understanding the role of the scapular depressors ensures that strengthening activities for such transfers exercise the correct muscles.

Shoulder Abduction and Scapular Stabilization

The sequence of muscle activation in shoulder abduction begins with stabilization of the scapula. This provides a stable base upon which the GH abductors can ground

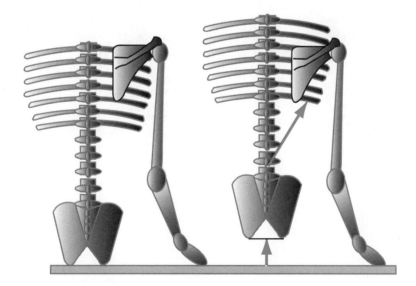

 FIGURE 7-6
Closed-chain scapular depression results in trunk elevation in a transfer from a wheelchair.

themselves and act on their distal attachments (humerus). Stabilization of the scapula relies on isometric contractions of muscles; subsequently, the concentric contractions of these muscles produce the scapular movements needed for complete shoulder abduction.

A basic concept in kinesiology explains the need for scapular stabilization. When a muscle contracts, it shortens; whether the origin or insertion moves depends on which moves most easily. (Recall Newton's discovery that the acceleration of an object relates to its mass.) The scapula has less mass than the entire upper extremity. Therefore when glenohumeral muscles contract, they will move the scapula unless other factors intervene.

All muscles that move the humerus at the glenohumeral joint require scapular stabilization first. Most, except for the pectoralis major and latissimus dorsi, originate on the scapula and insert onto the humerus. Without scapular stabilization, glenohumeral muscles that originate on the scapula would waste their excursion and move the wrong segment. Isometric contractions of the upward scapular rotators produce scapular stabilization, preventing downward scapular rotation when the supraspinatus and deltoid muscles activate to abduct the GH joint (Figure 7-7).

Elevation via Shoulder Abduction

With the scapula stabilized, glenohumeral muscles concentrically contract and successfully abduct the humerus at the GH joint. The supraspinatus provides pure abduction. The deltoid originates above the glenoid; this attachment and the relatively short moment arm for abduction result in a great proportion of the deltoid's force having a linear effect, directed parallel to the glenoid. Early in abduction, isolated concentric contraction of the deltoid elevates the humerus, impinging the structures between the humeral head and the acromion rather than abducting the humerus.

Three factors prevent undesirable elevation of the humerus in abduction. First, the supraspinatus originates medial to the glenoid rather than above, producing a linear effect directed into the glenoid fossa. Early activation of the supraspinatus results in pure abduction without elevation. Second, the combined pull of the infraspinatus, teres minor, and subscapularis directly opposes the elevation effect of the deltoid[1] (Figure 7-8). These smaller muscles pull mostly through the abduction axis and exert a downward linear pull on the humerus without interfering with abduction. Third, as abduction progresses, the linear component of the deltoid force directs into the glenoid, similar to the supraspinatus early in abduction, enabling continued abduction without humeral elevation.

Scapular stabilization, balance between upward and downward forces affecting the humerus, continued GH abduction, and upward scapular rotation combine so that an individual can raise their hand above their

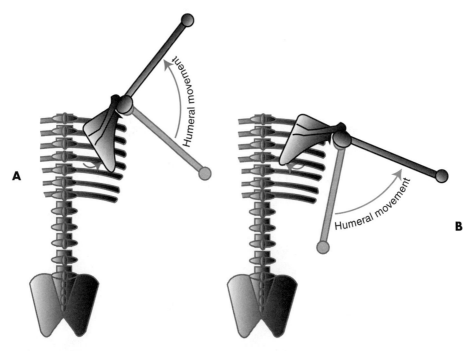

FIGURE **7-7**
Glenohumeral movement **(A)** with and **(B)** without scapular stabilization. Notice that the amount of humeral movement remains the same in each case.

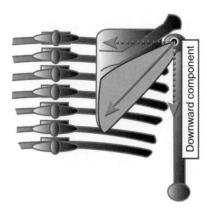

FIGURE 7-8
The infraspinatus, teres minor, and subscapularis (not visible from this view) pull the humerus downward and inward. The downward component of the force balances the elevating effect of the deltoid early in abduction.

head (Figure 7-9). **Scapulohumeral rhythm** describes these simultaneous GH and scapular movements (A Closer Look Box 7-6).

Rotator Cuff

Four muscles—the subscapularis, supraspinatus, infraspinatus, and teres minor—comprise the **rotator cuff**. We already have described their actions in different functions. This collective name arises out of the appearance and function of these muscles as a circular cuff securing the humeral head close to the glenoid fossa. The GH ligaments and rotator cuff muscles help stabilize the joint.

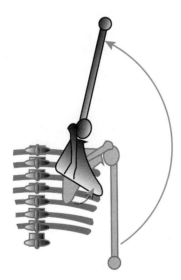

FIGURE 7-9
Elevation of the upper extremity through abduction requires both a glenohumeral and a scapular contribution.

The rotator cuff plays a critical role in stabilizing the GH joint when the hand holds objects that produce a downward force on the upper extremity.[1]

Although they stabilize the glenohumeral joint together, individual groupings of rotator cuff muscles demonstrate functional diversity, including two antagonistic, or opposing, actions. The supraspinatus primarily functions as a GH abductor. The infraspinatus, teres minor, and subscapularis have a common downward effect on the humerus, balancing the upward pull of the deltoid on the humerus early in abduction. The infraspinatus and teres minor externally rotate the humerus because of their locations posterior to the rotation axis. The anteriorly located subscapularis acts as an antagonist, internally rotating the humerus (Table 7-2).

Glenohumeral Subluxation

Normal GH joint stability involves a certain orientation of the glenoid and the superior joint structures—the joint capsule, supraspinatus, and posterior deltoid. The glenoid faces slightly upward because its inferior edge protrudes more laterally than its superior edge. As the pull of gravity moves the humeral head inferiorly along the glenoid, the humeral head moves laterally and downward. This movement stretches the superior joint structures, and their recoil prevents the humeral head from moving farther downward (Figure 7-10).

When the hand holds a weight, the supraspinatus contracts to provide increased support. The supraspinatus may contract to support the upper extremity even when the hand does not hold a weight.[1] (The correlation of subluxation with flaccid paralysis of the supraspinatus after a cerebral vascular accident [CVA], or stroke, verifies the role of the supraspinatus in the prevention of subluxation[3]).

After a CVA the GH joint commonly becomes partially dislocated (**subluxation**). Although severe spasticity may affect parts of the upper extremity, some GH muscles, like the supraspinatus, become essentially inactive. This shift in muscle balance combines with slight realignment of the scapula and causes the glenoid to lose its upward orientation; therefore the normal mechanism for securing the humeral head into the glenoid fails (A Closer Look Box 7-7).

Glenohumeral Dislocation

Shortening of the GH extensors/adductors also occurs commonly following a CVA. This limits both active and passive GH abduction, which occurs only when the adductors (antagonists to the motion) have sufficient length to provide distal excursion.

Spasticity causes the shoulder to assume an adducted, internally rotated position at rest, and it remains in this

BOX 7-6

A **CLOSER** LOOK

Elevating the Hand through Shoulder Abduction: A Biomechanical Perspective[4]

"Shoulder elevation" commonly refers to shoulder abduction that raises the hand above the head. Try not to confuse shoulder elevation with scapular elevation, a pure movement of the scapula only. Practitioners prefer the term shoulder elevation even though shoulder abduction sounds less confusing. Regardless of terms, raising the hand above the head involves complex coordination of clavicle, scapula, and humerus movements at sternoclavicular, acromioclavicular, scapulothoracic, and glenohumeral (GH) joints. While we focus on the hand, as the distal end of the chain, very little motion would occur without involving the most proximal joint (sternoclavicular). According to Donatelli, the clavicle elevates 4 degrees at the sternoclavicular joint for every 10 degrees of shoulder abduction. Without clavicular motion, elevation of the hand above the head proves impossible.

Most of our thinking about shoulder elevation (shoulder abduction) centers on the combination of movements at the scapula (in the sternoclavicular and acromioclavicular joints) and at the humerus (in the GH joint). The terms initial (0 to 60 degrees), middle (60 to 130 degrees), and final (140 to 180 degrees) describe the three phases of shoulder elevation.

During the initial phase of shoulder elevation, the scapula upwardly rotates 1 degree for every 3 degrees of GH abduction. In the "setting" portion of the initial phase (0 to 30 degrees), the GH abductors (mostly deltoid) produce a superior shear force countered by the subscapularis, teres minor, and infraspinatus muscles. This counterforce depresses the humeral head and provides some compression to the glenohumeral joint.

Practitioners focus on movements in the initial phase to strengthen a number of motor patterns following shoulder surgery. Intervention in this phase aids dynamic scapulothoracic stability and reduces the chances of compensatory shoulder movements resulting in unwanted "shoulder hiking" and impingement (jamming the humeral head into the more superior acromion). Specifics of these protocols include:

- Strengthening of humeral and scapular depressors (subscapularis, teres minor, infraspinatus, latissimus dorsi, lower trapezius)
- Manual therapy for scapular mobility
- Strengthening of upward scapular rotators (serratus and upper/lower trapezius) as well as retractors (middle trapezius, rhomboids)

According to Donatelli,[4] the following muscles contribute during the middle or critical phase of shoulder elevation (60 to 130 degrees):

- 43% deltoid
- 9% supraspinatus
- 25% subscapularis
- 22% infraspinatus and teres minor

The humeral head glides and rolls superiorly/inferiorly within the glenohumeral joint 1 to 2 millimeters. Glenohumeral abduction and upward rotation of the scapula occur nearly equally in this phase with the greatest scapular rotation taking place between 80 and 140 degrees. Involvement of the lower trapezius increases to assist with upward rotation of the scapula.

In the final phase (140 to 180 degrees), scapulohumeral rhythm consists of 3.5-degree abduction at the GH joint for every degree of upward scapular rotation. Note that both GH and scapulothoracic joints continue to contribute even though the ratio favors GH movement as it did in the initial phase. Full upward scapular rotation positions the glenoid directly inferior to the humerus, where it acts as a base of support.

position unless moved by an external force. Standard treatment protocols use daily range of motion exercises to prevent joint and muscle contracture. Once contractures have occurred, forcing the shoulder into abduction with aggressive range of motion can cause dislocation of the humeral head. Contracture of the pectoralis major

prevents distal excursion of its humeral attachment required for the normal arc of abduction. As the practitioner attempts passive abduction, the tight pectoralis major stabilizes the humerus at the point of the muscle's attachment. This shifts the axis of motion from the humeral head to the point of attachment of the

TABLE 7-2

Functional Diversity of Rotator Cuff Muscles

MUSCLE COMBINATIONS	ACTION
Infraspinatus teres minor subscapularis	Humeral head depression to balance upward pull of the deltoid early in GH abduction
Infraspinatus teres minor	External humeral rotation
Subscapularis	Internal humeral rotation
Supraspinatus	Humeral abduction

pectoralis major. The humeral head dislocates to follow this new arc of motion for abduction in which the elbow moves up and the humeral head down (Figure 7-11).

Mary Smith developed typical spasticity in her shoulder complex muscles following her CVA. Sometimes she appeared to forget she had a left arm as it fell off tables and the armrests of her wheelchair. Once while her grandson pushed the wheelchair, she cut her hand when her fingers got caught in the spokes.

Mary had a sizeable palpable subluxation and received treatment at a small hospital by an occupational therapy practitioner. The OT practitioner had learned the benefits of aggressive range of motion during his training, but had not kept up with current trends in shoulder rehabilitation. He would stretch Mary's arm into abduction despite her complaints. Mary often told her children that people at the hospital wanted to hurt her, but the family attributed this to the disorientation that often accompanies a CVA. The OT practitioner taught family

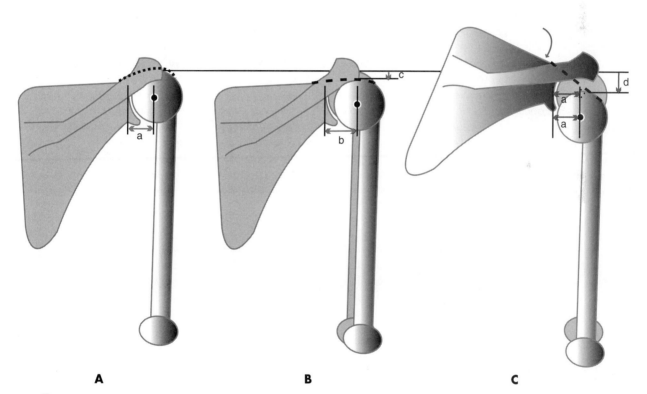

A   **B**   **C**

See the CD

FIGURE **7-10**

A, The humeral head rests in its most medial position when centered in the glenoid; distance *a* is minimal. **B**, Downward movement of the humerus due to gravity accompanies lateral tracking of the humeral head as it follows the lateral curvature of the glenoid (distance *b*). This increased distance between the glenoid and the humeral head stretches the superior soft tissue, which recoils and prevents further downward motion. Thus distance *c* between the acromion and the humeral head remains minimal. **C**, The scapula rotates increasingly downward, and the inferior glenoid moves out from under the humeral head. Downward movement no longer produces lateral tracking. (Distance *a* remains the same before and after the humerus drops.) Without lateral movement, the supportive tissues do not tighten and the humerus moves downward a greater distance (*d*), resulting in subluxation.

BOX 7-7

A **C L O S E R** L O O K

Glenohumeral Subluxation

Practitioners spend a great deal of time and energy trying to reduce GH subluxation. Stimulating the deltoid seems attractive because it immediately reduces glenohumeral subluxation by elevating the relaxed, adducted upper extremity. In many cases practitioners focus on the middle deltoid because in isolation this muscle quickly elevates the humeral head and reduces subluxation—but only during active stimulation as this is not the natural mechanism to prevent subluxation.

Basmajian and DeLuca[1] convincingly established the middle deltoid as "inactive even with heavy pulls on the arm. Other muscles running vertically from the scapula to the humerus, particularly the biceps and long head of the triceps, were conspicuously inactive as well." The two researchers[1] demonstrated that only the supraspinatus and the posterior fibers of the deltoid actively prevented subluxation. Because the middle deltoid does not normally hold the humeral head into the glenoid fossa, external stimulation of these fibers cannot reduce subluxation over time.

OT practitioners who stimulate the middle deltoid to reduce subluxation misinterpret research. Stimulation of the posterior deltoid and the supraspinatus, however, has proved effective in the reduction of subluxation.[5] Stimulation of these muscles is consistent with Basmajian and DeLuca's findings[1] and preferable to stimulation of the middle deltoid.

Basmajian and DeLuca[1] also explained that the superior joint structures—the joint capsule, supraspinatus, and posterior deltoid—combined with proper angulation of the glenoid all help prevent subluxation. If gravity's pull on the upper extremity forces the scapula to rotate downward and the glenoid to lose its orientation, the superior structures lose their effectiveness. In this way, downward movement of the humeral head replaces the normal lateral movement preventing the normal stretch and recoil of the superior structures (Figure 7-10). Successful prevention of subluxation involves improving an individual's scapular positioning primarily through strengthening of the upward scapular rotators.

Therapeutic concern often centers on decreasing pain attributed to subluxation. Two separate studies have demonstrated very little association between shoulder subluxation and pain after CVA.[2,7] In fact, more poststroke shoulder pain seems linked to limited external rotation than to subluxation.[7] Effective treatment strategies for the reduction of shoulder pain and the prevention of stretching in the shoulder capsule include support of the affected upper extremity and use of natural means such as lap trays and armrests to help individuals maintain that support.

members how to perform shoulder abduction, but they lacked his knowledge of anatomy and his skill level, so they often caused Mary more discomfort. Unaware of the growing possibility of dislocation, they continued to provide daily range of motion exercises believing it would ultimately help her regain some function.

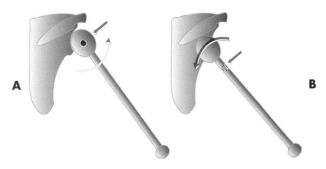

A   **B**

FIGURE **7-11**
Dislocation of the humeral head in the case of forced abduction with a tight pectoralis major.

As Mary's shoulder muscles contracted into typical spasticity patterns, it became harder and harder to get her shoulder abducted. Her family unintentionally aggravated this condition with aggressive stretching that increased spasticity because it stretched the shortened muscles beyond their elastic limits. Small muscle tears healed into inelastic scar tissue, yielding an even denser connective tissue contracture. Finally, a strong push toward abduction during daily ranging by a family member lead to dislocation of the humeral head.

The Elbow Complex and Forearm

Classification of the elbow as a hinge joint describes its basic flexion–extension function. However, the elbow moves in less obvious ways. The ulna and radius articulate with the humerus to form a combination of joints. Considering the elbow as a complex of joints more accurately reflects its ability to allow flexion, extension, and radial rotation for supination and pronation of the forearm.

The elbow's complex anatomical makeup makes it a relatively unforgiving joint when it comes to injury. The elbow's thin articular capsule responds in an exaggerated fashion to trauma that often results in joint contracture after the injury. Additionally, all three major upper-extremity nerves (radial, median, and ulnar) cross the joint within millimeters of the capsule, increasing the likelihood that neurological damage will accompany orthopedic trauma (A Closer Look Box 7-8).

ARTICULATIONS

Articulation between the humerus and ulna forms the medial portion of the elbow complex. This ulnotrochlear hinge has one degree of freedom and allows movement (flexion and extension) in only one plane around one side-to-side axis. Laterally, the radius articulates with the humerus to form a shallow ball-and-socket radiocapitular joint. The attachment of the radius to the ulna through the interosseus membrane prevents abduction and adduction of the radius. Thus movement only occurs at two axes, flexion/extension and rotation. (For in-depth coverage of the ligaments of the elbow, go to A Closer Look Box 7-9.)

The uniaxial proximal and distal radioulnar joints allow radial rotation for pronation and supination of the forearm. Proximally the radius spins around an axis at

BOX 7-8

A **CLOSER** LOOK

Orthopedic Elbow Injuries
The superficial nature of the elbow joint makes it vulnerable to a number of pathologies including septic bursitis. As it crosses the elbow joint the brachialis muscle is 96% muscle belly. This makes it susceptible to tearing during dislocations.

Posterolateral dislocation, the most common type of dislocation, often occurs in gymnastics, where the olecranon acts as a weight-bearing pivot. When the olecranon dislocates posteriorly the brachialis often tears. The healing process in this case and in many other elbow injuries typically involves extraneous bone deposition (heterotopic ossification) leading to severe bony joint contracture.

BOX 7-9

A **CLOSER** LOOK

Ligaments of the Elbow
A number of ligaments reinforce the elbow joint:
- Radial collateral ligament—this is a strong triangular band stretching over the lateral side of the joint. Its apex attaches proximally to the lateral epicondyle of the humerus.
- Annular ligament—it surrounds the radial head and joins to the base of the radial collateral ligament.
- Ulnar collateral ligament—this is the medial counterpart to the radial collateral ligament; its triangular shape consists of anterior–posterior and weak oblique bands with an apex on the medial epicondyle of the humerus. The ulnar nerve runs very close to this area, predisposing it to injury if the ulnar collateral ligament ruptures.

its center. Distally it spins in a larger arc around an axis closer to its ulnar edge. The shape of the radius and its two attachments to the ulna account for these different movements (Figure 7-12 and A Closer Look Box 7-10).

The radius curves laterally from proximal to distal. A line drawn from the center of the proximal radius runs along the ulnar edge of the distal radius. This line forms the axis for pronation and supination (see Figure 7-12, *B*). Ulnar attachments of the proximal and distal radius complete the design and guarantee the different movement arcs of these two ends.

Proximally, the annular ligament holds the radius close to the ulna and allows spinning within the ligament. Distally, the articular disk secures the ulnar edge of the radius closely adjacent to the ulna. This attachment causes the distal radius to spin around the ulna. (Notice on most articulated skeletons that the radius attaches to the distal ulna by way of a pin or screw through the center of the ulna, but proximally attaches by way of a screw through the center of the radius.) These different centers of rotation allow the radius to cross over the ulna in pronation so that it brings the hand from palm-up to palm-down.

MUSCLES FLEXING AND EXTENDING THE ELBOW

Elbow flexion occurs when muscle forces anchored on the forearm and directed toward the shoulder travel anteriorly to the side-to-side flexion/extension axis.

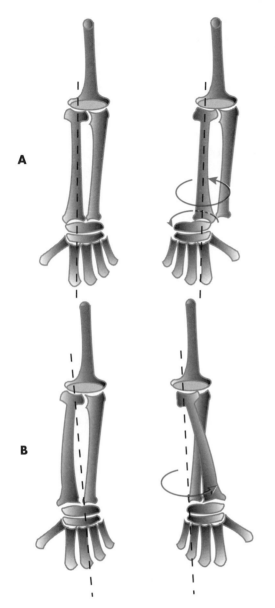

FIGURE **7-12**
Supination and pronation with a **(A)** straight radius results in disaster. **(B)** The slightly curved radius allows for movement.

BOX 7-10

ACLOSERLOOK

A Straight Radius
If the radius had the straight shape of the humerus with similar proximal and distal attachments, it would rotate around an axis within itself both prox- imally and distally, spelling disaster for pronation and supination of the hand. The hand would completely dislocate from the ulna to pronate and turn the palm down (see Figure 7-12, *A*). The curved design of the radius bends it away from its long axis (see Figure 7-12, *B*). This and its different proximal and distal attachments allow the radius to rotate around itself proximally and around the ulna distally. The ulna, wrist, and hand remain connected along the ulnar aspect as the radius brings the hand around the ulna.

Extending the Elbow Using the Shoulder

Bernice Richards shows off her new white convertible and its hand controls to the OT staff at the clinic. After watching her use elbow extension to brake, the OT intern asks, "How can Ms. Richards extend her elbows with C5 quadriplegia since the triceps receives innervation from C6 and C7, below the level of her lesion?"

His supervisor explains that the functional movements Bernice displays involve elbow extension linked with shoulder flexion. Bernice links elbow extension and shoulder flexion by planting her hand, stabilizing the chain's distal end so that shoulder flexion causes elbow extension. Because Bernice has muscle strength in her shoulders (via C5-innervated shoulder flexors like the deltoid), she can move both the shoulder and the elbow as long as she has her hand stabilized. Bernice loses the link between shoulder and elbow once her hand regains freedom in space, and she can no longer extend her elbow against resistance.

Once inside the clinic Bernice agrees to show the OT intern how she uses elbow extension to pull on her stockings. Sitting on the clinic mat, Bernice prevents her trunk from falling for- ward by planting her hands on the mat, performing a push-up motion.

The OT supervisor points out that Bernice externally rotates her humerus at the end of the extension movement when push- ing her trunk into a vertical position. This terminal external shoulder rotation produces a few more degrees of shoulder flex- ion and hyperextends her elbow (Movie 7-1). Because Bernice has 5 degrees or more of elbow hyperextension, she can hold the terminal elbow position using hyperextension as a lock. In hyperextension the weight of Bernice's upper trunk projects posterior to the elbow flexion/extension axis and creates an extension force, resisting elbow flexion. Bernice's ligaments

The biceps brachii, brachialis, and brachioradialis are the largest muscle masses in the anterior arm and serve this function. Muscles like the extensor carpi radialis longus and pronator teres, by virtue of their anterior locations and origins on the humeral epicondyles, assist in elbow flexion. Their attachments close to the flexion axis produce short moment arms for flexion, explaining their minimal function in this movement. The triceps, with posterior attachments travels posterior to the side-to-side elbow axis and serves as the major elbow extensor.

prevent further hyperextension, and her elbow remains stable in hyperextension as long as her trunk's weight projects posterior to the axis.

The OT supervisor compares Bernice's elbow hyperextension to a similar motion used by another client, 7-year-old Alex Fecteau. Alex has hip and pelvic muscle weakness due to Duchenne-type muscular dystrophy. When Alex stands, he hyperextends his knees and arches his spine backward, displacing his center of gravity and allowing him to bear weight with very little muscular effort. Both these motions conserve energy, using ligaments to counter gravity.

Inhibition of the Biceps

People with upper motor neuron syndromes such as CVA or traumatic brain injury often develop severe flexor spasticity in their upper extremities. This tightness on one side of a joint limits its antagonistic motion; for example, tight elbow flexors interfere with elbow extension. Lack of any movement on a regular basis results in shortening of tissues around the joint (joint and muscle contracture). Daily range of motion exercise can prevent contractures, but spasticity also makes completing such exercises difficult. Finding a way to inhibit muscle contractions resulting from spasticity greatly eases joint range of motion and helps prevent contractures.

Electromyographic (EMG) studies of normal muscle use in different movement combinations have proved applicable when reducing spasticity. An EMG recording of the biceps demonstrates strong activation of this flexor–supinator in combined forearm flexion and supination. Strong flexion with supination recruits the brachialis as a synergist for forceful elbow flexion.

The biceps drops in importance if the task requires elbow flexion with forearm *pronation*. Via EMG, we see a marked decrease in biceps activity accompanying forearm pronation even during continued elbow flexion. This makes sense considering pronation opposes supination, so the biceps must "give in" and be stretched while the pronators activate. Once the task requirement for supination disappears, the brachialis becomes the primary elbow flexor because it inserts only on the ulna and has no pronation or supination effect. Extrapolating from these EMG recordings, elbow flexion with forearm pronation inhibits the biceps. We use this information about motor programming to our advantage when positioning the forearm in pronation before attempting elbow extension against flexor spasticity at the elbow. This "pronation switch" turns off the biceps and decreases the resistance to passive extension.*

When Mary Smith arrived at Maple Grove Skilled Care Facility, she held her left arm flexed tightly against her body.

---

*Unpublished findings from EMG studies performed in the lead author's laboratory.

She refused to let any nurses or aides move her arm through passive range of motion, so the nursing supervisor contacted the OT department.

The OT practitioner explained to Mary that putting her arm through range of motion probably would alleviate some of her stiffness and soreness. He promised to try some new techniques that would make range of motion less painful than it had been in the past.

While they talked about Mary's family the OT practitioner gave Mary's left arm a gentle massage to gain her trust. He solicited her ideas about ways to decorate the clinic for the upcoming holiday season as he slowly and carefully pronated her left forearm to inhibit the biceps. The OT practitioner explained to Mary that in the past, staff might have attempted to extend her elbow with her palm up in supination, a position associated with increased activity in the biceps.

Afterwards the OT practitioner explained to the nursing staff how pronating Mary's forearm first inactivated her biceps, making elbow extension easier and more comfortable. He continued explaining that elbow extension in pronation stretched the tight biceps tendon even further because both of the biceps' antagonistic movements—extension and pronation—occur simultaneously. After this informal in-service, Maple Grove nursing staff adopted this technique and found daily elbow range of motion exercises easier and more beneficial for everyone.

PRONATION AND SUPINATION

Pronation and supination arise from forces that pull the radius across the forearm toward the ulna. Anterior forces (pronator teres and pronator quadratus) produce pronation; posterior forces (supinator) result in supination. The strongest supinator, the biceps, wraps around the radius like a string wraps around a top when the forearm pronates. Contraction of the biceps spins the top (the radius), producing supination (Figure 7-13). (Flexing the elbow to midposition clarifies this relationship and displays the most effective action.)

The brachioradialis functions as both a pronator and a supinator. Like the muscles previously described, the brachioradialis directs a force that pulls the radius toward the ulna. As the forearm pronates, the brachioradialis' force lies dorsal to the axis for pronation and supination and supinates the forearm to midposition. At midposition it loses this relationship, and its role as a supinator stops. With the forearm fully supinated, the brachioradialis directs a force on the volar (pronator) side of the axis and causes pronation to midposition (Figure 7-14). The direction of pull and its relationship to the axis help explain the brachioradialis' contradictory functions. The ability of the brachioradialis to assist in supination and pronation proves a great asset

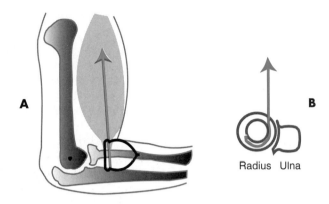

FIGURE 7-13
The biceps spins the radius like a top to produce essential rotation necessary for supination. **(A)** A side view and **(B)** a cross-sectional view of the radius and ulna.

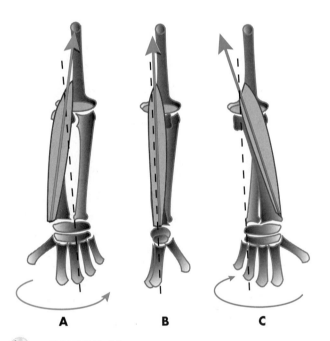

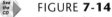

FIGURE 7-14
The brachioradialis changes its relationship with the pronation and supination axis as it moves the forearm. In this view, intersection of the axis (dotted line) by the force vector means the muscle produces movement. **A**, When the forearm supinates the brachioradialis pronates. **B**, With the forearm in a neutral position the brachioradialis has no effect. **C**, When the forearm pronates the brachioradialis supinates.

after loss of the biceps through musculocutaneous nerve damage or loss of the pronator through median nerve damage. (For in-depth coverage of nerve injury associated with the various muscles of the elbow and forearm, see A Closer Look Boxes 7-11 and 7-12.)

Isolation of the Supinator

Although not always active, the biceps has greater mass and strength compared to the supinator. Quieting the biceps to perform supination with only the supinator helps determine the function of the radial nerve. Because the biceps and supinator perform supination with two different nerves, the musculocutaneous and radial, respectively, if an individual supinates using only the supinator, we can conclude that the radial nerve is intact.

Eduardo Ybarra visits the hand-therapy clinic after cutting his forearm with a saw. The OT practitioner evaluating him needs to know whether the trauma has affected innervation to his supinator muscle. The OT practitioner knows two mechanisms for supination involving different muscles. Rapid supination and combined supination and elbow flexion against gravity activate the biceps. Slow supination with the forearm supported activates only the supinator. To isolate Eduardo's supinator, the OT practitioner positions Eduardo's forearm in a supported, flexed, and pronated position. She palpates the biceps tendon in the cubital fossa and instructs Eduardo to turn his palm up slowly. Under normal conditions, the supinator activates alone in this position. Without radial nerve function, the supinator remains inactive and the biceps substitutes for the missing action of the supinator. The OT practitioner does not feel any action in the biceps tendon and concludes that Eduardo's radial nerve has function distally at least as far as his supinator.

Function and Adaptation

Ergonomics concerns itself with active muscles during movement as well as how an activity changes under different conditions. Elbow flexors produce an upward force that supports the flexed elbow when the hand holds a weight, but at the same time this muscle force compresses the joint. The biceps force pulls the ulna upward against the humerus (**joint force**). Joint force varies even while supporting the same weight as a function of where on the forearm we hold that weight.

CARRYING A HANDBAG

Linda Valdez, a legal secretary recently diagnosed with rheumatoid arthritis, talks with her OT practitioners about the large handbag she carries. The handbag puts a hefty load on Linda's elbow flexors. The OT practitioner has some concerns that the reaction force resulting from strong contraction of the elbow flexors produced by her biceps may damage Mary's fragile elbow joint when she carries this handbag.

In Figure 7-15, Linda places a 5-kg handbag at her wrist, 20 cm from the center of rotation at the elbow joint *(A)*. She flexes her elbow to 90 degrees, and supinates her forearm. The biceps muscle operates at a moment

BOX 7-11

A C L O S E R L O O K

Nerves and Pathology around the Elbow

Entrapment of the median nerve in the forearm occurs most often where the nerve runs between the two heads of the pronator teres muscle (pronator syndrome). Motor and sensory symptoms occur in structures innervated by the median nerve distal to the pronator teres.

Anterior interosseus nerve (AIN) entrapment involves the motor branch of the median nerve in the forearm. Compression sometimes occurs at the fibrous arch of the origin of the flexor digitorum superficialis muscle and results in muscle weakness specific to the long flexor of the thumb (flexor pollicis longus), as well as to the index and middle fingers (flexor digitorum profundus). Owing to the importance of these muscles in grasp, an AIN entrapment impacts specific prehension patterns like three-jaw pinch (opposition of thumb pad to index and middle finger pads).

Fracture of the proximal humerus may result in radial nerve laceration as the nerve passes through the spiral groove in the humerus on its way to the forearm and hand. Loss of the wrist extensors (wrist drop) results and renders grip nearly nonfunctional.

Radial nerve entrapment occurs in radialtunnel syndrome, with compression of the nerve as it traverses the Arcade of Froshe. (The Arcade of Froshe is a fibrous arch formed by the two heads of the supinator;) At the Arcade of Froshe the deep motor branch of the radial nerve dives into the supinator muscle and exits to travel on the posterior side of the interosseus membrane where it becomes the posterior interosseus nerve (PIN). With enough inflammation and swelling, compression occurs proximal to the supinator. This leads to wrist drop similar to that caused by radial nerve damage in the spiral groove. Individuals experience pain in the area of compression, but have no sensory symptoms along the distribution of the radial nerve because only motor fibers travel in the nerve at this point. Damage at the spiral groove results in a full complement of sensory and motor symptoms because both motor and sensory fibers travel together more proximally.

Unfortunately during the first 4 to 6 weeks of radial tunnel syndrome the symptoms mimic lateral epicondylitis. Pain presents in the general area of the common extensor tendon. Provocative tests, such as those described in A Closer Look Box 7-12, often give false positive results. Proper treatment and a good prognosis depend on a clear and thorough differential diagnosis.

Cubital tunnel syndrome involves compression of the ulnar nerve where it passes between the medial epicondyle and the olecronon. Blows to the "funny bone" make us well aware of the path the ulnar nerve takes at the elbow! Scar tissue associated with constant pressure or repeated trauma to the medial side of the elbow leads to numbness and tingling along the ulnar sensory distribution (ring and little fingers). Eventually motor loss can include the intrinsic muscles of the hands affecting grasp.

BOX 7-12

A C L O S E R L O O K

Provocative Testing for the Elbow

Wartenberg's sign—test of ulnar nerve function

Place the hand palm-down, fingers spread on a table. Ask the individual to actively bring the fingers together. Inability to adduct the fingers suggests an ulnar neuropathy affecting the intrinsics of the hand.

Lateral epicondylitis test (Mills' test)—test for lateral epicondylitis ("tennis elbow")

This test localizes soft tissue soreness in the forearm. Fully extend the elbow and flex the wrist while palpating the lateral epicondyle. Consider pain at the lateral epicondyle of the humerus a positive test, indicating inflammation of the common wrist and finger extensor mass where it attaches at the lateral epicondyle (lateral epicondylitis, also known as "tennis elbow"). Note: this test puts stress on the radial nerve at the elbow and can alternatively indicate the presence of radial tunnel syndrome. Electrodiagnostic studies (electromyogram and nerve conduction velocity) performed by a physician help rule out radial nerve compression. This type of differential diagnosis helps ensure correct treatment.

Medial epicondylitis test—test for "golfer's elbow"

Palpate the forearm at the medial epicondyle during forearm supination and wrist extension. Interpret pain over the medial epicondyle as a positive test indicating inflammation of the common wrist and finger flexor mass where it attaches at the medial epicondyle (medial epicondylitis, also known as "golfer's elbow").

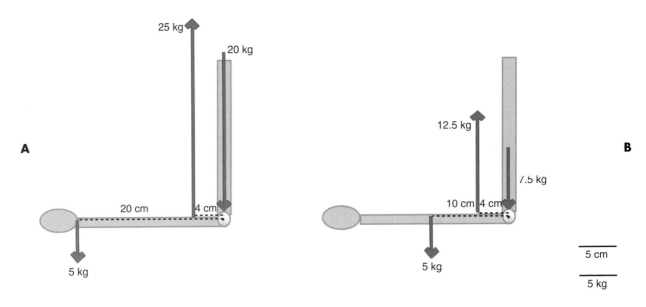

FIGURE **7-15**
Linda places her 5-kg handbag **(A)** at her wrist and **(B)** near her elbow. The biceps produces 25 kg of force when Linda holds her 5-kg handbag at the wrist **(A)**. The biceps force decreases to 12.5 kg when she places the handbag closer to her elbow.

arm of 4 cm through a line of application parallel to the long axis of her humerus. Linda carries the same purse closer to her elbow in Figure 7-15, *B*, 10 cm from the center of rotation at the elbow joint.

The resistance forces produced by Linda's handbag operate with two very different moment arms. How large a force must Linda's biceps muscle generate to counteract the torque produced by the weight of the handbag? From an ergonomic standpoint, how does moving the handbag closer to or farther from the joint affect the forces acting on her elbow joint? How large is the reaction force *(R)* at the ulnotrochlear joint?

To calculate absolute values of forces, we would need to include in the problem the weight of Linda's forearm and the extension tendency it produces. However, because we only want to know the relative effect of moving the handbag closer to Mary's elbow, we can simplify the problem.

The force of the biceps under each condition requires the equation for equilibrium of torques in opposite directions:

$$(5 \text{ kg} \times 20 \text{ cm}) = F \times 4 \text{ cm}$$

$$100 \text{ kg-cm} = F \times 4 \text{ cm}$$

$$100 \text{ kg-cm}/4 \text{ cm} = F$$

$$25 \text{ kg} = F$$

$$(5 \text{ kg} \times 10 \text{ cm}) = F \times 4 \text{ cm}$$

$$50 \text{ kg-cm} = F \times 4 \text{ cm}$$

$$50 \text{ kg-cm}/4 \text{ cm} = F$$

$$12.5 \text{ kg} = F$$

Linda's biceps contracts with greater force as she places the handbag closer to her wrist (Figure 7-15). While we usually focus on the biceps creating a tendency toward flexion, we also must keep in mind the way joint tissues experience this force. The upward biceps force pulls the ulna superiorly against the trochlea of the humerus, compressing the ulnar notch onto the distal humerus. No observed movement up or down indicates equilibrium; Newton said in this condition that the forces in opposite directions are equal. The matching downward force (reaction force or joint force) projects through the humerus, in opposition to the biceps force. The two forces meet at the joint surfaces. Determine the approximate value of the reaction force using the formula for equilibrium of upward and downward linear forces:

$$\text{force up} = \text{force down}$$

$$25 \text{ kg} = R + 5 \text{ kg}$$

$$25 \text{ kg} - 5 \text{ kg} = R$$

$$R = 20 \text{ kg downward}$$

$$12.5 \text{ kg} = R + 5 \text{ kg}$$

$$12.5 \text{ kg} - 5 \text{ kg} = R \qquad R = 7.5 \text{ kg downward}$$

Linda's biceps works twice as hard to hold the handbag at her wrist; the reaction force more than doubles.

The OT practitioner explains the danger of strong joint reaction forces and their destructive effect on Linda's fragile joints. He shows her how to protect her joints by moving even relatively light loads closer to the affected joints.

Summary

The more deeply we study the shoulder and elbow, the more information we discover. Our hands get where we want them to go because of sternoclavicular joint freedom and scapular movement. The rotator cuff muscles form a cuff but play a larger role than simply rotation. Scapular muscles sometimes move the trunk. The elbow can flex and extend because of muscles that move the shoulder. Heavy handbags create dangerous joint-reaction forces. All these mysteries become clear once we apply a few relatively simple concepts from biomechanics.

Applications

■ APPLICATION **7-1**
Muscle Function Simulations

Use duct tape to attach a string to the deltoid tubercle on the humerus of a model skeleton. Pull the string toward the (1) acromion lateral to the front-to-back axis, (2) distal clavicle anterior to the side-to-side axis, (3) midspine of the scapula posterior to the side-to-side axis, and (4) sacrum posterior and inferior to the side-to-side axis.

What happens each time? Which muscle does each new pull represent? In the last case, contrast the rotational effect on the humerus with that of the latissimus. In all cases, why do you have to pull so hard to effect movement?

■ APPLICATION **7-2**
Muscle Function Drawings

Prove to yourself that you can demonstrate muscle function by drawing the force of contraction in its proper relationship to the axis of motion. Draw the humerus, elbow, and ulna. Next, draw a force representing the pull of the brachialis on the ulna that produces flexion. Can you redraw the brachialis force as if the brachialis were surgically reattached to become an elbow extensor?

■ APPLICATION **7-3**
Limited Shoulder Strength

Hospital engineers plan to design door handles for use by all patients in the spinal cord unit. They have asked the OT department to help them determine how much force average patients have available to operate a door handle using shoulder flexors and abductors. Figure 7-16 depicts a 60-kg man with C5 quadriplegia and fair muscle grades in shoulder flexion. Some individuals on the unit have less shoulder strength, for example, poor grade strength in flexors and abductors allowing only 70-degrees flexion and 50-degrees abduction. The door handle the engineers have designed requires operation by a movement midway between shoulder flexion and abduction (scaption).

The muscle fibers of the anterior and middle deltoid lie approximately at a 30-degree angle from each other and 2 cm from the axis of motion in the glenohumeral joint. With the arm outstretched, the center of gravity for the entire upper extremity falls approximately at the elbow, about 30 cm from the shoulder joint in an average person.

7-3A. How much force will individuals with fair anterior and middle deltoid muscle grades have available?

7-3B. How much force will individuals with poor anterior and middle deltoid muscle grades have available?

7-3C. How much force can fair and poor strength ranges produce when anterior and middle deltoid fibers combine in midrange?

Discussion. What advantage (if any) does scaption, the range midway between shoulder flexion and abduction, gain? How can noninvasive methods, such as manual muscle testing and goniometry, assist in determining the amount of muscle force available for daily activities?

■ APPLICATION **7-4**
Loads on Upper-Extremity Joints

Keyboarding with an unsupported upper extremity may cause shoulder, elbow, and wrist fatigue. Although these joint positions do not seem extreme or awkward, gravity's pull on the forearm creates torques at each joint. *Nancy Grant,* an OT student working in a computer lab, weighs 50 kg. Determine the amount of torque gravity creates at her shoulder, elbow, and wrist joints (see Appendix B):

1. The upper extremity contains 4.8% of total body weight.
2. The forearm and hand contain 2.1% of total body weight.
3. The hand contains 0.6% of total body weight.
4. The moment arm for the combined center of gravity extending Nancy's shoulder is 7.7 cm.
5. The moment arm for the combined forearm and hand center of gravity extending Nancy's elbow is 6.8 cm.
6. The moment arm for the hand flexing the wrist is 2.3 cm.

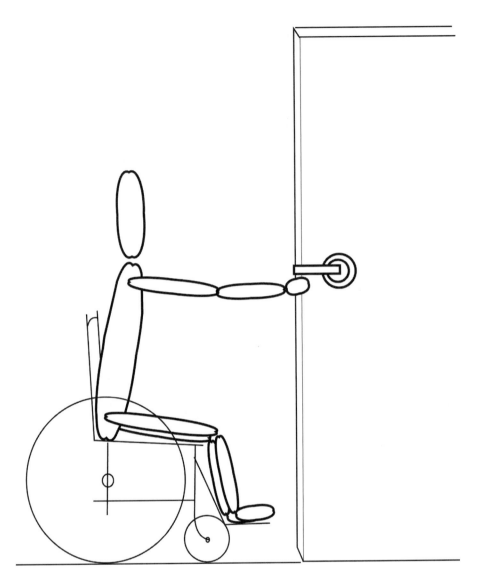

FIGURE **7-16**
The anterior deltoid muscle measures fair strength at 90 degrees of shoulder flexion.

Discussion. Interpret the requirements of the shoulder, elbow, and wrist joints in response to the tendencies created by gravity. How can the load on the muscles be reduced?

See Appendix C for solutions to Applications.

REFERENCES

1. Basmajian JV, DeLuca CJ: *Muscles alive: their functions revealed by electromyography,* ed 5, Baltimore, 1985, Williams & Wilkins.
2. Bohannon RW, Andrews AW: Shoulder subluxation and pain in stroke patients, *Am J Occup Ther* 44(6):507-509, 1990.
3. Chaco J, Wolf E: Subluxation of the glenohumeral joint in hemiplegia, *Am J Phys Med* 50:139-143, 1971.
4. Donatelli RA: *Physical therapy of the shoulder,* ed 4, St Louis, 2004, Churchill Livingstone.
5. Faghri PD, Rodgers MM, Glaser RM, et al: The effects of functional electrical stimulation on shoulder subluxation, arm function recovery, and shoulder pain in hemiplegic stroke patients, *Arch Phys Med Rehabil* 75(1):73-79, 1994.
6. Steindler A: *Kinesiology of the human body,* Springfield, Ill, 1973, Charles C Thomas.
7. Zorowitz RD, Hughes MB, Idank D, et al: Shoulder pain and subluxation after stroke: correlation or coincidence? *Am J Occup Ther* 50(3):194-201, 1996.

RELATED READINGS

Hall SJ: *Basic biomechanics,* New York, 1995, McGraw-Hill.
Nordin M, Frankel VH: *Basic biomechanics of the musculoskeletal system,* ed 3, Philadelphia, 2001, Lippincott Williams & Wilkins.
Williams PL, Bannister LH: *Gray's anatomy: the anatomical basis of medicine and surgery,* ed 38, New York, 1995, Churchill Livingstone.

LAB BOX

Find applied activities exploring concepts in Chapter 7 in the following laboratory exercises:

Topic	Laboratory
MMT and goniometry principles for shoulder, elbow and forearm	**Lab 3** Overview of ROM & MMT Additional Lab: MMT to Determine Neurological Level in SCI Motion CD
Differential effects of carrying a handbag closer versus farther away from the elbow	**Lab 4** Accessory Joint Motions/Muscle Excursion/Active & Passive Insufficiency/Max Assist Transfers
Effects of gravity on various upper extremity joints	
Movements of upper extremity associated with trunk movements	**Lab 6** Head, Neck, and Trunk: Curves, Movements, Measurements, Muscles
Articulations, scapula movement associated with upper extremity use, muscles affecting the scapula and humerus, scapulohumeral rhythm, differential functions of glenohumeral abductors, drawing muscle function	**Labs 7 & 8** Shoulder Complex: Scapular Movement, Differential Functions of Scapular and Glenohumeral Muscles, Differential Functions of Supraspinatus and Deltoid in GH Abduction
ROM and MMT of shoulder, torque range of motion of elbow (elbow flexion contracture)	**Lab 9** MMT & ROM of Shoulder; Elbow & Forearm: Torque Range of Motion

8

The Distal Upper Extremity

K E Y **TERMS**

Flexor Retinaculum
Carpal Tunnel Syndrome
Circumduction
Transverse Arch
Longitudinal Arch
Tenodesis Release
Tenodesis Grasp
Intrinsic Minus Hand

hapter 7 focused on the importance of the shoulder, elbow, and forearm by considering their many articulations, muscles, and movements. While these proximal upper-extremity segments provide reach and partial positioning, the wrist provides fine adjustments for placement and the hand grasps and manipulates to complete a task.

The same hand that breaks boards and cinder blocks in martial arts provides perfect intonation on a violin neck or manipulates a needle in microsurgery. The 15 joints in the thumb and fingers along with the transverse and longitudinal arches of the hand allow positioning that adapts to almost any shape. A multitude of muscles, each with its own discrete neural control, allows performance of a range of tasks, from a power grip for holding a hammer to delicate pressure for picking up an egg. We position our thumb pad opposite the pads of the other fingers precisely enough to grasp a single human hair. That same opposition movement locks the entire thumb around a rope tightly enough to support the body's weight.

The Wrist

Much more than a connection of the hand to the arm, the wrist positions the hand so that the long finger flexors and extensors can grasp and release objects. Although they do not attach to the fingers, synergistic actions of the wrist extensors and flexors working with finger flexors and extensors position the long finger muscles in an optimal length–tension range for forceful, effective prehension. More directly, combinations of wrist muscles act as agonists powering forceful wrist deviation for functions such as hammering and throwing.

Eight carpal bones, the distal radius, and the ulnar disk comprise the wrist. Framed proximally by the distal radius and ulnar disk, these bones articulate in a semicircular arrangement around the central capitate bone. Various ligamentous attachments arrange the carpal bones into an arch, the concave surface of which lies at the base of the palm. Its convex surface forms the back of the base of the hand. This osteofibrous structure, which provides a strong and stable attachment for muscles, provides a structural foundation for the palm's complex contours.

On the palmar surface the hook of the hamate and pisiform bone on the ulnar side connect through the **flexor retinaculum** (transverse carpal ligament) to the more radially placed scaphoid and trapezium. The concave shape

of the combined carpal bones and the fibrous roof provided by the flexor retinaculum make a carpal tunnel. This structure contains a large number of important neurovascular and tendinous structures that pass through to the hand. Because of such close quarters, swelling from inflammation accompanying compression of these structures results in **carpal tunnel syndrome** (A Closer Look Box 8-1).

ARTICULATIONS

The wrist is classified as a condyloid joint, allowing motion in two planes. Flexion and extension occur in the sagittal plane around a double side-to-side axis. These movements involve two separate pairs of articulations—the radius and ulnar disk with the proximal row of carpals and the proximal with the distal row of carpals[9] (Figure 8-1 and A Closer Look Boxes 8-2 and 8-3).

Abduction and adduction occur in the frontal plane around the anterior-to-posterior axis found in the capitate bone. Frequently, we call wrist abduction *radial deviation* and wrist adduction *ulnar deviation*. **Circumduction** describes a combination of movements. From a neutral position the wrist moves into extension, then in sequence into radial deviation, flexion, and ulnar deviation before it moves back into extension. Because circumduction involves more than one movement, it involves more than one axis, unlike true rotation in the forearm and arm. When we use paintbrushes and markers to draw circles, we demonstrate everyday examples of circumduction in action.

MUSCLES

Muscles named for their functions at the wrist contain the word *carpi* in their names and originate on or near the distal end of the humerus in association with the humeral epicondyles. The large area of muscle mass in the forearm produces force that the tendons transmit to stabilize the wrist and move the hand. Each muscle crossing the wrist functions at the wrist, even when named for a movement it produces in the hand (finger flexion and extension).

Muscle function depends on a muscle's relationship to the axes of motion, not its name. Tendons passing anterior to the wrist's side-to-side axis flex the wrist. They include flexors carpi radialis (FCR) and ulnaris (FCU) as well as the finger flexors digitorum superficialis and profundus.

BOX 8-1

A **CLOSER** LOOK

Carpal Tunnel Syndrome

Wendy Dabdoub noticed tingling (paresthesia) in her thumb, her index and middle fingers, and occasionally in her ring finger (median nerve distribution). (Like many people with peripheral neuropathy, she generalized the sensory symptoms to occur "in the hand" or generally on the "thumb side of the hand" even though with discrete testing only her thumb, index, middle, and half of the ring finger palmar surfaces yielded symptoms.) She associated this discomfort with her job. Wendy packs fruit for shipment, a job that involves repetitive, simultaneous wrist and finger flexion against resistance; others with similar duties echo her complaint. Holding positions for too long, grasping and releasing too frequently against resistance, or holding extreme or awkward wrist positions commonly lead to carpal tunnel syndrome.

Carpal tunnel syndrome has a variety of causes including medical conditions associated with tissue swelling and orthopedic problems. (The careful and definitive diagnosis of carpal tunnel syndrome often involves a team where a physician or surgeon relies on measurements made by a hand therapist. Additionally, although not always performed when carpal tunnel syndrome is suspected, a careful medical history can reveal concomitant medical problems more responsible for this disorder than what might appear obvious.[1]) Linda Valdez, who has rheumatoid arthritis, risks developing carpal tunnel syndrome, as does Henry Isaacs, who fractured his wrist in a fall at his skilled care facility. Although some risks seem obvious, careful determination of the cause of Wendy's condition remains elusive without a closer look at her workplace.

In Wendy's case the problem stems both from direct pressure on her median nerve and from overuse of the tendons of the flexor digitorum superficialis and profundus. Finger flexion in a position of wrist flexion puts direct pressure on the median nerve between the flexor retinaculum and the flexor tendons. As wrist and finger flexors activate in this awkward grasping function, the tendons squeeze the median nerve against the tight flexor retinaculum, and wrist trauma results. (See Closer Look Box Animation 8-1.)

Repeated finger flexion and extension with a flexed wrist forces Wendy's finger flexor tendons to travel back and forth on the edge of the flexor retinaculum. This friction inflames the tendons (tendonitis) and their sheaths (tenosynovitis), causing swelling in the wrist.

The carpal tunnel is a closed passage top to bottom and side to side and transmits a tight neurovascular bundle with little room to spare. Swollen tissues take up more room, squeezing the tunnel's contents. The cramped space puts direct pressure on Wendy's median nerve, decreasing its blood supply (ischemia). She first noticed the "pins-and-needles" sensation (paresthesia) on the radial half of her hand, the area of skin supplied by cutaneous branches of the median nerve. If continued, pressure could cause nerve damage affecting both the cutaneous and motor fibers of her median nerve. Malfunction of motor fibers or altered sensory feedback could lead to weakened grasp, a secondary symptom. Prolonged, poorly managed carpal tunnel syndrome can cause atrophy of the hand's thenar muscles.

Wendy and her employer took the most reasonable and responsible treatment course, reducing the damaging influence (overuse) by instituting "stretch breaks." Cutting the flexor retinaculum (carpal tunnel release surgery), to cure overuse, creates more room in the passage but destroys a normal anatomical structure and ignores the real cause of the problem. Returning to the harmful practices responsible for tendonitis and swelling easily leads to recurrence even following surgery. Job-site analysis and appropriate recommendations generated a more lasting solution.

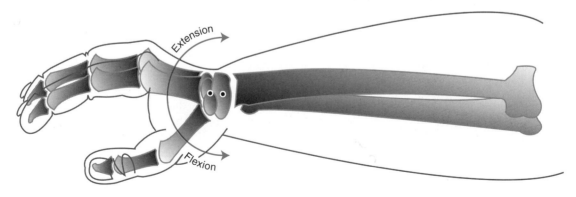

FIGURE **8-1**
Wrist flexion and extension occur at more than one side-to-side axis because of the complexity of the wrist articulation.

Tendons passing posterior to the side-to-side axis, traversing one of the dorsal compartments, extend the wrist and include the extensors carpi radialis longus (ECRL) and brevis (ECRB), extensor carpi ulnaris (ECU), and (finger) extensors digitorum, indicis, and digiti minimi. (See A Closer Look Box 8-4 for an elaboration of the dorsal compartments.) Although numerous digital muscles listed here do affect the wrist, this section concentrates first on muscles named for their wrist functions.

Pure wrist motions like flexion occur only with activation of paired wrist muscles. Just as bilateral contraction of the erector spinae cancels lateral flexion and produces vertebral extension, activation of both wrist flexors cancels radial and ulnar deviation and produces balanced flexion (Figure 8-2). Similarly, the radial and ulnar wrist extensors drive balanced wrist extension. Use of one, for example, the extensor carpi ulnaris, produces combined extension and ulnar deviation because the ulnaris, like the other wrist muscles, functions across two axes. Table 8-1 summarizes the functions of the wrist muscles with respect to their relationships to the two axes of motion. Loss of any one wrist muscle results in severe but predictable wrist imbalance.

Eduardo Ybarra cut his arm with a saw while making his son a rocking horse. The accident damaged his radial nerve near the elbow, and his extensor carpi ulnaris ceased to function. The OT practitioner expected to see weakness in wrist extension because Eduardo had one less muscle available. True to this expectation, when Eduardo extended his wrist, only his radial wrist extensors functioned, resulting in weakened wrist extension. In addition, unwanted radial deviation accompanied extension because the extensor carpi ulnaris could not cancel the deviation effect.

Eduardo's biggest problem, unbalanced, severely weakened ulnar deviation, originates from the loss of his extensor carpi ulnaris. Without this muscle, Eduardo's attempts at ulnar deviation result in flexion and ulnar deviation by the flexor carpi ulnaris. (The muscle's name—flexor carpi ulnaris, or flexor of carpus [wrist] on the ulnar side—describes its combined function in the absence of its partner.) Furthermore, Eduardo has only minimal ulnar deviation because the extensor carpi ulnaris supplies a stronger force in ulnar deviation. How can Eduardo lose one ulnar extensor and experience this great deficit in ulnar deviation?

Paul Brand, a renowned hand surgeon, together with colleague Anne Hollister demonstrated the true functions of wrist muscles.[4] Their work shows that many wrist muscles are named for functions quite different than those they actually perform.

Figure 8-3 provides Brand and Hollister's summary[4] of muscle function at the wrist based on moment arms for the various movements. The graph indicates the length of each wrist muscle's moment arm for flexion–extension and ulnar–radial deviation. Muscles with the longest moment arms for ulnar or radial deviation lie at the extreme positions of the x axis. The longest moment arms for flexion or extension stand at the

BOX 8-2

A **CLOSER** LOOK

Wrist Motions, Ligaments, and Problems—A Land of Acronyms

The wrist gains its stability from numerous ligaments including the scapho-lunate (S-L) and luno-triquetral (L-T) ligaments. These two primary ligaments stabilize the scaphoid, lunate, and triquetrum through the ranges of flexion and extension. Notice their names derive from their attachments, the more radial attachment named first in each case.

Wrist extension derives 50% from radiocarpal joint motion and 35% from midcarpal motion. Slight supination and radial deviation accompany extension. The separate contributions reverse in wrist flexion, with 35% radiocarpal and 50% midcarpal contributions. Slight ulnar deviation and supination accompany flexion.

Instability of the wrist results from thinning (attenuation) or rupture of either the L-T or the S-L ligament. Volar intercalated segment instability (VISI) occurs with L-T ligament damage, and frequently occurs with a fall. In this pattern the scaphoid and lunate flex during wrist flexion (S-L ligament intact) but the triquetrum extends due to the impaired L-T ligament. Use the mnemonic VISILTOUT, VISI instability pattern with the LT ligament OUT, to remember this condition.

Dorsal intercalated segment instability (DISI), the most common instability pattern for the wrist, involves rupture or attenuation of the S-L ligament. Opposite of the VISI pattern, wrist extension involves lunate and triquetrum extension, but scaphoid flexion. Remember DISISLOUT: DISI pattern with the SL ligament OUT.

BOX 8-3

A **CLOSER** LOOK

The Ulnar Side of the Wrist—Anatomy and Clinical Considerations
A triangular fibrocartilage complex (TFCC) supports the ulnar aspect of the wrist, in place of a synovial articulation between the triquetrum and the ulna. This complex ligamentous arrangement involves connections between the triquetrum, lunate, extensor carpi ulnaris, and the ulna itself to stabilize the ulnar wrist. The following structures comprise the TFCC:
Ligaments:
- Ulno-triquetral (UT) ligament
- Ulno-lunate (UL) ligament
- ECU and its tendinous sheath
- Proximal radio-ulnar ligament (PRUL)
- Distal radio-ulnar ligament (DRUL)
Cartilage:
- Articular disk
Bones:
- Triquetrum
- Lunate
- Distal ulna

The TFCC provides a shock absorber to the distal ulna. While the radius articulates directly with the scaphoid and lunate, the ulnar articulations with the triquetrum and lunate are less direct and involve more play via the TFCC. A firm ulnar attachment would severely restrict pronation and supination. The table below shows the dynamic nature of the TFCC and ulnar disk and the shock absorption properties yielded depending on position.

Shortening/Lengthening of Disk as a Function of Position	*Shock Absorption, % of Load Bearing*
Pronation: 2 mm of space available (disk is close-packed; ulna is in closest proximity to the triquetrum)	40 to 60 %
Neutral: 2 to 4 mm of space available	18 to 20%
Supination: 4 to 6 mm of space available (disk is loose-packed; ulna is furthest from triquetrum)	4 to 8%

BOX 8-4

A **CLOSER** LOOK

Know Your Compartments!
Multiple finger and wrist extensors travel through specific connective tissue bands in the dorsal wrist. Various injuries and surgeries refer to these compartments. Remember the six compartments and tendinous constituents of the dorsal wrist with the following numerical mnemonic by starting on the radial side and moving ulnarly: 221211. This identifies the number of tendons traveling through each compartment.
- APL/EPB (2)
- ECRL/ECRB (2)
- EPL (1)
- EDC/EIP (2)
- EDQ (1)
- ECU (1)

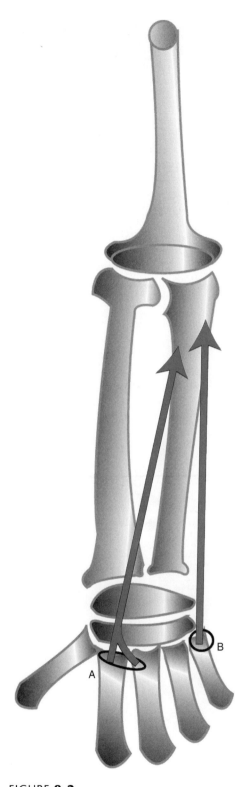

extreme positions of the y axis. The farther each muscle lies from the intersection, the greater its tendency to perform that function. (For a working exercise exploring Brand and Hollister's moment arm graph, refer to the Interactive Excercise animated Figure 8-3 on the CD and Evolve site).

The graph clarifies that each named wrist muscle produces two movements. Originally, anatomists named each muscle for the strongest action they believed it produced. The flexors carpi radialis and ulnaris function primarily as their names suggest, and as their longer moment arms for flexion rather than deviation indicate. The same holds true for the extensor carpi radialis brevis (ECRB).

The extensors carpi radialis longus and ulnaris fail to adhere to this naming scheme; each has a longer moment arm for deviation than for extension. In fact, the ulnaris has a moment arm for ulnar deviation more than four times its moment arm for extension. (Brand[5] suggests that a more appropriate name, such as *adductor carpi dorsalis,* would emphasize deviation instead of extension.) This graphic summary of each muscle's effect on the wrist explains why Eduardo's loss of the extensor carpi ulnaris creates a greater deficit in ulnar deviation than in extension.

BALANCE AFTER TENDON TRANSFER

Surgeons use Brand and Hollister's findings[4] to make decisions about the transfer of function from innervated to noninnervated muscles.

In Eduardo's case, a second injury resulted in the loss of all wrist extensor function. His surgeon suggested that Eduardo's pronator teres might replace his lost wrist extension. Eduardo's surgeon detached the pronator at its insertion, split it, and reinserted one side onto the distal ECRB tendon and the other onto the ulnar side of the fourth metacarpal.

A procedure like this involves extensive planning and a keen eye toward mechanics. Surgeons historically reinserted the pronator teres only onto the extensor carpi radialis brevis tendon distally because this tendon has a shorter moment arm for radial deviation than the extensor carpi radialis longus (ECRL). Brand and Hollister[4] note that the brevis, although less of a radial deviator than the longus, still has a substantial moment arm for deviation (see Figure 8-3). If the pronator attaches only to the ECRB insertion, wrist extension produces unwanted radial deviation, creating wrist imbalance.

Eduardo's surgeon followed one of Brand and Hollister's two suggestions[4] for balanced wrist extension. The ulnar insertion on the fourth metacarpal provides an ulnar deviation moment arm nearly equal to the radial deviation moment arm of the ECRB.

FIGURE 8-2
Activation of *both* the FCR (flexor carpi radialis) and the FCU (flexor carpi ulnaris) results in balanced wrist flexion. Activation of either alone produces partial wrist flexion with unwanted deviation in one direction or the other.

TABLE 8-1

Wrist Muscle Function Based on Relationships

MUSCLES	RELATIONSHIP TO AXIS	FUNCTION
FCU & FCR	Anterior to side-to-side axis	Balanced wrist flexion
ECRL, ECRB, & ECU	Posterior to side-to-side axis	Balanced wrist extension
FCU & ECU	Ulnar side of front-to-back axis	Balanced ulnar deviation
ECRL, ECRB, & FCR	Radial side of front-to-back axis	Balanced radial deviation
FCU	Anterior to side-to-side axis; ulnar to front-to-back axis	Wrist flexion with ulnar deviation; no pure movement possible
ECU	Posterior to side-to-side axis; ulnar to front-to-back axis	Wrist extension with ulnar deviation; no pure movement possible
ECRL & ECRB	Posterior to side-to-side axis; radial to front-to-back axis	Wrist extension with radial deviation; no pure movement possible
FCR	Anterior to side-to-side axis; radial to front-to-back axis	Wrist flexion with radial deviation; no pure movement possible

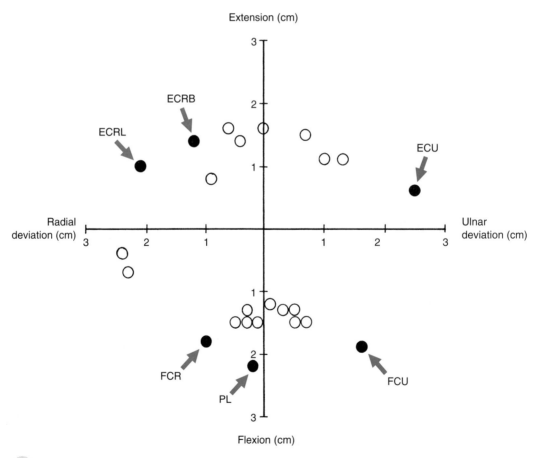

FIGURE **8-3**

Moment arms for the various wrist muscles (extensors and flexors) producing wrist flexion, extension, and deviation. *ECRB,* Extensor carpi radialis brevis; *ECRL,* extensor carpi radialis longus; *ECU,* extensor carpi ulnaris; *FCR,* flexor carpi radialis; *FCU,* flexor carpi ulnaris; *PL,* pollicis longus. (Modified from Brand PW, Hollister A: *Clinical mechanics of the hand,* ed 2, St Louis, 1993, Mosby.)

The two attachments cancel each others' deviation effects. Because both new insertions share the original extension moment arm of the ECRB, contraction of the pronator teres produces balanced wrist extension. Thus Eduardo regains balanced wrist extension through transfer of the pronator teres and now pronates relying more heavily on the pronator quadratus and brachiora-dialis (from a supinated position).

The Hand

The hand is composed of 19 bones (27, including the carpal bones); 18 intrinsic muscles, beginning and ending in the hand, share attachments to various sites on these bones with 18 tendons of extrinsic muscles. The extrinsic tendons transmit forces from the long finger flexor and extensors and the long thumb abductor, whose muscle bellies make up the fleshy part of the forearm. The majority of hand muscles cross two or more joints, and most extrinsic muscle tendons function across four joints, including the wrist.

Balance at the wrist through paired muscle contractions seems a simple feat compared to the balancing act between the long flexors and extensors and the intrinsic muscles. Truly, for all of their strength, the long flexors and extensors can do little without the refining moderation provided by the intrinsics.

Fingers conform to a wide variety of shapes, flexing to grasp objects and hold them against the resistance created by their weight. Muscles, especially extrinsic muscles, give and take in function. One relaxes, yielding in passive distal excursion as its antagonist contracts to produce movement through proximal excursion. In both grasp and release, the intrinsic muscles balance the effects of long flexors and extensors.

ARCHES

We tend to imagine the hand in action, grasping, opening with a cupped palm, or finely manipulating small objects; but even a relaxed hand yields valuable information about its structure. Splint fabrication that ignores the shape of the relaxed hand creates more difficulties for the wearer than the problem that originated a referral!

Hands have many creases, shadows, and curves (Figure 8-4) but no flat places. Two arches, oriented 90 degrees to each other, furnish the overall curved effect. The **transverse arch** curves from the radial to the ulnar side of the hand. Its apex, or highest point, lies near the head of the third metacarpal (Figure 8-5, *A*). The **longitudinal arch** curves from the wrist to the fingertips (Figure 8-5, *B*) with its highest point at the row of

metacarpal heads (2 through 5). Different lengths of the metacarpals and the corresponding metacarpophalangeal (MCP) joints result in lengthening of the arch at metacarpal number 3 and shortening at number 5. Failure to appreciate the short length of the longitudinal arch on the ulnar side of the hand results in splints that extend too far distally and block flexion of MCP joints 4 and 5.

Both arches change shape as the hand moves to manipulate objects, but its relaxed state provides the key to understanding hand structure. The radial and ulnar ends of the hand (metacarpals 1, 4, and 5) experience greater mobility than ligament-bound metacarpal heads 2 and 3 with the greatest freedom occurring in the thumb. Cup your hand or manually wiggle the fifth metacarpal head in alternating anterior and posterior directions to demonstrate the ulnar side's mobility. Regardless of mobility, hands do not relax into a boneless mass but instead relax into their arches. Forcing the hand into a flattened position with a splint damages the hand. Successful focus on any specific hand problem avoids disturbing the basic architecture of these normal arches.

ARTICULATIONS

The hand gets its freedom of movement from the serial arrangement of finger joints and nearly parallel arrangement of fingers. Metacarpals 1 through 5 articulate with the proximal phalanges of each finger at the condyloid MCP joints. These joints allow flexion and extension as well as abduction and adduction in digits 2 through 5. Because of the joint shape and arrangement of ligaments, full flexion of the MCP joints involves maximal stretch of the ligaments and limits abduction and adduction (Figure 8-6 and A Closer Look Box 8-5).

Individual phalanges articulate at the interphalangeal (IP) hinge joints. The thumb has one IP joint, but digits 2 through 5 exhibit proximal interphalangeal (PIP) joints between proximal and middle phalanges and distal interphalangeal (DIP) joints between middle and distal phalanges. These joints allow only flexion and extension, one less plane of movement than the MCP joints, but both proximal and distal IPs remain essential for finger-to-palm grasp. IP joints alone allow grasp between the digital pads and the distal palm. Working with both types of joints permits a whole-hand grasp that ranges in diameter from smaller than a broomstick straw to larger than a soda can. Normally the MCP and IP joints flex and extend together, but muscle imbalance caused by disease or injury can produce isolated and incongruous movement of MCP to IP joints.

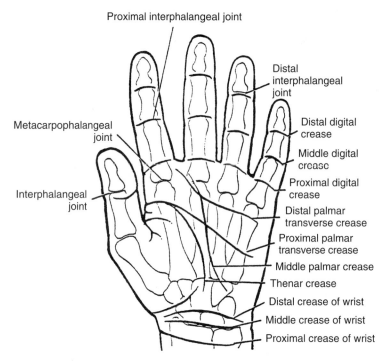

FIGURE **8-4**
Palmar skin creases relate to underlying wrist and digital joints. Metacarpophalangeal joints lie at the level of the distal palmar crease. (From Fess EE, Phillips CA: *Hand splinting principles and method,* ed 2, St Louis, 1987, Mosby.)

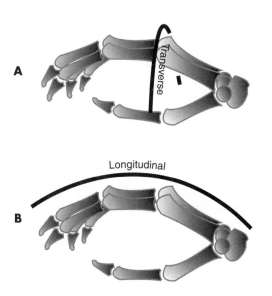

FIGURE **8-5**
The transverse **(A)** and longitudinal **(B)** arches.

The Thumb

The thumb acts like an extra index finger, one rotated nearly 90 degrees and attached directly to the wrist at a 30-degree angle from the palm (instead of in the same plane). Thumb joints differ from their counterparts in the other digits. The lone IP joint of the thumb, a hinge like all other IP joints, works with the MCP joint, a condyloid joint in appearance but an IP joint in function. Together the IP and MCP joints allow only flexion and extension of the distal and proximal phalanges.

The first metacarpal moves freely at the carpometacarpal (CMC) joint, found at the very base of the thumb. The CMC joint functions like a freer version of the MCP joints in the other digits. This saddle-shaped joint deserves special consideration because of its articulation with the distal surface of the trapezium bone. The proximal surface of the first metacarpal conforms to the saddle-like trapezium just as a person riding a horse conforms to its saddle. The thumb's CMC joint, not its MCP joint, can perform flexion–extension as well as abduction–adduction, allowing the less mobile MCP and IP joints to perform flexion and extension in many different positions in relation to the palm. Its proximal location and additional freedom of movement provide

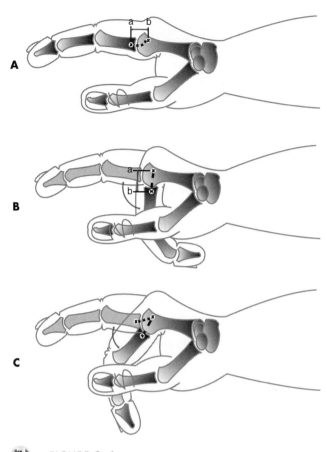

See
the
CD

FIGURE **8-6**

A, Points *a* and *b* lie close together in the extended position, resulting in a slack ligament. **B**, The points lie farther apart in metacarpophalangeal flexion, tightening the ligament. Immobilization in metacarpophalangeal extension allows the ligaments to shorten secondary to the inability of the joint to move and stretch daily. **C**, After immobilization, the tightening of the shortened ligament restricts metacarpophalangeal flexion as *a* and *b* become separated by the movement of the joint from extension to flexion. The index finger flexes more in **B** than in **C**, where tight ligaments limit flexion after improper immobilization in metacarpophalangeal extension.

BOX 8-5

A CLOSER LOOK

Tight Joint Positions

The close-packed joint position stretches ligaments tight, preventing further movement and compressing joint surfaces.[7] If the MCP and interphalangeal (IP) joints require immobilization (for example, after surgery or fracture), splinting uses the close-packed position— full MCP flexion and full IP extension. This position maximally stretches structures so that scar tissue assumes the length of the tissue in that position. Once the joint regains mobility, movement goes in the direction of tissue slack and scar tissue does not limit motion. Liken this to placing a Band-Aid on your elbow. Placing the Band-Aid lengthwise covering the olecranon in an elbow-extended position— a position with slack dorsal skin—results in tightness and limited motion into elbow flexion. Placing the same Band-Aid in a position of elbow flexion—with the skin stretched to the maximum amount by the position—allows both elbow flexion and extension into full range. The Band-Aid placed in a position of joint tension (flexion) means any movement out of this position goes toward greater slack. In this analogy, the Band-Aid represents the scar tissue.

Immobilization of the MCP in extension allows scar tissue to bridge the joint, connecting opposite sides in the slack position (see Figure 8-6). As the MCP flexes, adjacent points on opposite sides of the joint separate as usual because of the shape of the metacarpal head. However, because of scarring and shortening, tissue stretch reaches its limit early in the movement and passive insufficiency of the scar tissue prevents good functional range into MCP flexion (extension contracture). However, individuals with palmar burns often form skin contractures with the hand splinted in MCP flexion. Practitioners must weigh the greater likelihood of skin flexion contracture against that of joint extension contracture to determine appropriate intervention for the best functional outcome.

opposition, the ability to touch the thumb pad to the pads of the other fingers.

Because of the difference in orientation of the axes of motion, flexion–extension and abduction–adduction of the thumb occur in different planes than those of digits 2 through 5. Instead of a side-to-side axis for flexion and extension, the thumb flexes and extends around an axis oriented front-to-back in relation to the palmar and dorsal surfaces of the hand (A Closer Look Box 8-6). Thumb abduction–adduction revolves around

a side-to-side more than a front-to-back axis. Because of these different orientations, thumb movements differ from movements of the same names in the fingers (A Closer Look Box 8-7).

A complete discussion of thumb articulations must examine opposition, touching the palmar surface of the thumb to that of the other digits. Opposition involves movement of the thumb from the palm, around and

BOX 8-6

ACLOSERLOOK

Directional Terms

As anatomy and kinesiology students, we learn new directional terms for the body. Synonyms such as ventral for "anterior" and dorsal for "posterior" abound in descriptions of the hand and forearm. Some abandon the original terms because words like anterior and posterior lose their clarity as the hand moves around the body. The flexor tendons lie anterior to the MCP joints when the palm faces forward but posterior to these same joints in a rear-facing palm. Using "palmar" instead of "anterior," the flexor tendons always rest on the palmar side of the joints regardless of the hand's position in space. The following terms describe the forearm and hand. Learn all these synonyms because the ideal descriptive term differs with each situation.

Original Term	*Synonym*
Anterior	Palmar, volar, ventral
Posterior	Dorsal
Medial	Ulnar
Lateral	Radial
Adduction (wrist)	Ulnar deviation
Abduction (wrist)	Radial deviation
Manual digital rotation (digits 2 through 5) at the MCP (turning the palmar surface toward the thumb)	Supination of digit
Manual digital rotation at the MCP (turning the palmar surface from the thumb)	Pronation of digit

BOX 8-7

ACLOSERLOOK

Thumb Movements

Thumb movements differ from movements with the same names in digits 2 through 5 because of the thumb's different orientation on the hand. While flexion of digits 2 through 5 sweeps through the sagittal plane, thumb flexion occurs more in the frontal plane. Thumb abduction (entirely at the CMC joint) sweeps out in the same plane as flexion–extension of digits 2 through 5. We can gain more understanding of this phenomenon from kinesthetic learning than from looking at figures. (See Closer Look Box Animations 8-2 and 8-3 for help with this.)

Supinate your forearm, and lay the hand palm up on a table. Extend the thumb by stretching it out from the palm and touch the table. Think of thumb flexion as sweeping the palm clean. Move the thumb toward the palm and then onto it so that continuation of this flexion movement sweeps across and stays in contact with the palm. Remember that the axis sticks out of the CMC joint with a palmar–dorsal orientation. The plane of the movement is the plane of the palm.

Abduct and adduct the thumb in a position of forearm midpronation–supination (neutral) so that you are looking at the hand from the radial side. You should see your thumbnail and the side of the index finger. Adduction, the beginning point of abduction, occurs here with the side of the thumb closest to the fingers in contact with the palm and proximal index finger.

Maintain this thumb orientation without losing sight of the thumbnail and move your thumb from the palm. Performed with the left hand, full thumb abduction yields the L shape. This motion should form an arc in a plane nearly perpendicular to the palmar plane. The axis sticks out from the base of the first metacarpal (the location of the CMC joint).

then over to another digit so that the pad of the thumb is opposite to the pad of the other digit.

Opposition combines movements rather than producing a pure movement like flexion. Opposition involves thumb abduction from the palm, thumb flexion in this abducted position, and the appearance of thumb rotation. Kapandji's illustrations[7] describe pure rotation on an axis through the thumb, but Brand and Hollister[4] use the term *circumduction* through a cone-shaped path with an apex at the CMC joint (Figure 8-7). They describe opposition as thumb pronation; supination returns the thumb to the beginning, unopposed position.[4]

Regardless of the reference cited, some kind of rotation looks obvious during opposition. Notice that before you begin the opposition movement, you can see digital creases and finger pads in digits 2 to 5, as well as on the side of the thumb. Fingernails of the thumb and fingers remain out of view. Now touch the thumb to the little finger and watch the thumbnail come plainly into view. Circumduction, or thumb pronation, turns the thumb around and changes your view from the thumb's front and side to its back. Most importantly, this movement occurs at the CMC joint; therefore problems and rehabilitation of opposition limitations must focus proximally at the CMC joint and not at the more distal MCP joint.

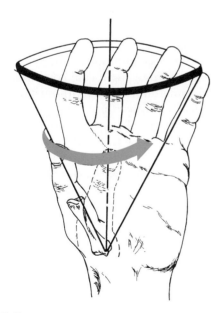

FIGURE **8-7**
Thumb movement occurs around a cone-shaped axis. (From Brand PW: *Clinical mechanics of the hand,* St Louis, 1985, Mosby.)

MUSCLES PRODUCING FINGER MOVEMENTS

Extrinsic Muscles

Important differences exist between the long flexor and extensor tendons. Anatomical differences, including cross section and tendon diameter derive from differences in function. The flexor tendons power various grips requiring varying degrees of strength and dexterity. Both the superficialis and the profundus act for strength. The profundus provides the force for any grip requiring distal interphalangeal flexion. The extensor tendons function primarily to open the hand, extending the fingers and flattening the transverse and longitudinal arches to efficiently release grasp of an object.

Because release of grasp requires less force, the extensor tendons generally exhibit three to four times less strength than flexor tendons. Six times thinner, injury occurs five times more commonly because of their less robust nature and the relative lack of dorsal subcutaneous skin coverage. Surgical repair of extensor tendon lacerations typically yields a result only 50% as strong as flexor tendon repairs. Injured extensor tendons need tendon graft replacements more frequently. (A Closer Look Box 8-8 contains the definitions of flexor and extensor tendon zones used for quick reference by surgeons and hand therapists when describing the locations and implications of specific tendon injuries.)

The tendons of the extrinsic flexors follow a path that includes a series of connective tissue pulleys serving two important functions (Figure 8-8). First, the natural tendency of the flexor tendons pulled tight across a semiflexed finger is to rise out of the concavity in the same way a bowstring pulled taut spans from one end of a bow to the other. This tendency of the flexor tendons to bowstring would obliterate the concavity of the palm during flexion unless constrained by the flexor pulleys. (This chapter explores the pathology of bowstringing later.)

Flexor pulleys also conserve excursion as another important function. Remember, a fundamental law of rotary motion dictates that points farther from the center of rotation (axis) of a segment move through a greater distance (Figure 8-9) as the joint progresses through its range of motion. The long flexor tendons attach at the distal end of each finger, far from more proximal joints such as the metacarpophalangeal and proximal interphalangeal. This results in potentially large amounts of excursion required to produce full range of motion. Paradoxically, full range at all three finger joints yields a surprisingly small amount of excursion. Upon close anatomical examination we find each flexor tendon travels through a pulley immediately after it crosses a joint. These pulleys act as anchors of the

BOX 8-8

A **CLOSER** LOOK

Know your Zones!

Flexor Tendon Zones

Zone I—The length traversed by the single FDP distal to the FDS insertion on either side of the middle phalanx.

Zone II—Traversed by the FDP and FDS tendons, from the level of the MCP joint (at the proximal edge of the A1 pulley) to the insertion of FDS (at the level of the A4 pulley). Considering the bifurcation of the FDS tendon and passage of the FDP tendon from underneath, zone II presents the most challenging area for hand surgeons to perform a tendon repair. Injury in this area presents greater risk of adhesion between the FDP and FDS tendons.

Zone III—The length of the FDS and FDP tendons from the distal edge of the transverse carpal ligament (flexor retinaculum) to the A1 pulley.

Zone IV—The area of the carpal tunnel—from the proximal to the distal edge of the transverse carpal ligament. Injury in this area presents greater risk of adhesion among the many structures traversing the carpal tunnel.

Zone V—The anterior compartment of the forearm—the area proximal to the transverse carpal ligament.

Extensor Tendon Zones

Zone I-II—Covers the area from the DIP joint to the middle phalanx. (Odd numbers for the extensor tendon zones lie at the joints.)

Zone III-IV—The PIP joint and the proximal phalanx. (This area includes the central slip and the lateral bands.)

Zone V-VI—Area of the MCP joint.

Zone VII—The extensor tendons at the dorsal wrist level (includes the six dorsal compartments).

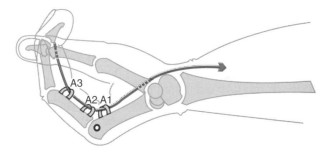

FIGURE **8-8**
Flexor tendons traverse a series of pulleys, three of which are shown in this figure. The pulleys maintain the concavity of the palm by preventing bowstringing of the flexor tendons. Pulleys also conserve muscle excursion.

tendons for function at a more proximal joint. Attachment close to the joint via the proximal edge of the pulley yields greater range of motion of multiple joints with relatively little excursion—a good thing considering the flexors digitorum superficialis and profundus have long tendons but short muscle fibers. (Figure 8-9 illustrates the different amounts of excursion necessary to move the same joint based on whether the tendon attaches closer to (via pulley) or farther away from the joint.)

Intrinsic Muscles—Interossei and Lumbricals

Just as the wrist muscles provide proximal stability and positioning during hand and finger use, intrinsic muscles of the hand render the long finger flexors and extensors effective in grasp and release. Despite their strength, the flexors digitorum profundus and superficialis, and the extensor digitorum communis produce severely abnormal movements without the balancing effect provided by intrinsic muscles.

The lumbricals typically surface first during hand dissections in the anatomy lab. Associated with MCP flexion through their origins on the flexor digitorum profundus tendon, they serve the opposite function distally owing to their insertions onto an expansion of the extensor digitorum tendon. (Observing their relationship to the axes they cross clarifies their complex functions.) Lumbricals travel anterior to the side-to-side axis for MCP flexion, producing flexion. Each lumbrical travels to the radial side of the digit and inserts onto the extensor digitorum communis tendon through an expansive arrangement of connective tissue called the *extensor expansion* (also called the *extensor* or *dorsal aponeurosis* or the *extensor* or *dorsal hood*). This connection posterior to the side-to-side axes allows the lumbricals to extend the IP joints.

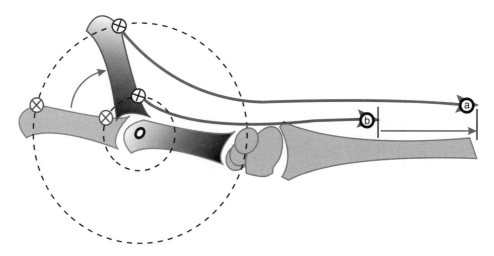

FIGURE **8-9**
Rotary motion dictates that proximal insertions move through less distance than distal insertions in the same segment movement. The greater the distance the insertion travels, the greater the muscle excursion necessary to move that insertion. Notice that tendon *a* exhibits more excursion than does *b*. Muscles functioning at more distal insertions require more excursion for movement unless the tendon passes through a pulley on the way to its insertion.

We think of the palmar and dorsal interossei primarily as finger abductors and adductors. Although these movements play a critical part in manipulation of objects, just as importantly the interossei act like the lumbricals to combine MCP flexion and IP extension.

The interossei originate on sides of the metacarpal shafts and partially insert onto the sides of the proximal phalanx of each finger. This course establishes a radial or ulnar relationship (depending on the finger) to the front-to-back axis at the MCP joint, where the interossei abduct or adduct. Each interosseus also inserts onto the extensor expansion, lending the interossei the same relationships to axes as the lumbricals and yielding the same functions, MCP flexion and IP extension.

The pennate fiber arrangement of the interossei and the two-to-one ratio of interossei to each finger result in greater strength than that of the lumbricals (Table 8-2).[6] The combined strength of the long finger flexors and intrinsics allows rock climbers to support their total body weight with only one or two fingers!

TABLE 8-2
Comparison of Interosseus and Lumbrical Cross Sections

DIGIT	INTEROSSEUS CROSS SECTION %*	LUMBRICAL CROSS SECTION %
Index finger	First dorsal = 3.2 First palmar = 1.3	First lumbrical = 0.2
Middle finger	Second dorsal = 2.5 Third dorsal = 2.0	Second lumbrical = 0.2
Ring finger	Second palmar = 1.2 Fourth dorsal = 1.7	Third lumbrical = 0.1
Little finger	Third palmar = 1.0 Abductor digiti minimi = 1.4	Fourth lumbrical = 0.1

(Modified from Brand PW, Beach RB, Thompson DE: Relative tension and potential excursion of muscles in the forearm and hand, *J Hand Surg* 6(3):209-219, 1981.)
*Values represent the percentage of total cross section (force capability) of all the muscles in the forearm and hand. Use them to compare one muscle with another. Notice that each interosseus has a higher percentage of force than each lumbrical and that each digit has two interossei and one lumbrical. The table includes the abductor digiti minimi because it serves as the "interosseus" for the fifth digit.

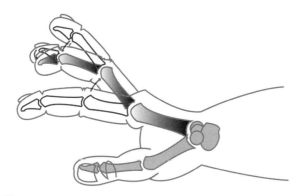

See the CD ▶ FIGURE **8-10**

Intrinsic minus hand consists of unchecked MCP extension by extensor digitorum and incomplete IP extension due to overextension of the MCP and subsequent tendon action of the long flexors on the IP joints.

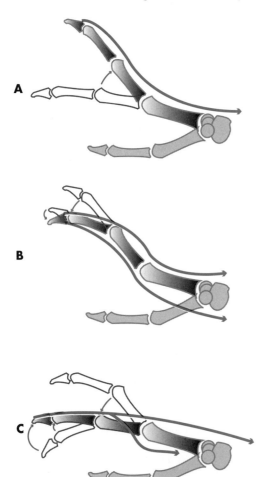

FIGURE **8-11**

Pull of the extensor digitorum alone (**A**) with simultaneous pull on the flexor digitorum profundus (**B**). Simultaneous pull of the extensor digitorum and the first dorsal interosseus and first lumbrical at their insertions onto the extensor expansion (**C**). In **C** the intrinsics correct the imbalance *without* the long flexors, which cannot correct intrinsic minus.

Although difficult to appreciate in a gross dissection (anatomy students often overlook the interossei in laboratory), the combined tension of the two interossei per finger provides the same amount of strength as a long finger flexor. The position of the interossei close to the axis of flexion–extension in the MCP joint limits their moment arm, but in no way diminishes their role in the total balance of hand function.

Two hand clinic clients demonstrate how the lumbricals and interossei work together. Yasmeen Harris, a 10-year-old girl, sustained serious injury to her right forearm after crashing through a storm door while playing tag. Surgeons reattached her tendons and median nerve, but the nerve did not fully regenerate. Zachary Larson, a 12-year-old boy, fractured his right elbow when he fell off a skateboard. Zachary crushed and stretched his ulnar nerve.

Yasmeen's median nerve damage paralyzed her first two lumbricals, releasing the long finger extensors from the balancing control of the lumbricals. While her ring and little fingers remained unaffected, Yasmeen's index and middle fingers exhibited MCP hyperextension and partial IP flexion. Unfortunately, children at school make fun of Yasmeen's "claw hand." Zachary's ulnar nerve damage paralyzed his interossei, causing a "clawing" appearance in all four fingers (2 through 5), with the greatest flexion in his ring and little fingers. With all four fingers involved, Zachary's nerve damage seems more extreme. Even Zachery's less involved index and middle fingers look more impaired than Yasmeen's.

Review the motor innervations of the interossei and lumbricals to appreciate the shared functions of the intrinsic muscles. The ulnar nerve supplies all the interossei and the lumbricals to the ring and little fingers. Ulnar nerve damage leaves the ring and little fingers with a total loss of intrinsic support and removes interossei force from the index and middle fingers, leaving only the lumbricals. Zachary's ring and little fingers have no intrinsic balance, while his index and middle fingers remain partially impaired. However, median nerve damage removes only the lumbricals to the index and middle fingers. Still supported by the interossei, Yasmeen's first two fingers display only mild impairment. Her ring and little fingers exhibit normal balanced function because they retain both interossei and lumbricals.

A fresh cadaveric dissection of the hand and forearm reveals the pure functions of isolated muscle contractions similar to those found in an **intrinsic minus hand** (Figure 8-10 and Movie 8-1). Pull on the extensor digitorum communis of the index finger and watch the IP joints extend and MCP joints hyperextend (Figure 8-11, *A*). Pull simultaneously on the flexor digitorum profundus in an attempt to correct MCP hyperextension with some flexion and see the characteristic claw created by MCP hyperextension and partial IP flexion (see Figure 8-11, *B*, and Movie 8-1). The long flexor has no effect on the MCP in this position and worsens the state of incomplete extension of the IP joints. Now pull instead on the first dorsal interosseus and first lumbrical at their insertions onto the extensor expansion to watch them immediately correct MCP hyperextension without causing IP joint flexion (see Figure 8-11, *C*).

This correcting influence of the lumbricals and interossei follows their definition as combined MCP flexors and IP extensors. A finger positioned in MCP hyperextension and partial IP flexion straightens to a pointing position (full extension) as soon as its lumbricals and interossei activate. Straightening requires MCP flexion (from hyperextension) and IP extension (from partial flexion). In other words, a straight finger occurs when the intrinsics' MCP flexion prevents MCP hyperextension by the extensor digitorum communis, correcting a claw before it occurs.

WRIST AND FINGER COORDINATION

The tendons of the long finger flexors and extensors originate in the forearm and cross the wrist to insert onto the fingers. Brand and Hollister[4] found that the finger muscles, through their long tendons, have overwhelming effects on the wrist (Figure 8-12). Many long finger flexors and extensors have moment arms for wrist flexion and extension as large as those of the wrist muscles themselves. A number of individual "slips" of the extensor digitorum communis can cause wrist deviation.

We must always remember that the finger muscles move both the fingers and the wrist unless the wrist has some form of stabilization. Moving two joints with one muscle has inherent problems because the individual excursion requirements of each joint movement can easily overcome the excursion capability of one muscle. Because the extensor digitorum communis (ED) extends the wrist, wrist stabilization via wrist flexors always accompanies ED activation. Otherwise the ED will run out of excursion at the wrist before completing finger extension. The same rule holds true of all finger muscles with moment arms at the wrist.

A look at Eduardo Ybarra's hand before surgery provides an example. Radial nerve damage paralyzed Eduardo's wrist and finger extensors, so he no longer can extend his wrist and fingers. Although the nerve damage had no direct effect on the finger flexors used in grasp (flexors are median and ulnar innervated), Eduardo experiences a severely weakened grasp. What causes Eduardo's grasp problems?

When Eduardo tries to grasp an object, his wrist flexes while his fingers encircle the object. He has so much wrist flexion that he cannot flex his fingers enough to close tightly around any object smaller than a tennis ball. Compare Eduardo's grasp pattern with your own to see

that wrist extension, not flexion, usually accompanies a forceful grasp. The tighter your grip, the more you extend the wrist, sometimes to 40 or 45 degrees (see Figure 8-13).

Active and Passive Insufficiency

Eduardo's difficulty with grasp exemplifies a common problem of multijoint muscles based on muscle excursion and its limitations. Every joint movement requires active muscle excursion, and muscles possess limited amounts of excursion. Because finger flexors cross multiple joints, without stabilization they flex each of those joints, including the wrist. Wrist flexion requires excursion, so when Eduardo's finger flexors contract to move his fingers, the excursion they use in unintentional wrist flexion gets subtracted, leaving a lesser amount available for finger flexion (Figure 8-13). Eduardo's grasping efforts result in incomplete finger flexion. The more Eduardo's unstabilized wrist flexes, the less excursion he has for his fingers.

In this way, active insufficiency (AI) occurs when a multijoint muscle acts at all its joints simultaneously. In addition to the long finger muscles, this concept applies to the biceps, triceps, quadriceps, and hamstrings (to name a few). (See Animations, Chapter 9, Biceps and Hamstrings Animations.) Determine the combination of joint movements leading to AI by identifying the muscle's function across each joint. For the biceps, AI occurs in combined shoulder and elbow flexion with forearm supination. In the finger flexors, simultaneous wrist and finger flexion exhaust the available excursion. Automatic motor programming to avoid AI consists of synergists stabilizing one or more joints in the chain to prevent movement, allowing the muscle to use its excursion at the targeted joint. In the wrist and hand, wrist extensors prevent wrist flexion by the long finger flexors, allowing them to use their entire excursion to flex the fingers.

"Insufficiency" also refers to inadequate strength capability. Strength capability encompasses the idea that tension (force) production relates to length. In passive stretch, an elastic fiber produces tension as its length increases. Active tissues like skeletal muscles create tension through shortening in concentric contraction. A muscle's length at the time of contraction affects its ability to produce force (Figure 8-14).

A muscle contracted across all its joints simultaneously attempts to produce force at its shortest length. The graph in Figure 8-14, *B* shows that shortened muscles produce less force. Therefore the combination of insufficient excursion and insufficient force produces active insufficiency.

Something else happens simultaneously on the other side of Eduardo's joints when his finger flexors encounter active insufficiency. On the extensor side, his

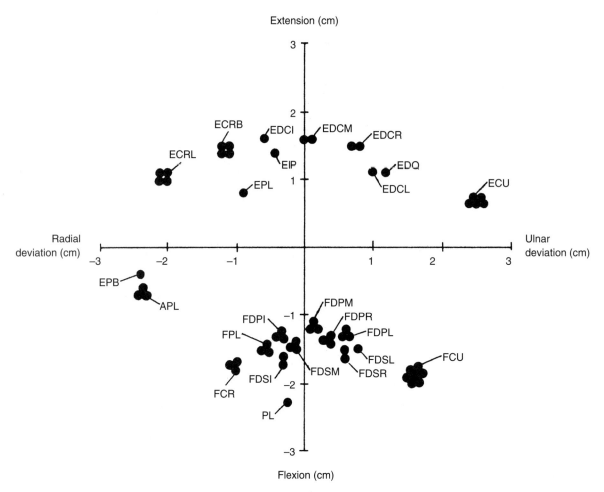

FIGURE **8-12**

This representational (not anatomical) diagram shows a simplified mechanical statement of the capability of each muscle to affect the wrist joint, whether or not its name designates function at the wrist. The positions of the tendons relative to the axes of flexion and extension and ulnar and radial deviation represent their moment arms at the wrist. The number of circles in a cluster indicates the tension capability of that muscle–tendon unit rounded to a whole number. *APL,* Abductor pollicis longus; *ECRB,* extensor carpi radialis brevis; *ECRL,* extensor carpi radialis longus; *ECU,* extensor carpi ulnaris; *EDCI,* extensor digitorum communis (index); *EDCL,* extensor digitorum communis (little); *EDCM,* extensor digitorum communis (middle); *EDCR,* extensor digitorum communis (ring); *EDQ,* extensor digiti quinti; *EIP,* extensor indicis proprius; *EPB,* extensor pollicis brevis; *EPL,* extensor pollicis longus; *FCR,* flexor carpi radialis; *FCU,* flexor carpi ulnaris; *FDPI,* flexor digitorum profundus (index); *FDPL,* flexor digitorum profundus (little); *FDPM,* flexor digitorum profundus (middle); *FDPR,* flexor digitorum profundus (ring); *FDSL,* flexor digitorum superficialis (little); *FDSI,* flexor digitorum superficialis (index); *FDSM,* flexor digitorum superficialis (middle); *FDSR,* flexor digitorum superficialis (ring); *FPL,* flexor pollicis longus; *PL,* palmaris longus. (From Brand PW, Hollister A: *Clinical mechanics of the hand,* ed 2, St Louis, 1993, Mosby.)

extensor digitorum communis experiences maximal stretch. Recall that movement resulting from concentric contraction of the agonists (finger flexors in this case) requires passive excursion of the antagonist (the extensor digitorum communis) stretched distally across the same joints. Unable to stretch across all its joints simultaneously, Eduardo's extensors experience passive insufficiency. Thus two mechanisms inhibit full finger flexion around an object—active insufficiency of the finger flexors and passive insufficiency of the finger extensors.

Understanding passive insufficiency can bring advantages to self-defense. An aggressor holds a weapon tightly with strong finger flexion and wrist extension. Grasping the aggressor's hand and forcing the wrist into flexion

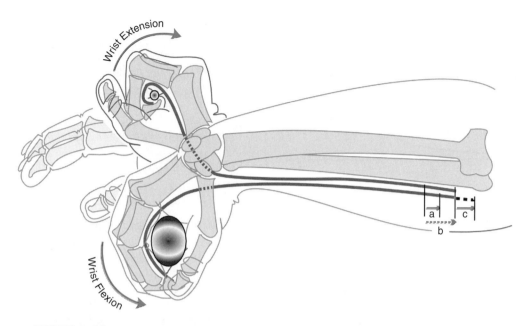

FIGURE **8-13**

The size of an object held in the hand differs greatly depending on the wrist position that accompanies grasp. Although not implied in their names, the finger flexors (FDP and FDS) have a flexion moment at the wrist. An unstabilized wrist results in wasting finger flexor excursion and leads to the hand's inability to grasp smaller diameter objects. Distance *a* represents the FDP excursion wasted in flexing the unstabilized wrist. The full excursion required for finger flexion (*b*) suffices for full finger flexion with the wrist extended but proves insufficient with wrist flexion. Additional excursion (*c*) would be required to fully flex the fingers with the wrist flexed.

maximally stretches the extensor digitorum communis. The tension created pulls the fingers into extension enough to reduce the force of the grip. Because the stretched extensor limits full wrist and finger flexion, the aggressor loses the grip on the weapon.

Tenodesis Grasp and Release

Passive insufficiency can have another advantage in tenodesis-type actions. The self-defense move previously mentioned forced wrist flexion to build passive tension in the extensor digitorum communis. This passive tension caused the fingers to extend slightly, reducing active flexion to grasp a handle. Consider the effect of passive tension on *relaxed* fingers. Active and passive wrist flexion stretches the finger extensors, producing enough tension (or tendon action) to pull the fingers into nearly full extension.

This wrist flexion and finger extension combination, called **tenodesis release**, occurs when the passive tension forces the fingers to extend and release an object. The name derives from tenodesis surgery, which shortens the long tendons of the fingers and attaches their proximal ends securely to bone. After surgery, the tendons reach passive insufficiency sooner in the movement. Tenodesis movements occur without surgery, but surgical shortening

increases efficiency because shorter tissues reach maximum stretch and build tension sooner than longer tissues. In tenodesis release, wrist flexion causes tension in the extensor digitorum communis. After surgery, less wrist flexion produces sufficient tension on the extensor to cause further finger extension.

Tenodesis grasp works on finger flexor tendons in the same way. Wrist extension stretches the flexor digitorum profundus, producing finger flexion. After a surgeon shortens the finger flexors and attaches them to bone, greater finger flexion accompanies the same amount of wrist extension, improving the grasp's efficiency.

Therefore tenodesis grasp and release occur without active contractions of the finger flexors and extensors. In each case, passive tension in the finger tendons, not active muscle contraction, causes the finger movement. (Go to the Evolve site to view a brief filmstrip showing tenodesis grasp and release in Movie 8-2.)

Bernice Richards calls her tenodesis grasp a "miracle grip." Because of her C5 quadriplegia, Bernice lost innervation to her finger flexors and extensors and wrist flexors and extensors. Shortly after she arrived in the spinal cord unit of the rehabilitation hospital, Bernice's OT practitioner noticed that she had a small amount of active wrist extension on the left side. This condition, known as "sparing," allows individuals with spinal

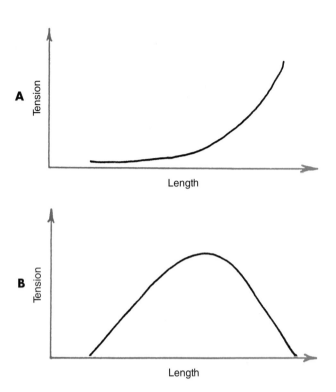

FIGURE 8-14

A, The general shape of the length–tension curve of a muscle under passive stretching. The muscle may require only a little tension to stretch near its resting length. The muscle requires more tension to stretch less as it nears its elastic limit. **B,** The general shape of active contraction of a muscle fiber. The muscle can produce its highest tension at its resting length. It produces less active tension if it contracts either at a shorter or more stretched beginning length. (From Brand PW, Hollister A: *Clinical mechanics of the hand,* ed 2, St Louis, 1993, Mosby.)

Basic Requirements for Tenodesis Grasp

Tenodesis provides a functional grasp in the absence of innervation to the actual grasping muscles (flexors digitorum superficialis and profundus). Often practitioners facilitate this through their understanding of biomechanics; however, they can also destroy its possibility for developing without a thorough understanding.

The basic requirements for tenodesis grasp:

1. Shortened finger flexors—As an alternative to surgical shortening a practitioner allows the long flexor tendons to decrease in length by extending the wrist only with the fingers flexed and flexing the wrist only with the fingers extended. This accomplishes maintaining joint movement while avoiding a passive insufficiency scenario (Movie 8-3). This second combination ensures shortening of the extensor digitorum for an effective tenodesis release.

2. Full wrist extension—the shortest finger flexors in the world will not provide grasp in the absence of wrist extension, needed to stretch the finger flexors. Maintaining wrist extension range of motion results from the above protocol.

3. Full finger flexion (MCP, PIP, and IP joints)—Providing full wrist extension to increase tension in finger flexor tendons in a hand with extension contractures of the MCP and IP joints yields a disappointing result. Using the protocol from requirement 1, maintain finger joint range of motion to provide the final requirement of successful tenodesis grasp.

---

cord injuries to perform isolated movements beyond the level of their lesion. Bernice took advantage of her spared innervation to develop sufficient strength to regain full active wrist extension.

Bernice's doctors originally thought she might need surgery to shorten her finger flexors enough to grasp effectively. OT staff members at the acute hospital where Bernice spent the days immediately after her accident understood how tenodesis grasp worked and were careful to move Bernice through the proper kind of passive range of motion (Movie 8-3).

These acute-care practitioners understood the importance of avoiding stretch in the finger tendons, allowing them to shorten over time after a cervical spinal cord injury. They took care to avoid stretching Bernice's long finger flexors while maintaining passive range of motion in her wrists. They passively extended Bernice's wrists and at the same time passively flexed her fingers. OT staff members only brought Bernice's fingers into full extension with her wrist simultaneously flexed. In this way, Bernice maintained extremes of joint range without experiencing tension in her tendons (Closer Look Box 8-9).

The OT staff members at the rehabilitation hospital took this technique one step further, allowing Bernice's flexor digitorum profundus to shorten so that even in full wrist flexion, her fingers maintained some flexion. The added shortening gives Bernice enough tension to hold a microphone in her left hand when she sings.

Extrinsic and Intrinsic Function

The fingers flex and extend to close and open the hand via alternate contractions of the flexor digitorum profundus and extensor digitorum communis. Activation of the long flexors and extensors requires synergistic activation of the wrist extensors for hand closure and wrist flexors for hand opening. Synergistic wrist movements prevent undesirable action of the long finger flexors and extensors at the wrist.

The role of the intrinsics remains less clear. Basmajian and DeLuca[3] believed the interossei activated any time IP extension accompanied MCP flexion. The lumbricals appeared active with IP extension regardless of MCP position and stayed most active in full IP and MCP extension at the end of hand opening. Basmajian and DeLuca[3] did not notice intrinsic functioning in hand closure. Brand and Hollister,[4] viewing the intrinsics from a surgical and functional perspective, emphasized the interossei as contributors to grip strength in a closed hand.

Clinical evidence provides a different interpretation of intrinsic function in hand closure. Vincent Pearson contracted an influenza virus several months ago. Subsequently, he developed Guillain-Barré syndrome, a neurological deficiency that paralyzed his intrinsic muscles. Vincent's intrinsic minus hands form characteristic MCP hyperextension and partial IP flexion when they open. The posture of his open hands reflects Basmajian and DeLuca's[3] summary of intrinsic muscle function, but Vincent's lack of intrinsic function has a noticeable effect on hand closure. When he reaches to pick up the newspaper, Vincent begins in MCP hyperextension and IP flexion. His fingers make a shallow sweeping motion as they roll the paper into his palm. Watching Vincent illustrates how poor intrinsic function drastically changes the ability to flex the fingers in a typical grasp.[8]

MUSCLES PRODUCING THUMB MOVEMENTS

The long flexors and extensor of the thumb cross many joints, as do the extrinsic muscles of the other fingers. Various wrist muscles balance the wrist as the thumb moves. The abductor pollicis longus has a long moment arm for wrist radial deviation (see Figure 8-12). Abduct your thumb and palpate the extensor carpi ulnaris tendon distal to the ulnar head. The activity you feel in the ECU tendon indicates how much work it takes to provide ulnar balance, preventing radial wrist deviation by the long thumb abductor.

Muscle combinations, or in some cases isolated muscles, move the thumb joints in specific ways. The IP joint of the thumb flexes only by the flexor pollicis longus. This flexor primarily functions at the IP joint during pinch. The flexor pollicis longus flexes the MCP and CMC joints, but the short flexor, short abductor, and thumb adductor play larger roles at these two joints.[4]

Two extrinsic extensors—the extensor pollicis longus and brevis—extend the thumb. The former extends the thumb at all joints and adducts the CMC joint. Because of median nerve damage, Yasmeen cannot oppose her thumb for grasp. She uses an adduction scissors grasp between her thumb and second metacarpal. The adduction effect of the flexor pollicis longus (spared because of its deep median innervation) works with the radially innervated extensor pollicis longus to generate enough adduction force to allow Yasmeen the ability to grasp most objects.

The third thumb extrinsic, the abductor pollicis longus, helps abduct the thumb but more effectively extends the CMC joint. Yasmeen's OT intern originally thought the radially innervated abductor pollicis longus would supply some abduction to her thumb until he discovered the inability of this muscle to bring the thumb away from her palm. More experienced OT practitioners note the role of the abductor pollicis longus to balance the strong thumb adductor, preventing the thumb from collapsing into adduction during pinch. This balancing function offsets its limited ability to abduct away from the palm.[4]

The thenar muscles—abductor pollicis brevis, opponens pollicis, and flexor pollicis brevis—generally seem to act as thumb-positioning muscles. The abductor pollicis brevis abducts the thumb, and the opponens pollicis pronates the first metacarpal in circumduction. The flexor pollicis brevis assists in pronation (flexor and pronator) and effectively flexes both MCP and CMC.[4] This flexor also fulfills a synergist role in pinch. Thenar muscle loss most obviously yields loss of opposition.

Stronger than the flexor pollicis longus, the adductor pollicis applies its force at a larger moment arm for CMC adduction than any muscle in the hand at any other joint.[4] This adductor acts as a flexor and supinator, sharing one and opposing another function of the flexor pollicis brevis (flexor and pronator).

Pinch

Brand and Hollister[4] termed adductor pollicis the "pinching muscle." It works with the flexor pollicis brevis to stabilize the first metacarpal, and together they provide a foundation for pinching power. This dual component of pinch involves MCP joint flexion and first metacarpal adduction at the CMC joint. The adductor pollicis and flexor pollicis brevis move and hold the base of the thumb so that the long flexor can flex the pad and tip of the thumb against other digital pads and surfaces. Tip and palmar (pad-to-pad) prehension result from this muscle combination.

Key pinch (lateral pinch) places the thumb pad against the lateral side of the index finger near the index proximal IP (PIP) joint. The flexor pollicis brevis and adductor pollicis work together on the thumb MCP and CMC joints, and the long flexor primarily operates the IP joint. The first dorsal interosseus, equally important in flexing and abducting the index MCP joint, stabilizes the index finger so that the thumb has something to pinch against. Brand and Hollister[4] suggest that digits 3 through 5 must flex to align themselves under the index finger as a brace in case the first dorsal interosseus fails.

Grasp

We identify grasp (prehension) patterns by their appearance. Cylindrical and spherical grasps hold objects of similar descriptions. Power grasps involve forceful grips on objects like hammers. Precision grasps, or pinches, require opposition of the thumb to the other digits, either tip-to-tip (tip prehension) or pad-to-pad (palmar prehension).

OT practitioners must identify which patterns require the thumb and, of those, which require opposition. For example, a scissors grasp (adduction of the thumb to the second metacarpal in a scissors motion) requires thumb adduction only, using primarily the adductor pollicis and ignoring the thenar muscles. Alternatively, in ulnar nerve loss, flexor and extensor pollicis longus provide scissor grasp. A hook grasp like that used to hold the handle of a suitcase requires no thumb use (Table 8-3).

Yasmeen has used a scissors grasp since her median nerve injury—loss of her median-innervated thenar muscles necessitated this built-in adaptive response. Zachary's grasp after ulnar nerve loss proves problematic (Figure 8-15), and he has fewer adaptive grasps available. This surprised his OT interns because they equated grasp with thumb opposition, mainly a median nerve function. OT practitioners reminded them of the role the ulnar-innervated thumb adductor plays in grasp. Figure 8-15, B shows the thumb position without the adductor pollicis' contribution to stabilize the first metacarpal.

TABLE 8-3	
Thumb Use in Grasp	
GRASP	THUMB USE
Spherical	Opposition
Cylindrical	Opposition
Power	Adduction against handle or opposition against flexed fingers (fingers flexed around handle)
Precision	Opposition
Hook	None
Scissors	Adduction

Zachary's loss of the interossei and the third and fourth lumbricals results in imbalance at the MCP joints of digits 2 through 5. Incapable of the deep sweep necessary to move around objects placed in the palm, the fingertips and volar metacarpal heads hold objects with point pressure (see Figure 8-15, B).

Pathological Conditions

Acute orthopedic trauma, nerve damage, and progressive connective tissue disease all disrupt hand function.

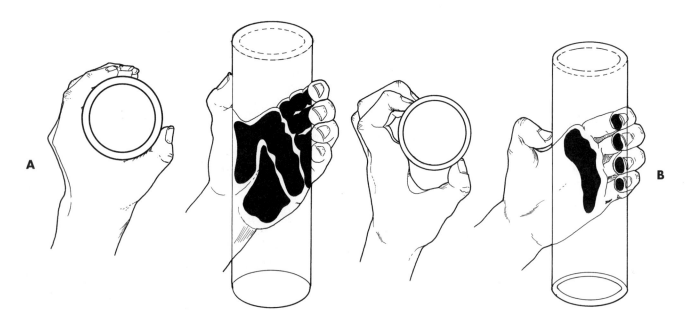

FIGURE **8-15**

A, A normal hand grasps a cylinder with the area of skin contact *marked in black.* **B,** A hand without ulnar-innervated intrinsic function limits the area of grasp to the fingertips and metacarpal heads can touch in grasp. (From Brand PW, Hollister A: *Clinical mechanics of the hand,* ed 2, St Louis, 1993, Mosby.)

We saw Vincent's intrinsic minus hand; now we see how changes in the relationships of forces to axes and muscle excursion requirements affect hand function in other individuals.

BOUTONNIERE AND SWAN NECK

Rheumatoid arthritis disrupted **Linda Valdez**'s extensor expansion, causing a condition called "boutonniere." Blunt trauma to the dorsal aspect of the PIP joint can cause similar connective tissue degradation. Regardless of cause, the mechanics of the problem remain the same.

When Linda flexes her finger, it stretches the extensor expansion over the dorsal aspects of her MCP and IP joints. A tear in the extensor tendon dorsal to the PIP joint causes her PIP joint to protrude through the expansion when passive tension develops in finger flexion. Just as a tear in the knee of a pant leg allows the pants to slip posteriorly on the knee in a deep-knee bend, the extensor expansion slips to the palmar side of Linda's PIP joint. The force of the digit extensor loses its moment arm for PIP extension. As the tendon slips palmarly with more finger flexion, it actually develops a moment arm for PIP flexion (Figure 8-16).

Linda bends her finger but cannot straighten it (extend the PIP). The more she tries to straighten her finger, the more the extensor digitorum communis flexes the PIP. Eventually, Linda hyperextends her distal IP (DIP) with excessive effort. She can passively extend her PIP and hold it straight, using the extensor. Passive extension reestablishes the dorsal relationship of the extensor to the PIP axis, and the muscle once again extends the PIP. Linda holds her finger straight until the next time she tries to flex her finger in a grasp, when the extensor expansion slips again and the problem reestablishes itself. If Linda decided not to passively extend her finger, allowing it to remain in flexion, she would develop a secondary joint flexion contracture.

"Swan neck," another biomechanical problem occurring in the finger, derives its name from a joint

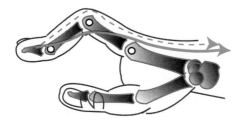

FIGURE 8-16
The extensor digitorum tendon's route in boutonniere. The normal path *(dotted line)* maintains a dorsal relationship to both interphalangeal joints and the metacarpophalangeal joint. The altered path *(solid line)* after palmar displacement lies anterior to the PIP axis, resulting in a proximal interphalangeal flexion moment.

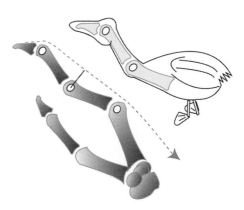

FIGURE 8-17
Configuration of joints in swan neck display an opposite pattern of flexion and extension than boutonniere. The name of this configuration was chosen because of its resemblance to a swan's neck.

misalignment resembling the head and neck of a swan (Figure 8-17). Think of swan neck as the opposite of boutonniere: PIP hyperextension with the surrounding joints (MCP and DIP) in flexion. In this problem, the extensor digitorum tendon gradually moves away from the PIP joint in a dorsal direction, increasing (instead of losing) its extension moment arm.

Not uncommonly, a person with rheumatoid arthritis can exhibit boutonniere in one finger and swan neck in another. Unlike boutonniere in which one can maintain the corrected position after passive range of motion using the other hand, passive correction of swan neck proves unsuccessful. Similar to boutonniere, swan neck develops into a joint contracture, an extension contracture, in this case of the PIP. The greatest impact involves a profound loss of the ability to move into grasp and conform to most shapes.

TRIGGER FINGER

Another problem involving the proximal interphalangeal joint and common in connective tissue diseases like rheumatoid arthritis is "trigger finger." The name derives from the position the finger assumes, resembling pulling a trigger. Again similarities to boutonniere come to mind because the complaint involves the same appearance—an inability to "straighten the finger." The mechanical cause differs, however, because trigger finger results from a problem involving the flexor instead of the extensor tendon.

The flexor tendons in trigger finger develop swelling along the synovial sheath, causing a tight fit and difficult passage through the series of pulleys that form a tunnel on the volar side of each finger. The thickened tendon slides proximally out of the tunnel as the finger flexes in grasp. Upon trying to extend the finger to release grasp, the swollen synovium bunches up at the entrance to the tunnel as the tendon glides distally, preventing distal excursion and therefore finger extension. Think of wearing a sweater and coat in the winter, with your arm as a tendon, a sweater as the tendon's synovial sheath, and a coat sleeve as the tunnel of pulleys. You can take your arm out of the coat without any problem (proximal excursion). When you place your arm back into the sleeve to put on the coat (distal excursion), your hand goes in, but as you push, the sweater bunches up and prevents your arm from gliding further into the sleeve.

ULNAR DRIFT/VOLAR SUBLUXATION

Linda's connective tissue disorder also creates ulnar drift. Ulnar drift occurs when the extensor digitorum communis tendon slips off the high, dorsal point of the MCP joint and moves toward the ulnar side (Figure 8-18). The digit or digits follow the drifting tendon, abducting or adducting at the MCP depending on the digit involved. With digits 2 through 5 involved, Linda's hand takes on a wind-swept appearance referred to as "wind-swept hand."

Appreciate the force relationship of the extensor digitorum communis tendon to the front-to-back axis for MCP abduction and adduction with ulnar drift. In its normal anatomical position the extensor digitorum communis has no moment for abduction and adduction because it pulls directly through this axis. After slipping ulnarly, the tendon develops a moment at this axis (see Figure 8-18). The index finger adducts toward the long finger; the long finger, abducts toward the ring finger. OT practitioners use the terms *ulnar deviation* and *ulnar drift* of the MCP to prevent confusion over abduction and adduction. The extensor still extends the finger, even though its moment arm decreases as it slips palmarly, falling down the MCP joint.

In some cases of long-standing ulnar drift the proximal phalanx slips palmarly off the metacarpal head (Figure 8-19). This happens for a number of mechanical reasons, including support failure in the dorsal structures. Because this semiflexed resting position places the lumbricals and interossei on slack, intrinsic contracture develops and worsens MCP volar subluxation.

In the absence of intrinsic contracture, the MCP joint extends passively after manipulation of the proximal phalanx in line with the metacarpal head. Failure to reduce subluxation before passive MCP extension can damage the joint further. Splinting the MCP into extension without reducing subluxation makes the situation worse. Passive extension of the MCP without reduction causes "tilting" (Figure 8-20) and damages joint surfaces.

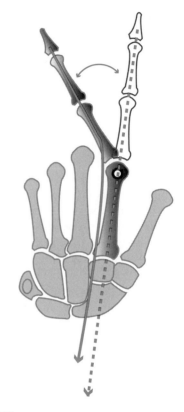

FIGURE **8-18**
Ulnar drift of the extensor digitorum communis tendon and the index digit at the metacarpophalangeal joint.

BOWSTRINGING

Iris Clark, a housewife with multiple sclerosis, cut the A1 and A2 pulleys of her right index finger while washing cracked glass. After her wound healed, she complained that she could not bend her index finger as far as the other fingers. The digital connective tissue pulleys (located proximal and distal to the MCP joint) keep the long flexor tendons in close proximity to the metacarpal and phalangeal bones. When Iris flexes her index finger, the palmar skin at the proximal digital crease elevates and webs out from the bowstringing of the long flexor tendons (Figure 8-21). Pressing on the skin over the tendons pushes the tendon back into its bed, increasing digital flexion.

Early mechanical inspection indicates that bowstringing increases the moment arm of the tendon at the joint. However, this longer moment arm proves useless because bowstringing uses up the muscle's limited excursion. In the case of a broken pulley, some amount of excursion associated with muscle contraction occurs before any observable joint movement. This amount of excursion pulls the tendon away from the bone through the broken pulley, creating the bowstring effect. The remaining excursion applies to motion, but remains inadequate to produce full range of motion.

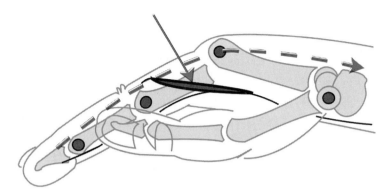

FIGURE **8-19**
Advanced ulnar drift at the MCP joints commonly leads to subluxation of the joint. Lacking the dorsal support provided by the central location of the ED tendon, the proximal phalanx moves volarly off of the metacarpal head. The finger assumes a flexed appearance (at the MCP), and because of the partial dislocation no longer extends. Secondarily, the intrinsics (lumbrical pictured here *indicated by arrow*) shorten as a result of myositic contracture, encouraging further volar subluxation and ultimate dislocation.

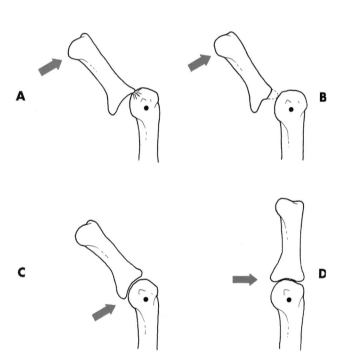

FIGURE **8-20**
The heavy arrows demonstrate force applied to a joint that has a partial subluxation, a block to free gliding, or both. **A** and **B,** Force applied with a long moment arm results in tilting without gliding and in eventual absorption of the lip of the phalanx. **C** and **D,** Force applied with a short moment arm (close to the joint) results in restored gliding. (Modified from Brand PW, Hollister A: *Clinical mechanics of the hand,* ed 2, St Louis, 1993, Mosby.)

Decreased range also occurs when a tendon or muscle that operates with a long moment arm inserts farther away from the joint. The more distal the insertion, the greater the distance a tendon must travel to move the joint (Figure 8-9). Because excursion remains limited and unchangeable, the available excursion now produces less range of motion, verifying Iris' complaint that she "could not bend her index finger as far as her other fingers" (Figure 8-21). (See Movie 8-3 showing the increased excursion requirement and moment arm in the case of bowstringing after pulley removal.)

JOINT CONTRACTURE AND TENDON ADHESION

Karen Wu, a 15-year-old high school sophomore, comes to the clinic complaining that her right middle finger does not straighten or bend all the way. The OT practitioner evaluating Karen's hand has a number of ideas about what could cause Karen's problem. Karen says that she broke her hand several months earlier. Because Karen lacks external scarring and her skin moves freely over the surface of her dorsum and palm, the OT practitioner concentrates on two very distinct possibilities— joint contracture and tendon adhesion.

The practitioner manipulates Karen's third finger to determine which condition causes her problem. Joint contractures involve the joint itself.

In the case of joint contracture, the position or movement of other joints in the sequence have no effect on movement of the joint with the contracture. Tendon adhesions, however, involve the tendon and do affect proximal and distal tendon excursion necessary for movement of all the joints the tendon crosses.

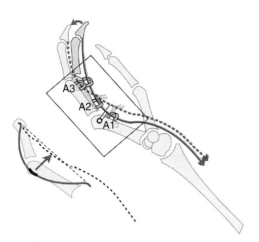

BOX 8-10

A CLOSER LOOK

FIGURE 8-21

The A1 and A2 pulleys normally hold the long flexor tendons close to the volar side of the metacarpophalangeal joint. Bowstringing of a tendon after these digital pulleys rupture changes the joint's mechanics. (The name derives from the appearance of a string on a bow; under tension the string naturally bridges the concavity of the bow rather than conforming to it.) Note that bowstringing of the long flexor tendon at the metacarpophalangeal joint increases the moment arm but results in wasting of excursion with less range of motion available for finger flexion (*indicated by curved, counterclockwise arrow at fingertip*).

Increased Range in Tendon Adhesion

Karen Wu needs a splint for the flexor tendon adhesion at her third metacarpal. The OT practitioner flexes Karen's MCP to create slack and check PIP extension when diagnosing the problem. Now the OT practitioner must splint the tendon under a mild stretch to attain the opposite motion. Because Karen's tendon crosses multiple joints distal to the point of adhesion, the OT practitioner must splint all the distal joints to produce a sufficient stretch. Consider what would happen if he splints only the PIP in as much extension as possible. After all, Karen can actively straighten her MCP and DIP joints, but not her PIP.

As soon as the OT practitioner places the PIP into the splint under tension, the MCP or DIP will curl into flexion. (PIP extension pulls the two surrounding joints into tenodesis flexion.) The end result extends the PIP, flexes the MCP and DIP, and leaves the flexor tendon in a relaxed, unstretched state. A successful splint puts all joints distal to the adhesion into extension. This splint places the entire flexor tendon under tension, and leaves no joints free to relieve it.

Karen's medical record shows she fractured the third metacarpal shaft 3 months ago, and the OT practitioner suspects flexor tendon adhesion at the site of the healed fracture may have caused Karen's problem. First, however, he must prove this theory.

Karen complains of limited ability to actively and passively extend her PIP. First, the OT practitioner positions Karen's MCP joint in flexion to create slack in the flexor tendon. He then attempts passive extension of the PIP.

If tendon adhesion caused Karen's problem, her PIP joint could move freely into extension. The slack created distal to the adhesion along the metacarpal shaft would allow the flexor tendon sufficient excursion for PIP extension (A Closer Look Box 8-10).

The OT practitioner successfully demonstrates full passive extension of the PIP joint while holding the MCP joint in flexion.

The OT practitioner verifies the adhesion by evaluating proximal flexor tendon excursion because an adhesion blocks both distal and proximal excursion of the adhered tendon. Active PIP flexion requires proximal excursion of the flexor tendon.

After checking Karen's passive PIP extension, the OT practitioner asks Karen to try flexing (bending) her finger. Karen cannot actively flex any distal joints, but the OT practitioner can move them passively into full flexion. Passive flexion verifies

proper joint function, and he concludes that an adhesion blocking excursion causes Karen's lack of active flexion.

If Karen had limited passive and active PIP extension regardless of MCP position and unlimited active joint flexion, the OT practitioner would diagnose Karen with PIP joint flexion contracture.

Of course, long-standing tendon adhesions lead to joint contractures. The possibility exists for an individual to have both. Practitioners often discover tendon adhesion only after beginning to see some movement gains in the treatment of a joint contracture.

Torque Range of Motion

OT practitioners have been measuring passive range of motion (PROM) since Bird T. Baldwin's work at the beginning of the twentieth century.[2] Most practitioners assume they have achieved some degree of accuracy with measurements using a goniometer, but PROM assessments in joints stiffened by edema or contracture prove especially vulnerable to inaccuracy. Disuse of any joint may result in contractures of skin, fat, or periarticular tissue. In these instances, PROM measurements depend on how much *force* the OT practitioner feels comfortable using to range the joint.

Torque range of motion tries to control and document the amount of force used in PROM evaluation. Passive ranging of a joint to the end point of motion demonstrates equilibrium of torques. Extending an MCP joint using some amount of force at a specific distance from the joint develops extension torque. The stiff tissue limiting this attempt creates a torque of flexion. Equalization of torques in each direction occurs at the end point of range.[4]

Sometimes the goniometer does not register change, yet the practitioner has the impression the joint moves more easily. Torque range of motion simply quantifies that feeling by measuring the force used to produce joint motion. Pulling on the segment with a small force gauge (Figure 8-22) allows measurement of force associated with degrees of joint motion. Hanging a known weight (force) on a segment provides an alternative type of PROM measurement (Figure 8-23).

These measurements allow OT practitioners to report both the range and the amount of force necessary to produce movement. These data generate a curve called a *torque-angle curve*, which reports the amount of force needed to bring the joint into different positions or joint angles (Figure 8-24). OT practitioners use these results to decide whether to continue therapy or try an alternative treatment (Figure 8-25).

Torque range of motion, involves a few simple but important procedures. Failure to follow these renders the measurement unreliable.

Fred Jackson, an engineer, visits the hand clinic after MCP joint replacement. He did not receive therapy immediately after the surgery as prescribed by his physician, so his hand has tightened into a dysfunctional flexion pattern. The OT practitioner

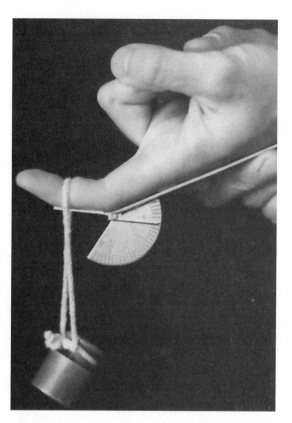

FIGURE **8-23**
One simple way to obtain a torque-angle measurement involves positioning the hand so that a hanging weight of, for example, 250 g, applied at a finger crease distal to the joint being ranged pulls at a right angle. (From Brand PW, Hollister A: *Clinical mechanics of the hand,* ed 2, St Louis, 1993, Mosby.)

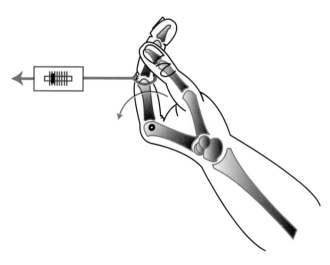

FIGURE **8-22**
A small "fish scale" force gauge quantifies the force involved in joint range.

who sees Fred on the first day determines that it takes 600 grams (g) to pull his MCP from 90-degrees flexion to 30-degrees flexion (60 degrees of extension). The next week a different OT practitioner documents that it takes only 300 g to move the MCP the same distance. The first therapist placed the force gauge loop on the PIP crease, giving her force a moment arm of 3 centimeters (cm). The second therapist placed the loop at the DIP crease, applying force at about twice the distance from the MCP axis.

The two OT practitioners could have avoided this miscommunication by either documenting where they applied the force gauge or converting the force to torque. Regardless of the name "torque-angle curve," most of these curves document force as read from the gauge because this seems simpler and faster than converting the force measurement to torque. In Fred's case, the conversion would have helped the clinic avoid a mistake in documentation. Conversion is simple; multiply the amount of force used by the moment arm. The first measurement converts to 1800 g-cm (600 g × 3 cm).

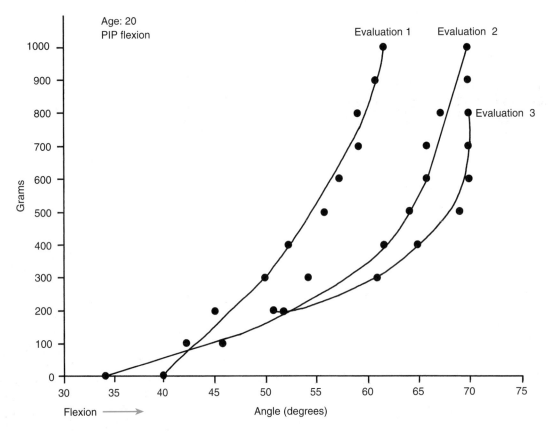

FIGURE **8-24**

This record of a patient's stiff finger shows three torque-angle curves, each one separated by 2 weeks of treatment. The last curve shows a vertical segment at high torque. This led to a decision to discontinue treatment due to lack of response. *PIP,* Proximal interphalangeal. (Modified from Brand PW, Hollister A: *Clinical mechanics of the hand,* ed 2, St Louis, 1993, Mosby.)

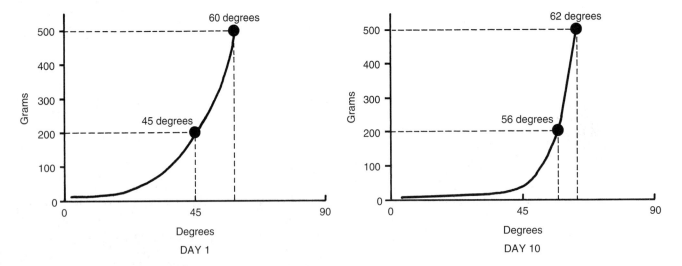

FIGURE **8-25**

The torque-angle curve of this stiff metacarpophalangeal joint shows a gentle, nonspecific curve. After 10 days of therapy, maximum flexion with a force of 500 g has increased only 2 degrees. But 200 g of force on day 10 produces 4 additional degrees of flexion due to less stiffness. The shape of the curve has changed to one typical of dense contracture, with a steep, straight terminal section. The 10 days of therapy improved the disuse contracture of the skin and fat but made no difference in the underlying connective tissue shortening. (Modified from Brand PW, Hollister A: *Clinical mechanics of the hand,* ed 2, St Louis, 1993, Mosby.)

The second also converts to 1800 g-cm (300 g × 6 cm) because the practitioner used less force at a longer moment arm. When OT practitioners prefer to record the force as it appears on the gauge, they must also document the moment arm to avoid confusion. Often practitioners follow a protocol that standardizes the moment arm by stipulating where to place the loop on the finger (i.e., "place loop at PIP crease to measure MCP extension").

Poor Fred has to undergo yet another failed evaluation before helping the clinic "clean up their act." As an engineer, Fred knows the importance of applying force gauges at 90-degree angles to prevent errors in measurement. He notes that the first therapist pulled the force gauge at a 90-degree angle to the proximal phalanx, the segment she moved. The third time Fred visits the clinic, an even less-experienced practitioner carefully places the loop at the level of the PIP crease but does not maintain a 90-degree angle. She records more force required for each position of extension and concludes Fred's MCP joint has worsened.

A force oriented at 90 degrees produces a pure rotary force (Figure 8-26, A, and A Closer Look Box 8-11). Orienting that same force at an angle other than 90 degrees wastes part of the force (Figure 8-26, B, and 8-27), because a pull along the segment has nothing to do with extending the MCP joint. (Remember that back

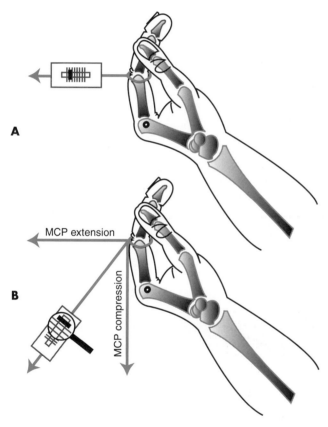

A

MCP extension

MCP compression

B

FIGURE **8-26**
Accurate measurement of the force required for passive joint movement relies on a 90-degree pull applied at a specified point on the moving segment. Here a force applied at the level of the PIP crease achieves passive metacarpophalangeal extension. (**A**) Pulling with a force oriented at an angle other than 90 degrees wastes the force in a linear effect, in this case, compression. The OT practitioner must increase the amount of force to passively range the joint. (Note the greater force reading under the magnifying glass [**B**] compared with the first force-gauge reading.) This additional force inflates the value, mistakenly representing an increase in joint stiffness. *MCP,* Metacarpophalangeal.

BOX 8-11

A **CLOSER** LOOK

Force Angles in Splinting
Fred Jackson wears a dynamic extension outrigger splint after MCP joint replacement surgery. He complains that one of the finger cuffs on his splint keeps slipping. The OT practitioner knows immediately that the rubber band attached to the cuff does not extend at a 90-degree angle to Fred's proximal phalanx. A force applied at 90 degrees to a segment pulls in the intended direction without causing the cuff to shift. If the cuff slips proximally, the force angles toward the hand, caused by a short outrigger (see Figure 8-26). Slipping distally implies a longer than needed outrigger. The OT practitioner adjusts Fred's splint to ensure a true 90-degree pull.

Because a dynamic force applied at an angle other than 90 degrees to the segment distributes a portion of the force into a linear component, part of the force results in compression or distraction of the joint instead of the intended rotary motion of the segment. In this scenario, the OT practitioner does not know how much force the splint actually administers in the intended direction to produce rotary joint movement. The linear component of the force pulls parallel to the segment, sliding the cuff from position. If the rubber band pulls with 200 g, some amount less than 200 g extends the MCP due to wasting of a portion of the 200 g in a linear direction. Instead of applying another rubber band to make up for the wasted component, the OT practitioner adjusts Fred's outrigger to pull at 90 degrees. Now all 200 g pull in the intended direction.

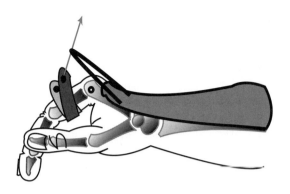

FIGURE **8-27**
Inaccurate outrigger adjustment causes dynamic force to pull at angles other than 90 degrees. In this case a short outrigger introduces a linear component of force, and the cuff slips proximally.

extensors pulling at far less than 90 degrees to the vertebral column produce more linear than rotary effect, resulting in much greater effort than you would think necessary to lift moderate amounts of weight.)

The Ergonomics of Grasp

Wendy Dabdoub works in a fruit-packing warehouse that requires constant handling of produce averaging 12 cm in diameter. A job-site analysis determines that Wendy applies 4.4 kilograms (kg) of force to maintain her grasp on the produce. Wendy demonstrates a full-hand grasp in the clinic (Figure 8-28, A). However, observation at her work site reveals that most of the time she holds the produce with a partial-hand grasp, making contact primarily with the distal phalanges of her fingers (Figure 8-28, B).

Measurements reveal that both grasps involve a position of 70 degrees of thumb abduction. Using a whole-hand grasp,

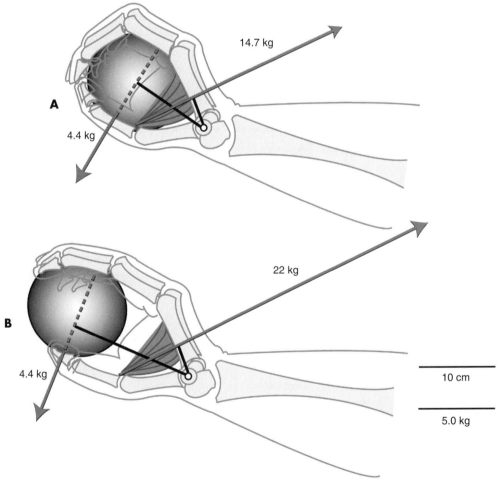

FIGURE **8-28**
Vector diagrams show force needed to maintain different grips. **A**, Whole-hand grasp.
B, Partial-hand grasp.

Wendy experiences resistance force equally along the palmar surface of her thumb, centered at the level of the proximal phalanx. The resistance orients approximately 90 degrees to the proximal phalanx, 10 cm from the CMC joint. With the partial-hand grasp, resistance force applies more distally, centered at the distal phalanx of the finger, 90 degrees to the finger pad and 15 cm from the CMC joint.

Her thumb maintains gripping force primarily through thumb adduction. The tendon of the adductor pollicis inserts on the base of the proximal phalanx. With the CMC in this abducted position, the combined fibers of the adductor tendon pull at a moment arm 3 cm from the axis for adduction (Figure 8-28).

To solve this equilibrium-of-torques problem use resistance (R), moment arm (MA), and the adductor pollicis (AP). Based on the equilibrium condition of torque created by the resistance (R × RMA) equal to torque created by the force of the adductor pollicis (AP force × muscle MA), we can determine the force of the adductor pollicis in each grasp.

Whole-hand grasp:

$$4.4 \text{ kg} \times 10 \text{ cm} = \text{AP force} \times 3 \text{ cm}$$

$$44 \text{ kg-cm}/3 \text{ cm} = \text{AP force}$$

$$\text{AP force} = 14.7 \text{ kg}$$

Partial-hand grasp:

$$4.4 \text{ kg} \times 15 \text{ cm} = \text{AP force} \times 3 \text{ cm}$$

$$\text{AP force} = 66 \text{ kg-cm}/3 \text{ cm}$$

$$\text{AP force} = 22 \text{ kg}$$

The partial-hand grasp requires the adductor pollicis exert more than 7 kg greater force than the whole-hand grasp because of the resistance's longer moment arm. For the same reason Wendy's finger flexors work harder. The added strain of the partial grasp aggravates Wendy's carpal tunnel condition, especially when combined with the wrist flexion movements necessary on her job. The OT practitioner educates Wendy about the damaging nature of a partial-hand grasp and encourages her to use a whole-hand grasp, and when possible, to pair the grasp with wrist extension.

Summary

The wrist and hand are amazing structures. Their functions help us clarify and elaborate our knowledge of anatomy. Grasp and manipulation require complex systems of balance. We learn to appreciate critical muscle balance at the wrist and MCP joints. Unless many muscles work together, hand function falters. Basic concepts of hand kinesiology form the foundation for clinical diagnosis and treatment.

Applications

■ APPLICATION 8-1
Balanced Wrist Function

Palpate your flexor carpi radialis and flexor carpi ulnaris tendons at the wrist, just proximal to the wrist flexion creases. Perform straight wrist flexion and note tension in both tendons. While holding this position, move the hand slowly toward ulnar deviation and note what happens. Why? Next, from ulnar deviations, slowly move back to flexion, then to radial deviation. What happens to the tension in each tendon? Why?

■ APPLICATION 8-2
Shorter Longitudinal Arch

Trace the outline of your hand with the palm up. Make sure your hand rests centered on the paper, with its ulnar border parallel to the paper's edge. Before lifting your hand off the paper, mark the location of the proximal palmar crease on the radial side and the distal palmar crease on the ulnar side. Take another piece of paper and cover your drawing. Slowly move the top sheet down, keeping the vertical edges together. Stop when you uncover one of the palmar crease markings. What do you notice?

See Appendix C for solutions to Applications.

REFERENCES

1. Atcheson SC, Ward JR, Lowe W: Concurrent medical disease in work-related carpal tunnel syndrome. *Arch Int Med* 158(14):1506-1512, 1998.
2. Baldwin BT: *Occupational therapy applied to restoration of function of disabled joints*, Washington, D.C., 1919, Walter Reed General Hospital.
3. Basmajian JV, DeLuca CJ: *Muscles alive: their functions revealed by electromyography*, ed 5, Baltimore, 1985, Williams & Wilkins.
4. Brand PW, Hollister A: *Clinical mechanics of the hand*, ed 2, St Louis, 1993, Mosby.
5. Brand PW: Relative tension of the muscles of the forearm and hand. Presented at *The insensitive hand: biomechanics of deformity*, Carville, La, 1987.
6. Brand PW, Beach RB, Thompson DE: Relative tension and potential excursion of muscles in the forearm and hand, *J Hand Surg* 6(3):209-219, 1981.
7. Kapandji IA: *Physiology of the joints*, ed 5, New York, 1982, Churchill Livingstone.
8. Smith LK and others: *Brunnstrom's clinical kinesiology*, ed 5, Philadelphia, 1996, FA Davis.
9. Soderberg GL: *Kinesiology: application to pathological motion*, Baltimore, 1986, Williams & Wilkins.

LAB BOX

Find applied activities exploring concepts in Chapter 8 in the following laboratory exercises:

Topic	Laboratory
MMT and goniometry principles for wrist and hand	**Lab 3** Overview of ROM & MMT Additional Lab: MMT to Determine Neurological Level in SCI Motion CD
Muscles and balance at the wrist, isometric torque curve of finger flexor strength as affected by wrist position, active and passive insufficiency	**Lab 10** Wrist and Hand: Synergistic Function of Wrist Extensors and Finger Flexors
Extrinsic and intrinsic function in the hand, effect of pulleys in the hand, passive insufficiency and tenodesis grasp, effect of various hand pathologies on active and passive range of motion	**Lab 11** Torque Range of Motion-Intrinsic Function-Tenodesis Grasp - Pulleys - Review of ROM Limitations
Traditional goniometry and torque range of motion in the case of a stiff PIP joint	
Prehension patterns and thumb use, normal and shallow digital sweep as a function of intrinsic muscles (and intrinsic minus condition), more on tenodesis grasp (and release)	**Lab 12** Prehension Patterns - Intrinsic Function and Digital Sweep- Tenodesis Grasp

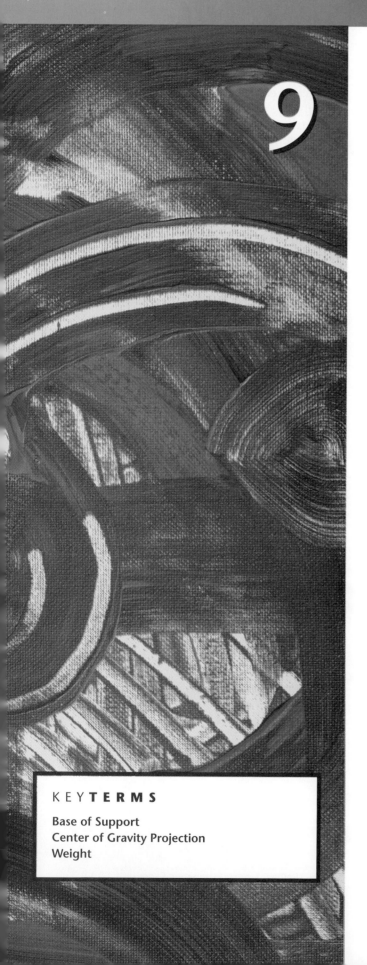

9

The Lower Extremity

K E Y **TERMS**

Base of Support
Center of Gravity Projection
Weight

*I*ndividuals walk in upright positions, leaving their hands free to explore and manipulate the environment. The lower extremities carry the **weight** of the body, moving it from place to place. Lower extremities also help maintain balance and equilibrium.

The lower extremities ground the body to the earth through a kinematic chain that includes the hip, knee, and ankle. Feet support our body's weight in part through the longitudinal arch lengthwise and the transverse arch widthwise, which together form the hollow between the heel and ball of the foot. These springlike arches absorb the forces created in standing and walking. In a way, similar to the butterfly's wings having effects at a distance, the foot's link to the ground below impacts posture in the vertebral column through the numerous muscles crossing multiple joints of the lower extremity.

Sitting proves no less dynamic. Closed-chain muscle actions across the hip stabilize the trunk in upright sitting and control leaning. Muscle lengths across the knee and hip directly influence sitting posture and serve as a primary focus in interventions for seating and positioning. Understanding the kinesiology of this region arms us with sound explanations of how knee position can lead to sacral skin breakdown when shortened hamstrings produce sacral sitting and kyphotic posture.

Movements and Muscle Use

HIP

As for all other joints, muscles function at the hip according to their relationships with the axes of motion. Flexors concentrically contract anterior to the side-to-side axis, initiating open-chain hip flexion (Figure 9-1). Flexors include the rectus femoris, sartorius, pectineus, tensor fasciae latae, and iliopsoas. The posterior hip extensors include the gluteus maximus and hamstrings (the biceps femoris, semitendinosus, and semimembranosus). Open-chain functions move the thigh in relation to the trunk at the hip joint. The same muscles adjust the verticality of the trunk through their pelvic attachments in closed-chain hip movements.

Closed-chain movements play large roles in the lower extremities because weight bearing stabilizes the foot. Each step of gait occurs with closed-chain ankle dorsi-flexion and hip extension pulling the body over the grounded foot. To sit upright in bed from a supine position, hip flexors bring the trunk toward the thighs in closed-chain hip flexion. While sitting, gravity's downward pull on the trunk causes closed-chain hip flexion or extension controlled by eccentric contractions of the hip extensors and flexors, respectively. Hip flexors

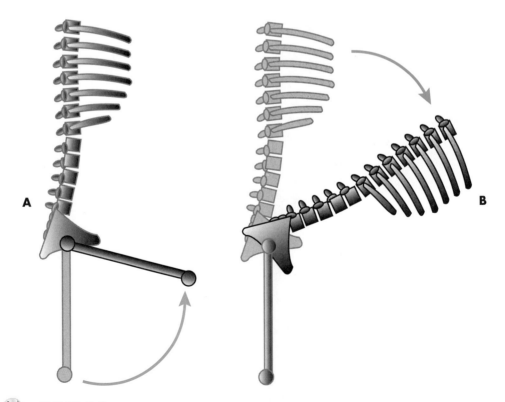

FIGURE **9-1**
Open-chain **(A)** versus closed-chain **(B)** hip flexion. (Review Figure/Interactive Exercise 4-10.)

counteract a posterior, extension pull by gravity. When gravity pulls the upper trunk anteriorly, hip extensors are activated and prevent forward movement of the trunk (closed-chain hip flexion). Control at the hip accompanies similar activation in the trunk flexors and extensors.

Besides moving the thigh or trunk, hip flexors and extensors influence the lumbar curve. The iliopsoas pulls anteriorly on its origins at the lumbar vertebrae and pelvic ilium to reinforce both the lumbar curve and anterior pelvic tilt associated with good posture. On the opposite side of the hip axis, the hamstrings affect pelvic tilt via their attachments to the ischial tuberosity. Tight hamstrings limit forward pelvic movement (closed-chain hip flexion) in toe touches, flattening the lumbar curve. (See Figure 9-2 and Animations 9-1 and 9-2 for toe touching with normal length and short hamstrings, respectively.)

Open- and closed-chain hip abduction and adduction interact with gravity's pull on the upper body at the hip in the frontal plane. The gluteus medius and gluteus minimus, together with the adductor group—the pectineus, gracilis, and adductors magnus, longus, and

brevis—maintain lateral stability of the pelvis and trunk over one leg as an individual walks, runs, and performs other movements. They also maintain active sitting balance in side-to-side and diagonal weight shifts. Closed-chain antigravity actions involve the two gluteal muscles pulling the trunk away from the body's midline, while the adductor group pulls toward the midline. Activation reverses when eccentric contractions control gravity's effect on the upper trunk.

Six small rotator muscles hold the femur firmly in the hip joint just as the rotator cuff muscles of the glenohumeral joint hold the humerus in place. The obturators internus and externus, gemellus superior and inferior, quadratus femoris, and piriformis all originate on the lower pelvis and insert onto or near the greater trochanter of the femur. The neck of the femur serves as a long lever arm, allowing the muscles to generate large amounts of torque. Open-chain movements by these six muscles laterally rotate the femur; closed-chain actions contribute to pelvic and trunk balance over the lower extremity.

Open-chain actions of the hip adductors also medially rotate the hip. They vary in length and attach along the shaft of the femur in front of that muscle's mechanical axis for rotation. Depending on the femur's position, hip abductors also have effective moment arms for medial rotation. Together, the medial rotators turn the thigh inward and assist in diagonal balance and weight shifts.

KNEE

The quadriceps femoris acts forcefully in kicking movements (open-chain hip flexion and knee extension). More frequently the quadriceps exhibits closed-chain knee extension, supporting the body weight against gravity in standing. Four muscles—the vastus medialis, vastus lateralis, vastus intermedius, and rectus femoris—comprise the quadriceps femoris. Of the four, only the rectus femoris originates on the pelvis, crossing the hip joint anteriorly. The others originate on the medial, lateral, and intermediate surfaces of the femur as their names imply. All four converge and insert into the central patellar tendon, enclosing the patella and attaching to the tibia. A multijoint muscle, the rectus femoris cannot simultaneously fully extend the knee and flex the hip (active insufficiency). It functions best as a knee extensor with simultaneous hip extension, as in the downward stroke of bicycle pedaling.

Posteriorly, the hamstrings flex the knee. Like the rectus femoris in front, the hamstrings cross two joints, and experience active insufficiency in simultaneous knee flexion and hip extension. The hamstrings avoid active insufficiency shortening during knee flexion because hip

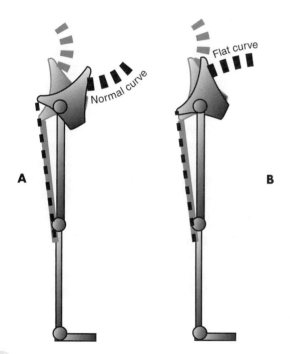

FIGURE **9-2**
A, Normal length hamstrings allow full flexion of the trunk and pelvis. **B**, Short hamstrings become stretched early as the trunk flexes onto the thigh. Once the hamstrings reach the limits of stretchability, they prevent further movement of the pelvis. Continued efforts to bend all must occur in the vertebral column through a reversal of the lumbar curve.

flexion by a synergist simultaneously produces hamstring stretch. The racing cyclist exemplifies this combination in the upstroke of the pedal, using her toe-clip attachment to the pedal and a strong hamstring-activated knee flexion with simultaneous hip flexion to pull the pedal up while the other foot pushes it down in a power stroke.

ANKLE

At the ankle the large triceps surae—the soleus and two heads of the gastrocnemius—courses posterior to the side-to-side axis and plantar flexes the ankle. The gastrocnemius originates on the distal femur, so it also flexes the knee. The gastrocnemius and soleus together insert onto the calcaneus through the tendo calcaneus, or "Achilles' tendon." These muscles support the weight of the body and provide enough force for an individual to stand on the ball of one foot while reaching high above the head (closed-chain plantar flexion). On the anterior side of the ankle side-to-side axis, the peroneus tertius and extensors hallucis longus and digitorum longus arise from the lateral tibia and assist the major dorsiflexor, the tibialis anterior.

While open-chain dorsiflexion and plantar flexion occur via their prime movers, closed-chain versions follow knee and hip motions during weight bearing. Moving from standing to sitting, closed-chain motions of the three joints (hip and knee flexion with ankle dorsiflexion) occur together. At each joint the antagonist contracts eccentrically to control gravity: hip and knee extensors and ankle plantar flexors control hip and knee flexion and dorsiflexion by gravity. The same muscles contract concentrically, providing the opposite motions at each joint when moving from sitting to standing.

Inversion and eversion movements help stabilize the foot on uneven ground and allow body weight to shift from side to side when an individual stands or moves. The tibialis anterior and tibialis posterior run medially across the ankle and pull the sole of the foot inward into inversion, or supination. Their insertions onto the medial tarsal bones help maintain the arches and distribute body weight to the lateral sides of the feet.

The peroneus longus and peroneus brevis pull the sole of the foot outward into eversion. These muscles originate on the fibula and insert onto the lateral tarsal bones. They distribute body weight onto the medial side of the foot by everting, or pronating, the foot during weight bearing.

The foot, like the hand, has a number of intrinsic and extrinsic muscles inserting distally onto its multiple phalanges. The lumbricals and interossei help maintain balance by flexing the metatarsophalangeal joints and extending the interphalangeal joints. They keep the toes in contact with the ground as we stand and move. The flexor hallucis brevis and extensor hallucis longus similarly balance the big, or great, toe. The flexor plays an important role in pushing the body forward during gait.

Intrinsic and extrinsic toe flexors, extensors, abductors, and adductors also help maintain balance by allowing the toes to grip the ground. With enough practice, toe muscles can produce movements similar to those of the fingers. For some individuals without upper extremities, the functional ability of the intrinsic and extrinsic toe muscles approaches that of the hand.

Balance

Unexpected encounters demonstrate the ability of our muscles to anticipate movement. After a surprising jolt or shove, the muscles adjust almost instantaneously. We see this anticipation at work when one step in a staircase is only a bit higher than all the others and causes us to stumble. Ancient Romans used this trick to protect their temples and palaces with long flights of such stairs. Invading armies, running too fast for their normal anticipatory mechanisms to function, would trip, giving the inhabitants a chance to defend themselves.

As the body moves in and out of various positions, muscle groups in the lower extremity continually respond to the body's changing center of gravity. The downward pull of gravity stimulates receptors in equilibrium reactions, which generate weight-bearing adjustments as an individual moves from standing to stooping to balancing the body on one foot. Drawing the projected force of gravity in any lower-extremity position establishes gravity's effect on each weight-bearing joint. We determine muscle forces responsible for balancing gravity's effect using the equilibrium of torques equation.

WEIGHT BEARING

The hip joint is a classic ball-and-socket joint in which the ball-like head of the femur sits firmly in the cuplike acetabulum of the pelvis. A series of ligaments form a tough, fibrous capsule that reinforces the joint. The iliofemoral ligament comprises the front of this capsule between the greater and lesser trochanters of the femur. The configuration of the hip permits motion around three separate axes—flexion and extension at the side-to-side axis, abduction and adduction at the front-to-back axis, and rotation at the up-to-down axis running from the femoral head to the condyles. The joints and bones of the lower extremity support the weight of the rest of the body and any added weight we hold or carry.

The curved bony architecture, muscles, and ligaments absorb and adapt to the large amounts of force and stress produced by movement in a gravity environment.

Balance at the Hip

The combined weight of the upper body—the head, torso, and upper extremities—interacts with gravity at the hip. Typically, gravity induces hip flexion, extension, abduction, or adduction because of the joint's three degrees of freedom. Direction depends on the upper body's alignment in relation to the hip joint. Gravity flexes the hip when the upper body's center of gravity falls anterior to the side-to-side axis, and the hip extensors (the hamstrings and gluteus maximus) equalize gravity's flexion torque to maintain upright posture.

Gravity extends the hip when the upper body center of gravity falls posterior to the side-to-side axis. Flexion torque of the the pectineus, iliopsoas, and rectus femoris balance this posterior sway. In each case, gravity causes closed-chain hip movement, and the trunk flexes or extends toward the femur as opposed to the femur flexing or extending toward the trunk. These balancing acts involve isometric muscle contractions that counteract gravity, so no movement occurs.

Crystal Turner, a 4-year-old girl with Down syndrome, has low muscle tone and experiences difficulty achieving upper-body balance at the hip. Because of her weak abdominal muscles and hip flexors, Crystal locks her knees in extension and leans backward when she stands upright. This position places her upper body's center of gravity slightly behind the hip joint. Crystal's iliofemoral ligament balances the extension effect of gravity and prevents extension beyond the upright position (Figure 9-3).

Even with weak hip flexors, Crystal controls forward bending by shifting her weight slightly forward. The hip extensors eccentrically contract to control her upper body as it bends forward in closed-chain hip flexion. Via concentric contraction, these extensors return her upper body to an upright position with closed-chain hip extension. She can stop at any point and hold the position with an isometric contraction of the hip extensors. Crystal's hip extensors maintain her upright posture in much the same way they do in an individual with normal muscle strength and tone since the hip extensors always interact with gravity to lower and bring the upper body erect. Only the last step, slight overextension of the hip, differs from normal muscle use.

Because of her muscle weakness, backward inclination of the trunk provides a safe position for Crystal. In spite of weak hip flexors, she leans forward in closed-chain hip flexion with control and recovers from leaning. However, for Alex Fecteau, a 6-year-old boy with newly diagnosed muscular dystrophy, the same adaptation fails when applied to the opposite side of the hip. Alex has weak hip extensors, and because posterior ligaments tighten and stabilize the hip only at the very end of the hip-flexion range, he cannot incline his trunk forward and expect ligaments to provide stabilization. Once Alex's center of gravity moves anterior to his

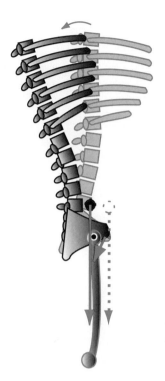

FIGURE **9-3**
The anterior hip ligament (iliofemoral ligament) helps maintain upright posture when hip flexors are weak or absent.

hip joint, gravity-induced, closed-chain hip flexion accelerates downward until passive stretch of the hamstrings and posterior hip capsule finally halt gravity's flexion torque. Alex must use his available upper-extremity strength to "climb up" the thighs into erect posture (Gower's sign), a maneuver recognized as a classic early symptom of muscular dystrophy.[1]

To understand gravity's effect on the hip's front-to-back axis for abduction–adduction, stand on one foot. Lean on the weight-bearing leg, shifting gravity's projection lateral to the abduction and adduction axis, and feel isometric contractions of the pectineus, gracilis, and three hip adductors in the medial thigh (Figure 9-4). As weight shifts toward the non-weight-bearing leg, gravity pulls the body into closed-chain hip adduction. Feel the hip abductors, gluteus medius and tensor fasciae latae, activate to balance gravity's adduction torque once the center of gravity projects to the adductor side of the axis. Closed-chain hip adduction has a ligamentous checkpoint in the iliotibial tract. The ligament itself balances against gravity and tolerates about 20 degrees of hip adduction without active contraction of the tensor fasciae latae to balance gravity's effect (Figure 9-5 and A Closer Look Box 9-1).

Gravity and Muscle Use

In Figure 9-6, **Iris Clark**, who weighs 60 kg, balances on her right foot to reach into an overhead cabinet. Even with

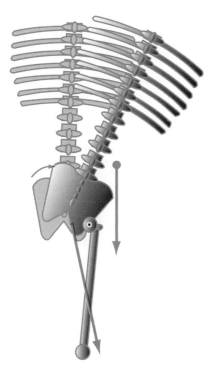

FIGURE **9-4**
Isometric contraction of the hip adductors balances gravity's abduction torque (abduction moment) at the front-to-back hip axis.

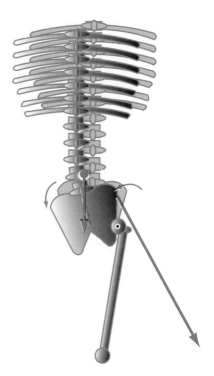

FIGURE **9-5**
Closed-chain hip adduction (pelvic obliquity) by gravity occurs in the absence of a sufficient contraction of the hip abductors. The lateral hip ligament prevents further hip adduction. The *arrow* represents the optional contraction of tensor fasciae latae to balance gravity's closed-chain adduction torque instead of relying on the ligament.

BOX 9-1

A **CLOSER** LOOK

Orthopedic Hip Problems
The head and neck of the femur form an angle of about 125 degrees to the shaft called the neck-shaft angle. Bone formation with a neck-shaft angle greater or less than 125 degrees affects the alignment of the entire lower extremity distal to the hip. Coxa valga, a neck-shaft angle greater than 125 degrees, results in a bowlegged appearance. The original problem begins where the proximal femur connects to the pelvis at the hips (os coxae), but evidence of the problem appears in distal lateral projection of the femurs (valga). Coxa vara, an angle less than 125 degrees, produces a "knock-kneed" appearance because the distal femurs project medially.

The same terms describe opposite effects at the knee (genu). Genu vara describes medial projection of the distal tibia associated with a bowlegged appearance. While they represent opposite problems at two different joints, coxa valga and genu vara both describe a bowlegged appearance. Similarly, coxa vara and genu valga both describe a knock-kneed appearance.

---

the outstretched right arm, her center of gravity projects downward on the adductor side of the front-to-back hip axis, producing a closed-chain adduction tendency. The hip abductors contract isometrically to balance this effect.

In this position, her body weight produces an additional torque, a torque equal to that of the abductors and the weight of the reaching extremity. Specific moment arms help determine the force requirement of the hip abductors. Iris' center of gravity lies to the left of her spine at about lumbar vertebra 3 (L3), approximately 8 cm from the hip axis. The hip abductors exert their combined force 5 cm from the hip axis. The right upper extremity's segmental centers of gravity lie at various distances from the hip joint—45 cm (hand), 40 cm (forearm), and 25 cm (upper arm).

The weight of Iris' head, trunk, and left extremity generates an adduction tendency equal to hip abduction combined with the right upper extremity's tendency to lean the trunk to the right in closed-chain hip abduction (see Figure 9-6, *B*). Calculate the force the hip adductors must exert:

$$60 \text{ kg} \times \text{cm} = (0.4 \text{ kg} \times 45 \text{ cm}) + (0.9 \text{ kg} \times 40 \text{ cm}) + (1.6 \text{ kg} \times 25 \text{ cm}) + (5 \text{ cm} \times \underline{\hspace{2em}} \text{ kg})$$

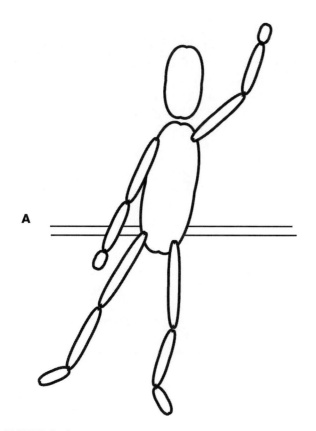

FIGURE 9-6
A, The hip abductors maintain balance at the hip when Iris reaches overhead and to the side. **B**, The hip abductors exert 77.2 kg to maintain balance in this overhead reach.

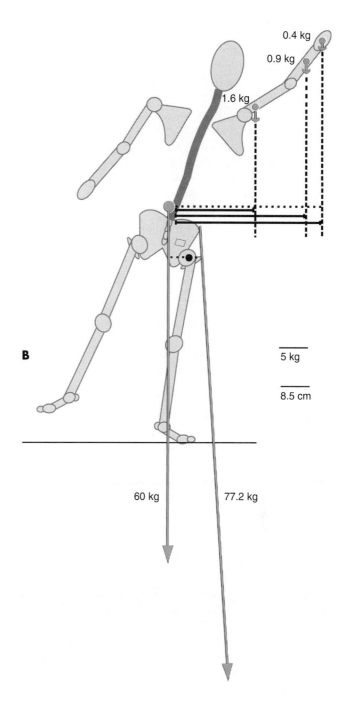

$$480 \text{ kg cm} = (18 \text{ kg cm} + 36 \text{ kg cm} + 40 \text{ kg cm}) +$$
$$(5 \text{ cm} \times \underline{\hspace{1cm}} \text{ kg})$$

$$480 \text{ kg cm} - 94 \text{ kg cm} = 5 \text{ cm} \times \underline{\hspace{1cm}} \text{ kg}$$

$$386 \text{ kg cm}/5 \text{ cm} = 77.2 \text{ kg}$$

Iris' outstretched right arm decreases the amount of force her hip abductors need because its weight combines with the force of the hip abductors to abduct the right hip. Stretching her left hand out would shift her body's center of gravity farther from the spine, creating a longer moment arm for hip adduction. Then Iris' hip abductors would have to increase their force to match the added adduction tendency. If Iris put her left hand on the countertop, weight bearing would create an upward reaction force that would decrease her body's adduction torque on the hip joint. Iris' hip abductors would contract less forcefully to balance her body at the hip joint, making their job easier. Thus upper extremities help maintain balance and decrease the amount of lower-extremity effort.

Since multiple sclerosis often compromises balance reactions, the occupational therapy practitioner performing Iris' kitchen evaluation explains the importance of placing her hand on a countertop (or cane) to correct for reaching movements. He draws a quick diagram that explains how Iris can make use of this information to prevent falls.

Balance at the Knee and Ankle

The same closed-chain analysis applies to ligament stretch, recoil, and isometric muscle contraction acting on the knee and ankle. The knee, a condyloid joint, allows flexion and extension at the side-to-side axis and rotation around the up-to-down axis. Gravity primarily affects the side-to-side axis.

Crystal projects her upper body's center of gravity anterior to the knee's side-to-side axis by assuming lordosis and slightly hyperextending her knees. With this adaptive posture, her center of gravity creates an extension moment balanced by the posteriorly placed knee ligaments and knee flexors, the hamstrings and gastrocnemius. Because her knee's ligaments prevent extension beyond the upright, knee-extended position and her iliofemoral ligament prevents hip extension, Crystal can "hang on" her ligaments to stand. As long as the ligaments remain intact, Crystal stands upright, even on one leg (unilateral weight bearing), with minimal or no muscle contraction.

As in the hip, no ligament balances against gravity-induced knee flexion. When the upper body's center of gravity projects posterior to the side-to-side axis, isometric extensor contractions balance the knee. The quadriceps femoris, attaching onto the tibia distally through the patellar tendon, balances against knee flexion through its proximal attachments on the femur and pelvis.

At the ankle, two muscle groups balance movement at the side-to-side axis for dorsiflexion and plantar flexion. When gravity falls anterior to this axis, posteriorly placed plantar flexors—the gastrocnemius, soleus, and tibialis posterior—activate. When gravity projects posteriorly, ankle dorsiflexors—the tibialis anterior and long toe extensors—equalize gravitational torque on the other side of the axis (A Closer Look Box 9-2). In a standing position, these muscle contractions produce closed-chain movements with muscles acting on their origins to pull the body forward or backward over the ankle.

Lower extremity movements in weight-bearing link movement at one joint with the others. Closed-chain ankle dorsiflexion, knee flexion, and hip flexion occur together in a deep-knee bend. The angle decreases between the dorsum of the foot and the lower leg, just as it does in open-chain dorsiflexion (Figure 9-7). Just as eccentric contraction of the knee extensor (quadriceps) controls knee flexion with gravity, eccentric contraction of the plantar flexor controls ankle dorsiflexion in a deep-knee bend.

Concentric contractions also produce closed-chain movements at the ankle during fine adjustments for balance in weight bearing. Dorsiflexors shorten and pull the tibia forward toward the dorsum of the foot. Slight knee flexion sometimes accompanies this adjustment. Plantar flexor contractions pull the tibia backward, and the knee extends.

During open-chain plantar flexion, the toes point as the forefoot moves in relation to the ankle. During closed-chain plantar flexion, the body stands on its toes.

BOX 9-2

A CLOSER LOOK

Toe Extension in Balance
Stand straight up, feet together, and sway backward just enough that you begin to lose your balance. Notice that your toes curl (toe extension) up as you try to stop yourself from swaying too far backward. What purpose does this serve?

Toe extension indicates projections of your body's center of gravity behind the ankle's axis for dorsiflexion and plantar flexion. The dorsiflexors pull the body forward at the ankle (closed-chain dorsiflexion). Newton's law states that the segment with the least mass moves first. Before the dorsiflexors, including the long toe extensors, pull the entire lower extremity forward onto the foot, the toes extend. If you lean back too far for the dorsiflexors to be effective, taking a step back to increase your base of support helps you maintain balance.

Toes, the distal ends of the lower-extremity chain, plant and stabilize, so the entire body including the heel moves in relation to the toes and metatarsal heads.

Gravity and Muscle Use
We demonstrate closed-chain plantar flexion when we reach toward an overhead cabinet. We examined the effect overhead reaching had on Iris' hip joint earlier, but now we consider its effect on her ankle. Gravity's projection determines responsive muscle activity for maintaining upright posture at the ankle. Iris weighs 60 kg (Figure 9-8, A), and most of that weight shifts onto the ball of her right foot as she reaches high above her head. We can assume that Iris' center of gravity lies slightly to the left of her spine at about L3. It projects downward posterior to the metatarsal heads, producing a force vector for closed-chain dorsiflexion. This vector has a moment arm of 8 cm (from Iris' **center of gravity projection** to the location of the pivot point at her metatarsal heads [Figure 9-8, B]). The gastrocnemius and soleus muscles produce equal torque toward plantar flexion to support Iris' weight.

Because the force of gravity acting on the body falls closer to the axis of motion than the force of the muscles acting against gravity, mechanical advantage belongs to the plantar flexors. The plantar flexors work almost twice as far from the axis (pivot) as Iris' body weight in this example of a second-class lever. Equilibrium of

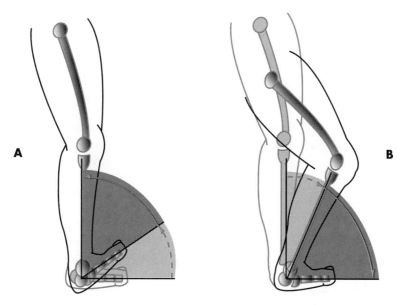

FIGURE **9-7**
The decreasing angle indicates **(A)** open-chain dorsiflexion and **(B)** closed-chain dorsiflexion.

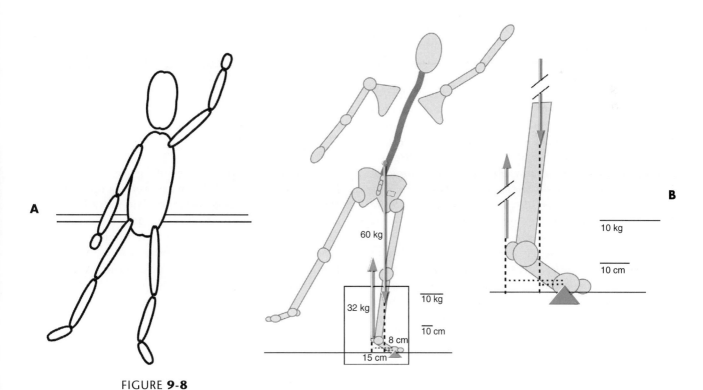

FIGURE **9-8**
A, As Iris reaches into an overhead cabinet, she shifts her weight onto the ball of one foot, which involves plantar flexion of the weight-bearing ankle. **B**, The gastrocnemius and soleus exert 32 kg to produce closed-chain plantar flexion and raise the total body weight onto the balls of the feet (metatarsal heads).

torques helps determine how much muscle force Iris needs to balance on her toes:

$$60 \text{ kg} \times 8 \text{ cm} = \underline{\hspace{1cm}} \text{ kg} \times 15 \text{ cm}$$

$$480 \text{ kg cm} = \underline{\hspace{1cm}} \text{ kg} \times 15 \text{ cm}$$

$$480 \text{ kg cm}/15 \text{ cm} = 32 \text{ kg}$$

Because of their longer moment arms, Iris' muscles exert about half the force of gravity to raise her body's weight.

TOILET TRANSFERS AND THE LOWER EXTREMITY

The hamstrings originate on the ischial tuberosity of the pelvis and continue inferiorly crossing the hip and knee to attach onto the tibia. Together with the gluteus maximus, they extend the hip as the quadriceps femoris extends the knee when an individual stands from a sitting, stooping, or bending position.

Sitting on a toilet of standard height usually demands hip flexion of 90 degrees or more. Since hip flexion stretches the hamstrings, they begin their hip extension contraction at a poor length for tension development. This length–tension disadvantage worsens when leaning forward into even more hip flexion to shift weight while preparing to stand from a toilet. Lack of armrests, assisting the individual to push off, further increases the difficulty.

Mary Smith's balance problems make her especially fearful during toilet transfers, so she avoids leaning forward and tries to stand from an erect sitting posture (Figure 9-9). In the erect position, her center of gravity projects directly through the base of support (toilet) but far behind her transitional base (feet on the floor). Mary must move forward a considerable distance to balance over her transitional base of support. Without this forward movement, Mary begins weight bearing on her feet before she has projected her center of gravity through that transitional base, causing her to fall backward.

The OT practitioner spends some time developing Mary's trust before asking her to lean forward when attempting to stand (Figure 9-10). Mary's head moves over her knees so that her body's center of gravity projects closer to her transitional base of support before she begins to stand. Even with overstretched hamstrings, this makes standing easier on the knees and reduces Mary's risk of falling backward between her feet and the toilet.

Consider the equilibrium torques at Mary's knees at the instant she begins standing and weight bearing through her feet. Her upper-body weight produces torque toward knee flexion balanced by Mary's quadriceps (especially on her right side) producing equal torque toward knee extension. The erect sitting posture (Figure 9-9) places Mary's center of gravity 33 cm from the axis of motion in her knee. The forward-leaning position (Figure 9-10) places her center of gravity 22 cm from the axis of motion at her knee. With this shorter moment arm, Mary's upper-body weight produces less knee flexion torque, and her quadriceps generate less force to extend her knees when she stands.

How much more force do Mary's quadriceps generate when she stands from an erect sitting posture as opposed to a forward-leaning sitting posture? With knees flexed to 90 degrees, the quadriceps operate at a 5-cm moment arm. Because only Mary's upper-body weight produces knee-flexion torque, subtract the weight of her lower extremities from her total 70-kg weight (see Appendix B, Table B-1). Each upper leg comprises 9.7% of her total body weight, each lower leg comprises 4.5%, and each foot comprises 1.4% (round the product):

$$2(0.097 + 0.045 + 0.014) \times 70 \text{ kg} = 21.84 \text{ kg}$$

$$70 \text{ kg} - 22 \text{ kg} = 48 \text{ kg} = \text{weight of body flexing the knee}$$

Calculate the force Mary's quadriceps must produce when she stands from an erect sitting posture:

$$48 \text{ kg} \times 33 \text{ cm} = 5 \text{ cm} \times \underline{\hspace{1cm}} \text{ kg}$$

$$1584 \text{ kg cm}/5 \text{ cm} = \underline{\hspace{1cm}} \text{ kg}$$

$$316.8 \text{ kg}$$

Calculate the force Mary's quadriceps must produce when she stands from a forward-leaning sitting posture:

$$48 \text{ kg} \times 22 \text{ cm} = 5 \text{ cm} \times \underline{\hspace{1cm}} \text{ kg}$$

$$1056 \text{ kg cm}/5 \text{ cm} = \underline{\hspace{1cm}} \text{ kg}$$

$$211.2 \text{ kg}$$

Mary needs approximately 100-kg greater quadriceps force when she stands from an erect as opposed to a forward-leaning sitting posture. The extra force produces an unnecessary strain that Mary cannot handle. Leaning forward clearly gives a superior advantage, but Mary's quadriceps still must exert considerable force for her to stand from a forward-leaning sitting posture.

Individuals with weak quadriceps like Mary's benefit from leaning forward and using armrests to push themselves up when they stand from sitting positions. Placing the hands on armrests allows closed-chain scapular depression and elbow extension to contribute to the effort. Closed-chain elbow extension and scapular depression each produce upward trunk movement. Another important adaptation, the raised toilet seat, reduces the torque of the upper body at the knees, reducing work load on the quadriceps (A Closer Look Box 9-3).

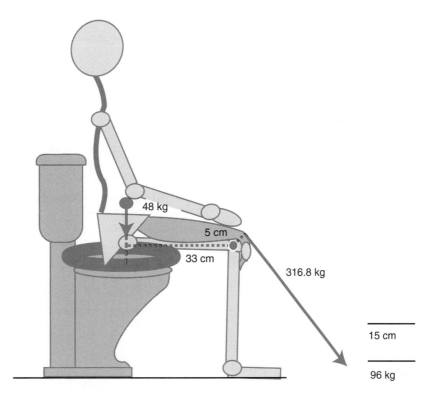

FIGURE **9-9**
Mary tries to stand from an erect sitting posture. Her quadriceps muscle produces 316.8 kg of force to balance the downward pull of gravity on the upper body.

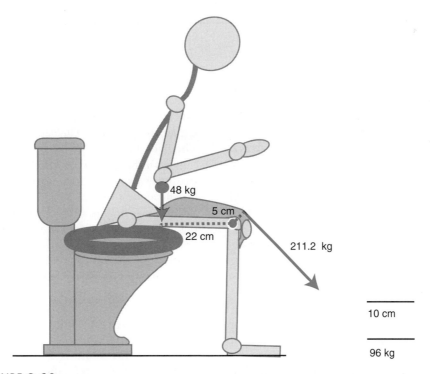

FIGURE **9-10**
Mary leans forward before standing. Her quadriceps produce 211.2 kg of force to balance her upper-body weight.

A **CLOSER** LOOK

Benefits of Raised Toilet Seats

Raised toilet seats prevent the erect upper body from developing a longer moment arm when an individual sits on the toilet. When the individual stands, the upper-body weight projects through the knee axis, so no flexion moment exists at the knee. Sitting causes the upper body to move backward in relation to the feet and knees, and the moment arm for knee flexion increases to maximum length in full sitting position (hips and knees flexed to 90 degrees).

The raised toilet seat allows the individual to sit with less than 90 degrees of hip and knee flexion, preventing development of the upper body's long moment arm for knee flexion. Standing from this raised position involves less quadriceps force because the upper-body weight pulls down with a shorter moment arm at the knee and produces less knee-flexion torque. Raising sofa and chair legs onto blocks approximates this result, but such efforts get dissipated by soft, sinkable cushions.

Wheelchair Adjustments Affecting Stability and Pressure

Wheelchairs provide a number of adjustments for comfort, fit, and stability. Even "bare minimum" models like those preferred for cost savings in long-term care settings provide a few adjustments for leg length. Staff often neglect simple adjustments like footrests. Many individuals in long-term care facilities, hospitals, and rehabilitation centers rest their feet at two different heights and varying degrees of internal or external rotation. Footrest adjustment affects pressure distribution, stability in positioning, and comfort. Adjusting footrests requires the use of one wrench and a few minutes of time, but this small amount of effort produces big gains for the wheelchair user.

Low footrests place excessive pressure on the posterior thighs, threatening venous return from the leg and foot as well as normal and shear forces on the skin and subcutaneous tissue. Low footrests promote posterior pelvic tilt as the buttocks slide forward. Posterior pelvic tilt leads to sacral sitting posture, reversed lumbar curve, and pressure sores on the sacrum and lumbar spines.

High footrests shift pressure distribution from the posterior thighs to the ischial tuberosities, also promoting posterior pelvic tilt as increased hip flexion pulls the ischial tuberosities forward through the hamstring link.

Recall that hip flexion stretches the hamstrings. With short hamstrings additional hip flexion from high footrests pulls the pelvis into posterior tilt, leading to sacral sitting posture and a rounded lower back. Both effects promote the development of pressure sores through excessive normal and shear forces on tissue overlying the ischial tuberosities.

Correctly adjusted footrests place the hips near 90 degrees and position the posterior thighs in contact with the seat or cushion surface, bearing some but not excessive weight. Remember to readjust the footrests when using seat cushions.

We rotate footrests so that the feet rest in a neutral forward position whenever other footrest adjustments are made. Toes rotated inward or outward usually cause discomfort and appear awkward. When footrest rotation moves far enough out of alignment, individuals often opt to cease using their footrests, creating the same problems associated with low footrests. (See A Closer Look Box 9-4 for a checklist of wheelchair adjustments and their effects.)

Normal Gait and Variations

People write entire books about walking. This section describes an overview of the *gait cycle* for a broad understanding of the joint movements and muscle activation patterns. Practitioners interested in designing interventions around gait problems should pursue reading, continuing education, and consultation with physical therapy practitioners who have expertise in this area.

The phrase *gait cycle* describes the sequence of motions occurring in normal walking. A full gait cycle encompasses the series of motions occurring between the time one lower extremity makes contact with the floor until it makes contact again. The gait cycle consists of two phases. The first, the stance phase, includes initial contact of the heel with the ground, loading of the body's weight onto the lower extremity for midstance and terminal stance, and lifting of the heel off the ground into preswing. The swing phase begins as the toe leaves the ground, continues as the lower extremity accelerates into midswing, and ends after it decelerates into terminal swing.

During initial contact and loading in stance, the knee and hip extensors stabilize the supporting lower extremity to carry the weight of the body. Dorsiflexors eccentrically contract to prevent the foot and toes of the supporting extremity from slapping the ground. Hip stabilizers (abductors) like the gluteus medius maintain the body's alignment over the supporting leg to balance gravity's pull toward closed-chain hip adduction while the weight shifts medially onto the inside of the supporting foot. By midstance ankle dorsiflexion continues as the plantar flexors eccentrically prevent the

BOX 9-4

A **CLOSER** L O O K

Positioning

Consider the three pelvic movements/positions (tilt—in sagittal plane, obliquity—in frontal plane, and rotation—in transverse plane) and the adverse effect in each of the following scenarios:

- Cushion/seat too deep: posterior pelvic tilt
- Footrest too low: posterior pelvic tilt
- Unilateral hip extension contracture: pelvic obliquity or pelvic rotation; in either case, misplacement occurs on the side with the hip extension contracture; a left hip extension contracture yields obliquity when the left iliac crest is higher than the right or rotation with the left side is protracted
- Sling upholstery hammocking: pelvic obliquity and increased weight on one ischial tuberosity or on both trochanters
- Seat too wide: lack of support, increased risk of scoliosis
- Attempting to position knees forward in case of unilateral hip adduction contracture: pelvic rotation with protraction of the iliac crest opposite the side of contracture
- 70-degree footrests with very short hamstrings bilaterally: posterior pelvic tilt
- Lack of lumbar support with flexible spine: reversed lumbar curve and posterior pelvic tilt
- Lumbar support with fixed lumbar kyphosis: no change in vertebral curves; lumbar pad pushes pelvis forward, resulting in decreased weight distribution to the posterior thighs; increase pressure on spinous processes and ischial tuberosities.
- Increased back recline with axis at the level of the upper lumbar area: support for anterior pelvic tilt
- Increased back recline with seat-level axis versus tilt-in-space: recline leads to closed-chain hip extension, posterior pelvic tilt, and sliding out; tilt-in-space maintains 90-degree hips and good pelvic position

body from falling forward at the ankles. Hip stabilizers, including the tensor fasciae latae and iliotibial band, help to balance the upper body over the supporting extremity.

In terminal stance the plantar flexors support the body weight while the momentum of the swinging leg helps propel the body forward. Hip stabilizers maintain balance over the supporting extremity, and weight remains on the inside of the foot for added stability. The flexor of the great toe provides the individual the power to push. As weight shifts during preswing, the erector spinae, lower abdominals, and hip abductors contract to stabilize the trunk and counterbalance pelvic movement. Plantar flexors and toe flexors provide a final push before the stance leg leaves the ground.

Hip flexors pull the swinging leg off the ground to initiate a forward progression and continue that activity throughout the swing. In initial swing the dorsiflexors concentrically contract to ensure the toes and foot clear the ground. Dorsiflexors continue into midswing while the erector spinae on the swing side counterbalance the trunk's lateral flexion tendency as the upper body sways slightly toward the stance side. The iliopsoas brings the leg forward into terminal swing while the hip extensors eccentrically contract to control the swing's momentum.

Knee extensors keep the leg straight in preparation for heel strike, and dorsiflexors keep the foot from slapping the ground on contact.

RUNNING

Running follows a sequence similar to normal gait except that both feet come off the ground immediately after terminal stance on one side and before initial contact on the other. Raising the body off the ground and propelling it with greater speed demands more muscle force Consequently, the lower extremity and spine must absorb greater impact forces.

JUMPING AND HOPPING

Jumping and hopping require greater muscle force from the knee and hip extensors as well as plantar and toe flexors to propel the body into the air. The same muscles absorb the returning weight through eccentric contractions as hip, knee, and ankle joints move into flexion and dorsiflexion upon and after impact. Strong hip stabilizers maintain balance over one leg when hopping.

CRAWLING AND CLIMBING

The sartorius runs diagonally from the ilium to the proximal medial tibia. It flexes the hip and knee while externally rotating the femur, as in cross-legged sitting or highland dancing. Active in normal gait movements, the sartorius functions more fully in the simultaneous hip and knee flexion found while crawling, marching, or climbing stairs. In crawling or climbing, the sartorius positions the legs so that the quadriceps and gluteus maximus gain the ideal position for propelling the body forward or upward.

Biomechanical Analysis

Every time we consider movements and the muscles used we analyze these actions with biomechanical analysis. Our recent discussion of gait, for example, used information obtained from biomechanical analysis. Often, computer analysis uses sophisticated equipment to provide multiple views of an activity. Electromyographic recordings monitor muscle activity by recording the actual electrical event of muscle activation.

OT practitioners generally use visual analysis to determine the joints, their movements, and the muscles used in these movements. Analysis allows identification of problematic links in ineffective function. For example, careful observation of someone experiencing difficulty eating might yield the discovery that this individual's lack of extreme supination, typically necessary for this task, presents a barrier to independence. Ultimate improvement hinges on identifying limited supination as the problem. Use of a different grip pattern might remove the need for supination in hand-to-mouth movements and restore an individual's independence in eating.

Initial attempts at biomechanical analysis often seem overwhelming. Indeed, only electromyographic analysis definitively confirms muscle use in activity. Nonetheless, clinically relevant biomechanical analysis holds an important place in OT practice.

Determining muscle activation in the context of activity performance requires consideration of each movement of the activity in relation to the resistance encountered. Does the movement occur against or with gravity? Does the movement occur against some resistance greater than gravity's pull? Does the movement occur rapidly? Each question helps the OT practitioner make an educated guess about the muscle groups responsible for movement.[2]

Figure 9-11 summarizes a form for biomechanical analysis. Find a copy of the referenced article for a thorough presentation of the process used to complete the form in Appendix G. We use this process to analyze daily activities such as donning shoes and socks to identify specific, problematic joints or muscle groups.

George O'Hara lives in a group home. His caretakers have noticed more dependence on others for dressing after a recent hospital admission for pneumonia. The OT practitioner observes George cross one leg over the other to reach his foot when he dons his shoes and socks.

To analyze this activity, determine which lower-extremity movements he uses and identify hip flexion and hip external rotation (Table 9-1). Analyze hip flexion from left to right across the form. Move back to the left of the form, and begin the process for the next movement observed. Stay focused on one movement to narrow the options. Proceed through all other joints involved, one segment at a time.

Beginning the process with hip flexion, estimate the percentage of full range of motion used to identify any extreme of joint range. In this case, crossing one leg uses more than 50% of hip flexion in the crossed-leg position (50% or 90 degrees being necessary for sitting). Indicate this percentage by marking >50% in the table and placing an asterisk in the box to highlight an extreme. Individuals experience difficulty in aspects of tasks requiring extreme joint motions. Identifying extremes helps locate problematic links.

Next, discern the active muscle group by asking several questions. Is the motion (hip flexion) rapid or resisted by an external object or force? George dons his socks and shoes without experiencing either. Does the movement (hip flexion) occur with or against gravity? Movements against gravity require concentric activation of the agonist named for the motion. Eccentric contraction of the antagonists controls movements when gravity provides the main force for movement. George flexes his hip against gravity, so he uses his hip flexors in concentric contraction.

Consider what happens with this same hip flexion when George lies supine in bed to don his socks. Initial hip flexion occurs against gravity, but once the hip flexes past 90 degrees, gravity assists this motion and his hip extensors act as the active group in eccentric contraction. If George had weak hip flexors, the supine position would allow them to contract through less range—0 to 90 degrees instead of 0 to more than 90 degrees of flexion. Furthermore, if George donned socks in bed, he could bring his hip up while he lay sideways, never having to contract weak hip flexors against gravity's resistance.

After identifying the motion and active muscle group, analyze the muscle contractions necessary to hold a position. George holds his hip flexed as he manipulates and places the shoe or sock on his foot. Ask the same questions as before to determine the active muscle group. Does he hold this position (hip flexion) against some

SEGMENT		INITIAL MOTION			HOLDING POSITION			
MOTION/ POSITION OBSERVED	% ROM	RESISTED OR RAPID	GRAVITY ASSISTS/ RESISTS	AGONIST GROUP/ CONTRACTION TYPE (CON OR ECC)	RESISTED	GRAVITY EFFECT	ISOMETRIC AGONIST	REP
V FLEX *Reaching for foot*	*50%*	*No*	*Assists*	*Extensors/ECC*	*No*	*Promotes flexion*	*Extensors*	*No*
V EXT *Returning from flexion*	*N/A*	*No*	*Resists*	*Extensors/CON*	*N/A*			
V L-ROT *Turning to reach right foot*	*<50%*	*No*	*No*	*Left rotators/CON*	*No*	*None*	*Left rotators*	*No*
S PRO *Reaching forward*	*>50%*	*Slight resistance at end*	*Slight assist*	*Protractors/CON*	*Slightly*	*Little if any*	*Protractors*	*No*
S RET *Pulling sock*	*N/A*	*Resisted*	*N/A*	*Retractors/CON*	*N/A*			
GH FLEX *Reaching forward and placing sock*	*<50%*	*No*	*Resists*	*Flexors/CON*	*No*	*Promotes extension*	*Flexors*	*No*
E FLEX *Positioning- Pulling sock-*	*<50% 50%*	*No Resisted*	*Resists N/A*	*Flexors/CON Flexors/CON*	*No N/A*	*Promotes extension*	*Flexors*	*No*

FIGURE **9-11**
Format for clinical biomechanical analysis of donning socks. Analysis of motion involving the vertebral joints, scapula, glenohumeral, and elbow joints. *ROM*, Range of motion; *CON*, concentric; *ECC*, eccentric; *REP*, repetition; *V FLEX*, vertebral flexion; *V EXT*, vertebral extension; *V L-ROT*, vertebral left rotation; *S PRO*, scapular protraction; *S RET*, scapular retraction; *GH FLEX*, glenohumeral flexion; *E FLEX*, elbow flexion; and *N/A*, not applicable. (Modified from Greene D: A clinically relevant approach to biomechanical analysis of function, *Occup Ther Pract* 1(4):44-52, 1990.)

external resistance? Does he hold this position (hip flexion) against gravity?

Gravity causes hip extension, so George's hip flexors may appear active. However, George crosses one leg and rests it instead of holding his foot in the air with isometric contraction of the hip flexors. Gravity pulls his hip into extension, but the thigh of his supporting lower extremity matches that force. George's OT practitioner concludes that hip flexors need not contract to maintain his observable hip flexion.

We perform some movements against gravity via contraction of one muscle group but maintain that position with isometric contraction of the opposite group:

Xavier Morales works under his car and reaches, extending his elbow to pick up a wrench from the floor. Lifting the wrench,

Xavier's elbow flexes against gravity. Past 90 degrees, gravity helps flex the elbow. Xavier uses his elbow flexors to bring the wrench into position, but he holds it in position against gravity's flexion effect with his elbow extensor. Xavier's elbow extensors stay active as long as he uses the wrench. In other words, his extensor maintains his elbow flexion.

Practitioners rarely perform formal, written biomechanical analyses, but problem-solving based on biomechanical analysis of activity proves valuable in OT practice. Practitioners commonly analyze activity, but their familiarity with the process and their intuitive approach render the endeavor indiscernible to unfamiliar observers. Even OT students who realize the importance sometimes wonder why they "have to write it all out" in school. Visual analysis involves a lengthy thought process that requires practice and attention.

TABLE 9-1
Biomechanical Analysis of the Donning of Socks and Shoes

SEGMENT		INITIAL MOTION			HOLDING POSITION			
MOTION/POSITION OBSERVED	% ROM	RESISTED OR RAPID	GRAVITY ASSISTS/ RESISTS	AGONIST GROUP/ CONTRACTION TYPE (CON OR ECC)	RESISTED	GRAVITY EFFECT	ISOMETRIC AGONIST	REP
H FLEX Lifting of one leg to cross over other	>50% *	Neither	Resists	Hip flexors/CON	N/A	N/A	N/A	No
Holding of position during donning of socks and shoes	>50% *	N/A	N/A	N/A	No	Hip extension while support of other lower extremity holds hip flexion	None	No

H FLEX, Hip flexion; *ROM,* range of motion; *CON,* concentric; *ECC,* eccentric; *N/A,* not applicable; *REP,* repetition.
*Indicates extreme joint movement.

Writing out the analysis illustrates the steps involved. Step by step, biomechanical analysis becomes as easy as it looks.

Summary

Most individuals think of the lower extremities solely in terms of walking; however, the lower extremities do more than just transport the body from place to place. Muscles at the hip produce closed-chain actions that move and position the trunk for reach. They also balance the trunk at the hip in sitting and maintain the center of gravity projection through the **base of support** in standing. The weight shifts required in sitting, standing, and walking involve lateral trunk flexion and extension, forward flexion, and inclination of the trunk through closed-chain abduction, adduction, flexion, and extension of the hip.

Biomechanical analysis provides a tool for the understanding of function through systematic determination of movement, position, and muscle activation. Biomechanical analysis concentrates on details—components of movement and positioning. Ultimately, biomechanical analysis and a heightened understanding of the musculoskeletal system through kinesiology enrich the clinical perspective. An informed view leads to more effective problem-solving. Through adaptation, we, as OT practitioners, can transform or reincorporate impaired function so that the tasks essential for role performance keep individuals actively engaged at home and in their communities.

Applications

■ APPLICATION **9-1**
Muscle Shortening During Hip Flexion
Place the heel of your hand on the anterior pelvis (anterior superior iliac spine) and the fingertips just distal to the anterior hip crease. In this position your hand represents the deep hip flexors (iliopsoas). Lift one foot off the ground using hip and knee flexion. While you flex the hip, keep your fingertips in one place on the anterior thigh and allow the fingers to flex as the proximal thigh approaches the trunk. This simulates the shortening of the hip flexors.

Put the foot down again, allowing your fingers to extend with the moving thigh. With the hand still in place, bend over at the hip with a straight back, as if to stretch the hamstrings. What happens to the fingers in this movement? How do these two movements—lifting the foot versus bending over—compare?

■ APPLICATION **9-2**
Open- and Closed-Chain Hip Abduction
Use your hand to mark the origin and insertion of a hip abductor. Place your left hand on the lateral aspect of the left hip with the heel of your hand on the iliac crest and your fingertips over the trochanter. Stand on your right foot and raise your left leg into abduction, foot out to the side of the body. Watch the fingers curl as the lateral thigh comes up. Now, stand on the left leg with your left hand still in place, allowing your right foot to leave the ground as you lean and bend to the left. What happens

to the fingers in this movement? How do these two movements—abduction of the left leg to the side versus leaning and bending to the left—compare?

See Appendix C for solutions to Applications.

REFERENCES

1. Behrman RE, Kliegman R, Arvin AM: *Textbook of pediatrics,* ed 15, Philadelphia, 1996, WB Saunders (CD-ROM).
2. Greene D: A clinically relevant approach to biomechanical analysis of function, *Occup Ther Pract* 1(4):44-52, 1990.

RELATED READINGS

Calliet R: *Low back pain syndrome,* ed 2, Philadelphia, 1968, FA Davis.

Calliet R: *Understanding your backache: a guide to prevention, treatment, and relief,* Philadelphia, 1984, FA Davis.
Hockenberry J: *Moving violations, war zones, wheelchairs, and declarations of independence,* New York, 1995, Hyperion.
Luttgens K: *Kinesiology: scientific basis of human motion,* ed 9, New York, 1996, McGraw-Hill.
Nordin M, Frankel VH: *Basic biomechanics of the musculoskeletal system,* ed 3, Philadelphia, 2001, Lippincott Williams & Wilkins.
Pedretti LW, Early MB: *Occupational therapy practice skills for physical dysfunction,* ed 5, St Louis, 2001, Mosby.
Trombly CA, Radomski MV: *Occupational therapy for physical dysfunction,* ed 5, Baltimore, 2002, Lippincott Williams & Wilkins.
Wiktorin CH, Nordin M: *Introduction to problem solving in biomechanics,* Philadelphia, 1986, Lea & Febiger.
Williams PL, Bannister LH: *Gray's anatomy: the anatomical basis of medicine and surgery,* ed 38, New York, 1995, Churchill Livingstone.

LAB BOX

Find applied activities exploring concepts in Chapter 9 in the following laboratory exercises:

Topic	Laboratory
Toilet transfers – foot placement and leaning forward	**Lab 2** Stability, Balance, Wheelchairs, Min Assist Transfers
Hip, knee and ankle in positioning; wheelchair adjustments affecting posture, stability and pressure	**Lab 13** Positioning in a wheelchair
Biomechanical Analysis	**Biomechanical Analysis Lab**

Appendixes

English to Metric Conversions

Throughout history, most cultures have required a commonly understood system of weights and measurements that allows for sharing of information and trade goods. Like those of the Babylonians, Egyptians, and Romans, the English system of weights and measures developed from body measurements. The more variable digit, palm, span, and cubit became a more uniform inch, foot, and yard through royal decrees. This system was used wherever English was the language of trade from the seventeenth through nineteenth centuries.

In the early eighteenth century, the French attempted to establish a uniform system of measurement that would be used throughout Europe and European territories. The British refused to be involved in developing the new system; therefore it was developed entirely by French academicians. The new system was based on the meter, a measurement that was {1/10,000,000} of the distance from the North Pole to the equator on a line passing through Paris.

A great deal of resistance to the new system emerged, even in France, but by the nineteenth century the system caught on among scientists because units of measurement reliably could be reproduced. The system was revised and modernized by the General Conference of Weights and Measures in 1960. It is called *Le Systeme International d'Unites* (International System of Units), which is abbreviated as SI.

Because this metric system is used by most of the world, it is the system of measurement used throughout this book. Table A-1 gives the most common conversions needed in biomechanical analysis.

TABLE A-1
Common british to metric conversions

BRITISH UNIT	×	= SI UNIT	×	= BRITISH UNIT
Length				
Inches (in)	2.54	Centimeters (cm)	0.3937	Inches
Feet (ft)	0.3048	Meters (m)	39.37	Inches
Yard (yd)	0.9144	Meters		
Mile	1.609	Kilometers (km)		
Mass				
Pounds (lb)	0.4536	Kilograms (kg)	2.205	Pounds
Slug	14.594	Kilograms		
Force				
Pound	4.4482	Newtons (N)	0.2248	Pounds

Body Segment Parameters

Measurements of the human body are needed to solve most problems in biomechanics. Whenever possible, actual measurements should be taken. However, statistical research data are used for proportional weight and center of gravity in each body segment because actual measurement cannot be made on living subjects.

The primary data for average body weights and centers of gravity were taken from a study done on eight elderly male cadavers.[*] These data have been revised by other researchers to make allowances for differences in age and gender; however, Dempster's data continue to

be widely used. Adaptations of these data, presented in Table B-1 and Figure B-1, give estimates adequate for most problem solving in the OT clinic. More exact data may be obtained by consulting bioengineers or human factors specialists.

Figure B-1 provides the percentage of distance from either end of each body segment to that segment's center of gravity. These measurements are used to determine moment arms in problems involving torque. Table B-1 gives the proportional weight of each body segment, also used to calculate torque.

TABLE B-1

Proportional percentages of body segments to total body weight

BODY SEGMENT	% OF TOTAL BODY WEIGHT
Head and neck	7.9
Trunk with head and neck	56.5
Upper arm	2.7
Forearm	1.5
Hand	0.6
Thigh	9.7
Lower leg	4.5
Foot	1.4

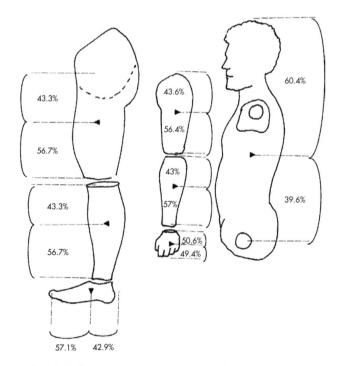

FIGURE **B-1**
Center of gravity for each body segment as a percentage of distance from the end of the segment.

[*]Dempster WT: *Space requirements of the seated operator,* WADC technical report 55-159, Fairborn, Ohio, 1995, Wright-Patterson Air Force Base.

Solutions to Chapter Applications

Chapter 2 Solutions

■ APPLICATION **2-1**
Appreciating Mass and Gravity

The atomic number for lead is 82 (from the periodic table); the atomic number for aluminum is 13. The difference in weight is proportional to the different atomic numbers. Gravity's effect is to accelerate each element to the ground at a rate of approximately 10 kg-m/sec^2; therefore the difference in weight is due only to the difference in mass.

■ APPLICATION **2-2**
Identifying the Active Muscle

1. The triceps should be stiffer than the biceps. If you are unsure, palpate these muscles directly on the skin so that clothing will not interfere with touch.
2. Again the triceps is active. The biceps remains quiet. Be sure to use only the strength necessary to do the task. Unnecessary straining leads to contraction of muscles surrounding the joint, which may skew results.
3. The triceps still is active.
4. The triceps long head origin-to-insertion distance increases as the elbow flexes, and the muscle lengthens as it contracts. These actions do not appear to make sense from an anatomical perspective. A muscle contraction that occurs when the muscle elongates is an eccentric contraction. The weight of the book pulls the elbow into flexion, and the contraction of the triceps controls the effect of the book on the elbow. We see eccentric contractions whenever we control the effect of gravity (moving slowly downward).
5. When you hold the book steady, this involves an isometric contraction of the triceps. The length of the triceps (as implied by the unchanged origin-to-insertion distance) is unchanged.
6. When you raise the book up, the origin-to-insertion distance shortens. Because the triceps again is active and shortened, the action is a concentric contraction. We see concentric contractions when we move against the effect of gravity (moving upward).

Regardless of elbow motion, the elbow extensors are active throughout these movements. The situation is the same with a push-up. Which muscle is active throughout the elbow motion in a pull-up?

Chapter 3 Solutions

■ APPLICATION **3-1**
Creation of a Mobile

The answer depends on the objects used in the mobile. Generally, an object is balanced if it assumes any position in which it is placed.

■ APPLICATION **3-2**
Scale Drawing of Your Lab Partner

Refer to Appendix B and Table 3-1 to determine this solution.

■ APPLICATION **3-3**
Vector Indicating Gravity's Effect on a Laundry Basket

Decide on a scale for a drawing of the vector; for example, 5 kg (or 50 N) equals 1 cm. (Note that only in a scale for a drawing is a measure of weight equal to a measure of distance.) Figure C-1 shows the weight of the basket drawn as a vector. The vector indicating a half-full basket of laundry would be half as long.

■ APPLICATION **3-4**
Force of Gravity Acting on a Spoon

To find the center of gravity for the spoon, balance it on a finger. The point at which the spoon balances is its center of gravity. Indicate this center with a dot on the drawing. In the figure the spoon's center of gravity lies at the junction of the handle and the bowl of the spoon.

In Figure C-2 the arrows point directly downward regardless of the angle of the spoon. The center of gravity remains the same no matter how an object is positioned. Gravity always pulls toward the center of the Earth. The vector's length remains the same in each diagram because it indicates the actual force gravity exerts on the spoon.

■ APPLICATION **3-5**
Force of Gravity Acting on Spoons of Different Weights

Draw a diagram of each spoon. To find each spoon's center of gravity, balance the spoon on a finger as before. The center of gravity, which is affected by weight distribution, may differ by several centimeters from the

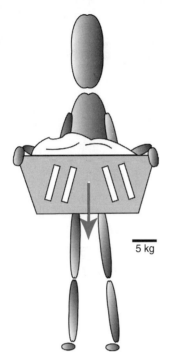

FIGURE **C-1**
A vector representing 10 kg points directly downward from the center of this laundry basket.

previous exercise. Individual spoons must be balanced to find each one's center of gravity.

The spoon with the built-up handle weighs 0.02 kg more than the regular spoon. (This is indicated in Figure C-3 by a slightly longer arrow.) Gravity vectors point directly downward regardless of the angle of the object itself. The vector originates at a different point in the length of the spoon due to the greater mass on the

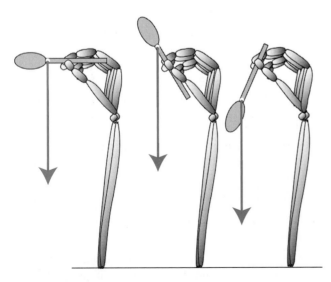

FIGURE **C-2**
Regardless of the spoon's position, the vector representing gravity always points directly downward.

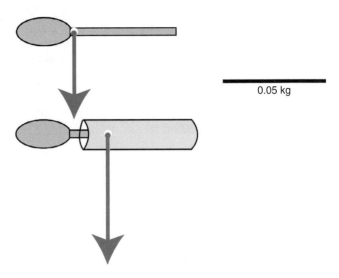

0.05 kg

FIGURE **C-3**
The extra weight of the built-up handle shifts the spoon's center of gravity from the bowl of the spoon.

handle end in the adapted spoon. For the best comparison, keep vectors to scale and indicate the proportions on the diagram.

Chapter 4 Solutions

■ APPLICATION **4-1**
Adding Forces and Establishing Equilibrium
Determining the amount of force is a simple problem of addition and subtraction based on the idea that downward forces must equal upward forces. The idea is represented as a formula by the equation $\Sigma F = 0$. Thus the summation of forces in each direction (up and down) equals zero. Put another way, $F_{up} = F_{down}$. Set up the equation with values of all the forces involved and solve for the unknown amount:

$$x = 3.5 \text{ N} + 5 \text{ N} + 3 \text{ N}$$

$$x = 11.5 \text{ N directed upward}$$

Stated as the summation of forces, assign the positive sign to all forces in one direction and the negative sign to all forces in the opposite direction (see Figure 4-2):

$$\Sigma F = 0 = 3.5 \text{ N} + 5 \text{ N} + 3 \text{ N} - 11.5 \text{ N}$$

■ APPLICATION **4-2**
Adding Forces
Add the 60-N force of the wrist weight to the 70-N force of the bucket of sand for total downward weight:

$$60 \text{ N} + 70 \text{ N} = 130 \text{ N}$$

A graphic representation should show the two vectors drawn in line, one starting where the other ends (see Figure 4-13, *B*). Using a scale of 10 N = 0.5 cm, the resultant force measures 6.5 cm, the combined length of both vectors. Spiros must exert more than 130 N of upward force.

■ APPLICATION 4-3
Finding the Resultant Force
Subtract the 40-N upward force from the 60-N downward force of the cast. Henry uses slightly more than 20 N of force to lift his arm.

$$60\ N - 40\ N = 20\ N$$

■ APPLICATION 4-4
Combining Forces
George's vector is 225 N to the right. Raul's vector is oriented upward at a right angle to George's so that it meets the diagonal line, representing the 350 N of force it takes to move the cart.

Use the Pythagorean theorem to determine an absolute value for Raul's vector:

$$a^2 + b^2 = c^2$$

$$a^2 + 225^2 = 350^2$$

$$a^2 + 50,625 = 122,500$$

$$a^2 = 122,500 - 50,625$$

$$a^2 = 71,875$$

$$a = 268\ N$$

Draw the parallelogram with a scale of 50 N = 1 cm (see Figure 4-17). George's vector measures 4.5 cm long oriented to the right. The diagonal vector is 7 cm long oriented upward and to the right at about 45 degrees to George's vector. Raul's vector measures 4.7 cm long oriented upward. Raul must push more than twice as hard this time to move the cart.

■ APPLICATION 4-5
Determining Force Capability
For a general idea, estimate the bulk of the biceps muscle by palpating it and grasping it between your thumb and index finger. (You may need to apply some resistance to make it easier to see and feel the muscle.) Remove your hand and hold the contour of the fingers representing the shape of the muscle. Trace this on paper and close the circle with a curved line. Find the cross section by measuring the height and width of the circle and multiplying them. (Use centimeters because centimeters are the units of the constant provided in this example.) Multiply the cross section by the constant for vertebrate skeletal muscle, 100 N/cm².

■ APPLICATION 4-6
Determining Excursion
Measure the length of the long head of the triceps from the infraglenoid tubercle to the olecranon with the upper extremity in full shoulder and elbow flexion. Divide this number by 2 to find the muscle's approximate maximal excursion.

■ APPLICATION 4-7
Drawing Vectors Indicating Contractions
Figure C-4 shows the three vectors drawn correctly. Each begins at the insertion and demonstrates a force directed proximally because in each case it is the insertion that moves. In all three conditions the same weight is used, and all three forces differ in amount. The three magnitudes indicate overcoming the weight in a concentric contraction (see Figure C-4, *A*), holding the weight in an isometric contraction (see Figure C-4, *B*), and lowering the weight in an eccentric contraction (see Figure C-4, *C*). Therefore the longest vector indicates the concentric contraction.

Chapter 5 Solutions

■ APPLICATION 5-1
Effort Needed To Open and Close a Valve
You probably noticed more effort was needed to turn on the water when you held the lever closer to the connecting screw than when you held it toward the end of the lever. The connecting screw is the center of rotation, the axis. The placement of your fingers determines the distance of the force from the axis; thus the lever length from the screw to your finger placement is the moment arm.

■ APPLICATION 5-2
External Torque Produced by a Barbell
Figure C-5 shows an elbow flexed in four positions— 30, 60, 90, and 120 degrees. All the segments and force vectors are drawn to scale. Draw the moment arms using the method described in this chapter. Notice that for many of the elbow positions, you move the T square along the force and never reach a point at which you can draw a perpendicular between the force and the axis. When this occurs use a dotted line to extend the force in the direction needed to draw the perpendicular distance. To estimate the length of the moment arm, measure with a ruler and convert to the scale shown.

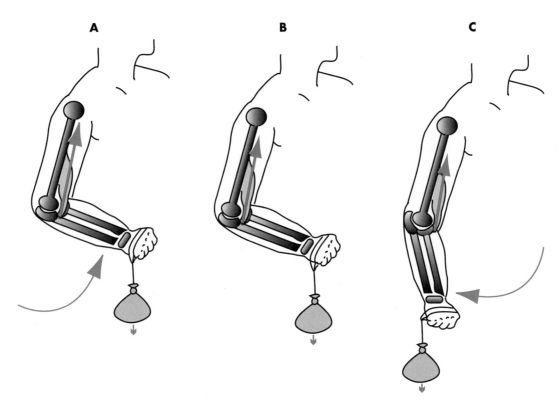

FIGURE **C-4**
Each vector begins at the insertion and demonstrates a force directed proximally in a
concentric contraction **(A)**, an isometric contraction **(B)**, and an eccentric contraction **(C)**.

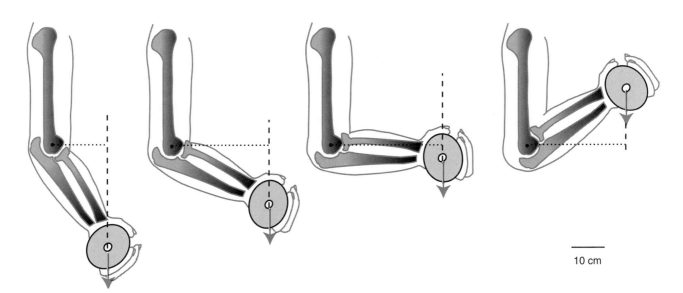

10 cm

FIGURE **C-5**
The factors involved in external torque. Vectors and moment arms are drawn to scale.

Converting kilograms to newtons, multiply the length of the moment arm by the force of the barbell to obtain the value of the torque produced by the barbell. The following equations demonstrate the torque present at elbow positions of 30, 60, 90, and 120 degrees of flexion, respectively:

$$50 \text{ N} \times 17 \text{ cm} = 850 \text{ N-cm}$$

$$50 \text{ N} \times 30 \text{ cm} = 1500 \text{ N-cm}$$

$$50 \text{ N} \times 34 \text{ cm} = 1700 \text{ N-cm}$$

$$50 \text{ N} \times 30 \text{ cm} = 1500 \text{ N-cm}$$

External torque changes throughout the range of motion as the length of the moment arm changes.

■ APPLICATION 5-3
Force Produced by the Biceps

Figure C-6 shows four figures representing the four ranges of motion. Lines representing the distance to the biceps tendon and the force of the biceps are drawn to scale. The biceps pulls directly upward and parallel to the humerus. Each elbow position can be set up as an equilibrium equation because we know from the previous application how much torque is created by the 5-kg weight. The following equations illustrate the torque present at elbow positions of 30, 60, 90, and 120 degrees of flexion, respectively. Answers to these equations have been rounded:

$$141.7 \text{ N} \times 6 \text{ cm} = 850 \text{ N-cm}$$

$$187.5 \text{ N} \times 8 \text{ cm} = 1500 \text{ N-cm}$$

$$200 \text{ N} \times 8.5 \text{ cm} = 1700 \text{ N-cm}$$

$$250 \text{ N} \times 6 \text{ cm} = 1500 \text{ N-cm}$$

The biceps moment arm changes throughout the range of motion. The biceps force changes to match the torque created in the opposite direction by the barbell. Internal torque usually operates in response to external torque. Supporting a weight held in the hand translates into creating enough torque internally to match the effect of the external torque operating at the same joint, the elbow in the opposite direction.

■ APPLICATION 5-4
Balance Needed To Hold a Tray of Food

The torque produced by the sandwich must equal the torque produced by the soft drink. Again, use the equilibrium formula, in which *MA* is moment arm:

$$(0.5 \text{ lb} \times 6.0 \text{ inches}) - (1.0 \text{ lb} \times \text{drink MA}) = 0$$

$$3.0 \text{ inch-lb} = 1.0 \text{ lb} \times \text{drink MA}$$

$$\text{drink MA} = 3.0 \text{ inches}$$

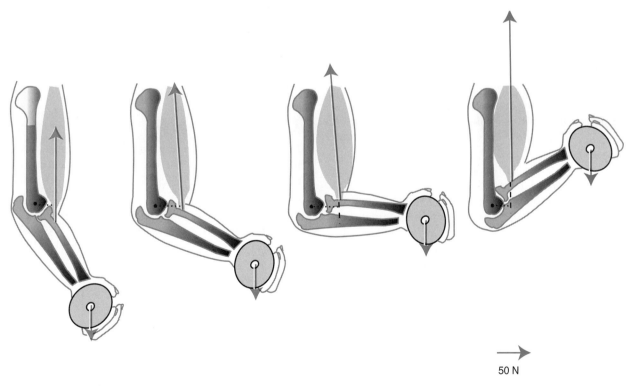

→
50 N

FIGURE **C-6**
The factors involved in internal torque. Vectors and moment arms are drawn to scale.

Chapter 6 Solutions

■ APPLICATION **6-1**
Upper-Extremity Reach

Reaching forward with both hands involves forward trunk flexion, a movement initiated by the trunk flexors, controlled by eccentric contraction of the extensors, and assisted by gravity. Holding the position while reaching requires an isometric contraction of the extensors. In each case, bilateral contractions are involved.

Reaching to one side involves lateral flexion. As in the previous case, the movement is initiated by one side and controlled and maintained by the opposite side.

Reaching straight up requires that the trunk extensors extend in a bilateral contraction. This is such a common position that we overlook its contribution to reach. Try reaching up with trunk flexion to feel the difference.

Reaching the right upper extremity across to the left side of the body involves rotation of the anterior trunk to the left. Remember that turning involves a unilateral contraction of the transversospinalis, in this case the right transversospinalis.

■ APPLICATION **6-2**
Open- and Closed-Chain Hip Movements

Long sitting is usually less comfortable than crossed-legged sitting because long sitting maximally stretches the hamstrings (passive insufficiency).

Moving into a crossed-legged position involves open-chain hip flexion because the distal end of the chain (the foot) moves freely in space as the hip flexes and externally rotates with knee flexion. Moving into long sitting is a closed-chain movement because the distal end of the lower-extremity chain is stabilized. Achieving the position involves hip flexion, but movement of the proximal attachments (origins) of the hip flexors causes the trunk to flex over the lower extremity.

Reaching for the toes in long sitting brings the hip extensors (hamstrings) to the end of their excursion. At some point even the longest hamstrings find their limit and prevent further hip flexion by pulling distally on the ischial tuberosities. (Distal is in the opposite direction from which the ischial tuberosities move in closed-chain hip flexion.) Once pelvic motion ceases, hip flexion stops. Continued forward motion to touch the toes involves vertebral flexion in the lumbar area. If the hamstrings are short, hip flexion stops even sooner in this effort and a greater degree of lumbar flexion is necessary.

■ APPLICATION **6-3**
Stance

When Paul bends over his treatment table, it produces the same types of forces as when Nancy bends over the sink. Paul's erector spinae must work twice as hard as when he stands erect. Placing his foot on a step stool changes the dynamics of posture. The stool introduces a counterforce with a vector that operates at a greater distance from the L5 disk than from Paul's center of gravity. Even a small amount of force can produce a sizable countertorque because of its longer moment arm. The same principle was at play when Nancy placed her hand on the side of the sink to support her upper body.

L5 DISK PROBLEM (CHAPTER 6)

In Figure C-7 the compressive and shear forces can be calculated with graphics and mathematics.

Graphic Solution

Draw the L5 disks at 30 and 70 degrees to the horizontal plane. The force of the weight of the body (400 N) lies 90 degrees to the horizontal plane. This weight line forms the hypotenuse of a right triangle that has the disk surface as its base. The right triangle has an angle that corresponds to the angle of the disk on the horizontal plane, that is, 30 or 70 degrees. The vector lying perpendicular to the base of the triangle represents the compressive forces operating on the disk surface from the weight of the body. The vector connecting these first two vectors lies along the base of the disk surface and represents the shear forces operating on the disk. Draw the diagram to scale so that the measurements estimate the compressive and shear forces operating on the disk. Remember that the compressive weight of the body must be added to the compressive force of the erector spinae. Through this addition the total compressive force that acts on the intervertebral L5 disk may be obtained.

Mathematical Solution

A right triangle representing the upright position has a hypotenuse of 400 N and one angle of 30 degrees. A second right triangle representing the bent position has a hypotenuse of 400 N and one angle of 70 degrees. The compressive force (C_W) of the weight of the body lies adjacent to this angle, and the shear force (S) lies opposite to this known angle. Use sines to determine sides opposite the angles and cosines to determine sides adjacent to the angles:

$$S = 400\ N \times \sin 30\ degrees$$

$$S = 200\ N\ standing$$

$$S = 400\ N \times \sin 70\ degrees$$

$$S = 376\ N\ bending$$

$$C_W = 400\ N \times \cos 30\ degrees$$

$$C_W = 346\ N\ standing$$

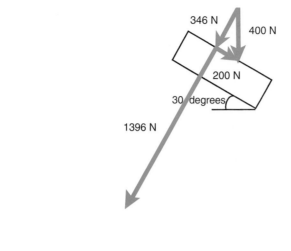

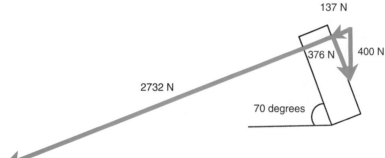

FIGURE **C-7**
The parallelogram method of adding forces provides a graphic solution in attempts to determine compressive and shear forces operating on a disk.

Total compression = 1396 N + 346 N

Total compression = 1742 N standing

$$C_W = 400 \text{ N} \times \cos 70 \text{ degrees}$$

$$C_W = 137 \text{ N bending}$$

Total compression = 2732 N + 137 N

Total compression = 2869 N bending

Chapter 7 Solutions

■ APPLICATION 7-1
Muscle Function Simulations

1. Pulling from the deltoid tubercle toward the acromion lateral to the front-to-back axis simulates contraction of the middle deltoid and produces humeral abduction at the glenohumeral joint.
2. Pulling toward the distal clavicle anterior to the side-to-side axis simulates contraction of the anterior deltoid and biceps long head, which together flex the humerus at the glenohumeral joint.
3. Pulling toward the midspine of the scapula posterior to the side-to-side axis simulates extension of the humerus by the posterior deltoid at the glenohumeral joint.
4. Pulling inferiorly and posteriorly toward the sacrum simulates extension of the humerus by the latissimus dorsi at the glenohumeral joint. The string pull differs from the actual pull of the latissimus because the string fails to show the latissimus' rotational effect on the humerus. The latissimus runs medial to the humerus and inserts on its anterior side. This medial relationship to the rotation axis and posterior pull of the latissimus results in internal humeral rotation. The string used in this application, like the latissimus, originates on the posterior side. Unlike the latissimus, the string moves to the lateral side of the humerus, placing it on the opposite side of the latissimus' rotation axis. A posterior pull lateral to the rotation axis results in external rotation of the humerus.

Notice that it takes considerable force to produce upper-extremity movement with the pull of a string. The string has a very short moment arm, and gravity acts on the upper extremity with a long moment arm. The muscles simulated must generate great magnitudes of force against even small amounts of resistance.

■ APPLICATION **7-2**
Muscle Function Drawings

Refer to Figure C-8. Notice that the segments are drawn as simple rectangles; no fancy artwork is necessary. Also notice that the force vector of the reattached brachialis (Figure C-8, *B*) continues straight, even though the muscle curves around the elbow. Its new inferior and posterior relationship to the elbow's side-to-side axis extends the elbow.

■ APPLICATION **7-3**
Limited Shoulder Strength

Solve this problem by determining the amount of force available in the anterior and middle deltoid fibers. Combine these forces using the parallelogram method. The resultant force is the amount of power available for operation of the switch.

7-3A: Fair Muscle Grades. Calculate the force of the anterior and middle fibers of the deltoid muscle by using equilibrium of torques. The force from the anterior and middle deltoid fibers (*D*) is angled upward and laterally. The force of gravity acting on the arm is valued at 30 N (*R*). The formula, in which *MA* stands for moment arm, is as follows:

$$(R \times RMA) = (D \times DMA)$$

The arm's approximate weight (2.88 kg) is derived from 4.8% of 70 kg. At 90 degrees the arm's center of gravity lies 30 cm from the axis of motion. Remember to convert centimeters to meters and kilograms to newtons:

$$(30 \text{ N} \times 0.30 \text{ m}) = (D \times 0.02 \text{ m})$$

$$9.0 \text{ N-m} = D \times 0.02 \text{ m}$$

$$D = 450 \text{ N}$$

Fair-strength anterior and middle deltoid muscles each can produce 450 N of force.

7-3B: Poor Muscle Grades. The moment arms (*MA*) for 50 degrees of shoulder abduction by the middle deltoid and for 70 degrees of flexion by the anterior deltoid are the sides of a right triangle opposite the angle of the joint. The lengths of these sides are calculated through the use of sines:

$$\sin 50 \text{ degrees} = \frac{\text{opposite side}}{30 \text{ cm}}$$

$$\text{Opposite side} = 30 \text{ cm} \times 0.7660 = 23 \text{ cm}$$

$$\sin 70 \text{ degrees} = \frac{\text{opposite side}}{30 \text{ cm}}$$

$$\text{Opposite side} = 30 \text{ cm} \times 0.9397 = 28 \text{ cm}$$

The force of the anterior deltoid is determined based on the equilibrium of torques—gravity producing extension

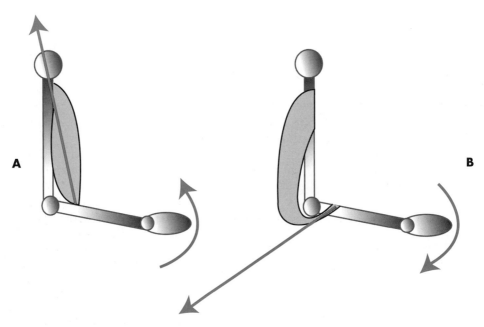

A **B**

FIGURE **C-8**
The brachialis in its anatomical **(A)** and surgically transferred **(B)** positions.

torque and the anterior deltoid producing flexion torque. In the following equation, $D_{anterior}$ stands for the force of the anterior deltoid. Remember to convert centimeters to meters and kilograms to newtons:

$$30 \text{ N} \times 0.28 \text{ m} = D_{anterior} \times 0.02 \text{ m}$$

$$8.4 \text{ N-m} = D_{anterior} \times 0.02 \text{ m}$$

$$D_{anterior} = 420 \text{ N}$$

The force of the middle deltoid is determined based on the equilibrium of torques—gravity producing adduction torque and the middle deltoid producing abduction torque. In the following equation, D_{middle} stands for the force of the middle deltoid. Again, remember to convert centimeters to meters and kilograms to newtons:

$$30 \text{ N} \times 0.23 \text{ m} = D_{middle} \times 0.02 \text{ m}$$

$$6.9 \text{ N-m} = D_{middle} \times 0.02 \text{ m}$$

$$D_{middle} = 345 \text{ N}$$

7-3C: Combined Muscle Fibers. The fair-grade anterior and middle deltoid fibers each pull with a force of about 450 N at an angle of approximately 30 degrees from each other measured at the insertion. These forces make up two sides of a parallelogram. The resultant force is a diagonal connecting the opposite corners. Calculate the resultant force by drawing a graphic representation or using mathematics. A drawing of the parallelogram is essential for a graphic solution and helpful for a mathematical one.

Graphic Solution. The vectors representing the forces of the anterior and middle deltoid fibers are at a 30-degree angle from each other. Complete the parallelogram by drawing the remaining two sides as dotted lines. The line that runs between the deltoid forces and extends to the opposite corner is the resultant force of the two portions of the deltoid that hold the arm in the position between flexion and abduction. Draw the vectors to scale and use the same scale to measure the resultant force and to approximate the force available to operate a switch.

Mathematical Solution. When both sets of muscle fibers pull with equal force, the resultant force divides the parallelogram into two equal triangles. Connecting the ends of the two 450-N forces forms a line that bisects the resultant force and produces two right triangles, each with a hypotenuse of 450 N and one angle of 15 degrees. The base of each triangle is the side adjacent to the 15-degree angle and has a value half that of the resultant force (*R*). Use cosine to determine the value of the

adjacent side, the combined forces of the anterior and middle deltoids with fair muscle strength producing flexion and abduction:

$$\cos 15 \text{ degrees} = \frac{\text{Adjacent side}}{\text{Hypotenuse}}$$

$$\cos 15 \text{ degrees} = \frac{(R/2)}{450 \text{ N}}$$

$$R/2 = 450 \text{ N} \times \cos 15 \text{ degrees}$$

$$R/2 = 450 \text{ N} \times 0.9659$$

$$R/2 = 435 \text{ N}$$

$$R = 870 \text{ N}$$

When an individual has poor muscle strength, the two portions of the deltoid are pulled with different amounts of force. Again the resultant force divides the parallelogram into two equal triangles. Draw a line from the end of each force to form a 90-degree angle with the resultant force. This forms two unequal right triangles with respective hypotenuses of 345 and 420 N. In the following equation, $R_{anterior}$ is the resultant force of the anterior deltoid and R_{middle} is the resultant force of the middle deltoid. Determine the combined forces producing flexion and abduction:

$$\cos 15 \text{ degrees} = \frac{R_{anterior}}{420 \text{ N}}$$

$$R_{anterior} = 420 \text{ N} \times 0.9659$$

$$R_{anterior} = 406 \text{ N}$$

$$\cos 15 \text{ degrees} = \frac{R_{middle}}{345 \text{ N}}$$

$$R_{middle} = 345 \text{ N} \times 0.9659$$

$$R_{middle} = 333 \text{ N}$$

$$R = 406 \text{ N} + 333 \text{ N}$$

$$R = 739 \text{ N}$$

Discussion. Both poor and fair muscle grades produce nearly double the amount of force available in the midrange position between shoulder flexion and abduction. Placing a switch in this midrange position maximizes an individual's available muscle strength. Generally, individuals use motions that combine muscle groups to increase their power in activity. In muscle testing, combination motions often are referred to as "substitutions" because they use the strength of two or more muscles or muscle groups and do not give a true picture of individual muscle strength. Awkward or unusual movements in activity are often the result of the combination of muscle groups to assist weaker muscles.

In designing adaptive equipment, calculate approximate values of muscle force by using manual muscle testing and joint range through goniometry. Calculate force for fair muscle grades using the body weight to estimate the weight of the body part being lifted. Calculate force for poor muscle grades by measuring the available range of motion, then measuring or calculating the distance of the body part's center of gravity from the axis of motion. For good and normal muscle grades, add extra weight at the center of gravity for the body part being lifted and calculate the maximum amount of force available for movement. These estimates and calculations help us as OT practitioners design and solve problems involving adaptive equipment.

■ APPLICATION 7-4
Loads on Upper-Extremity Joints

First, determine the combined centers of gravity for the humerus, forearm, and hand, which create extension torque at the shoulder, and for the forearm and hand, which create extension torque at the elbow (Figure C-9). Find the center of gravity for the hand where it creates flexion torque at the wrist. Draw the upper extremity on a grid, determine the coordinates, and plot them as shown in Chapter 3 (Figure C-10).

Torques created at each joint are calculated with the standard torque formula, weight times moment arm. Multiply the weight of the upper extremity (the arm, forearm, and hand) by the moment arm for the combined effect of the center of gravity at the shoulder axis. Then multiply the weight of the forearm and hand by their combined moment arm. Finally, multiply the weight of the hand by its moment arm. Remember to convert kilograms to newtons:

$$24 \text{ N} \times 7.7 \text{ cm} = 184.8 \text{ N-cm of extension torque at the shoulder}$$

$$10.5 \text{ N} \times 6.8 \text{ cm} = 71.4 \text{ N-cm of extension torque at the elbow}$$

$$3 \text{ N} \times 2.3 \text{ cm} = 6.9 \text{ N-cm of flexion at the wrist}$$

Each tendency created by gravity must be matched, exactly and in the opposite direction, by a muscle force at each joint. A series of equilibrium formulas yields exact amounts of force required. (Remember that muscle contractions are constant as long as the arm holds its position.) The solution is simple: Provide supports, such as arms on desk chairs and keyboard pads. If the chair is adjustable and lined up so that it supports the forearm at the level of the keyboard, expensive solutions may be unnecessary. If the computer operator uses the supports, less muscle activation is necessary.

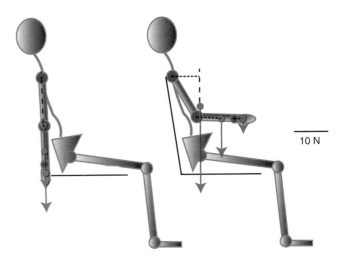

FIGURE **C-9**
No torques exist with the arm at the side because all the weight pulls through the shoulder, elbow, and wrist axes. When the upper extremity is suspended forward to type, various torques are created—extension by weight of the upper extremity at the shoulder, extension by weight of the forearm and hand at the elbow, and flexion by weight of the hand at the wrist. All must be balanced by muscle contractions producing equal torques of flexion at the shoulder and elbow and of extension at the wrist.

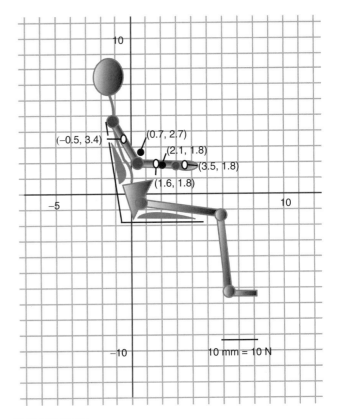

FIGURE **C-10**
Coordinates show the various centers of gravity affecting the shoulder, elbow, and wrist.

Chapter 8 Solutions

■ APPLICATION **8-1**
Balanced Wrist Function

As you move from straight wrist flexion toward ulnar deviation, notice that the flexor carpi radialis tendon softens a bit. This tendon, a radial deviator, must relax as it is pulled distally to allow ulnar deviation. Meanwhile, a contraction begins in the extensor carpi ulnaris to balance ulnar deviation. The opposite reaction occurs as you move into flexion and then radial deviation. The flexor carpi radialis and ulnaris tendons work together in pure flexion to balance each other's deviation effects. Radial deviation requires that the ulnaris yields as the radialis deviates. Activity picks up in the extensor carpi radialis longus to hold the wrist in radial deviation. As the two deviators work together, they cancel their opposite effects as flexors and extensors. (Note that if you try too hard, the muscles may go into static contraction. Try to think only of the movement. If necessary, have another person move a hand in the same direction and observe.)

■ APPLICATION **8-2**
Shorter Longitudinal Arch

If you drew your hand parallel to the edge of the paper, you should uncover the radial marking (proximal palmar crease) first. Because the palmar creases line up with the MCP joints, this action locates the second MCP distal to the fifth. The distal border of a volar splint should follow a line that connects these two creases. Any splint

extending beyond this line interferes with MCP flexion as rigid splint material distal to the MCP joints blocks the proximal phalanges in their flexion arc.

Chapter 9 Solutions

■ APPLICATION **9-1**
Muscle Shortening during Hip Flexion

The fingers of the hand should curl (flex) as the movements occur. Both movements have the same effect on the fingers because both are hip flexion. In the open-chain movement, the thigh moves closer to the pelvis. The approximation of the insertion to the origin causes the fingers to flex, representing the shortening of the muscle fibers. In the closed-chain motion, the pelvis (origin) approaches the thigh (insertion). This indicates slackening of the hip flexors because eccentric contraction of the hip extensors (hamstrings and gluteus maximus) controls closed-chain hip flexion with gravity.

■ APPLICATION **9-2**
Open- and Closed-Chain Hip Abduction

This activity mimics the hip flexion application in a different plane. Closed-chain hip abduction on the weight-bearing side usually is accompanied by lateral flexion of the trunk, which also occurs in the frontal plane. Distinguish vertebral movement from hip movement and realize that both occur.

Review of Mathematics

Working with Variables in an Equation

When an equation contains an undetermined value, isolate this variable on one side of the equal sign. Add, subtract, divide, or multiply equally on both sides of the equation so that the numbers on one side cancel and leave the variable to stand alone:

PROBLEM 1

$$8x = 48$$

$$x = \frac{48}{8}$$

$$x = 6$$

When numbers and values in an equation involve addition and subtraction and multiplication and division, isolate these different functions with parentheses and move the values within parentheses as a whole:

PROBLEM 2

$$0.3x + 0.25 \times 4 - 16 = 0$$

$$0.3x + (0.25 \times 4) - 16 = 0$$

$$0.3x = 16 - (0.25 \times 4)$$

$$0.3x = 16 - 1$$

$$x = \frac{15}{0.3}$$

$$x = 50$$

When numbers and values in an equation are isolated by parentheses, solve the functions to remove the parentheses:

PROBLEM 3

$$5\,(x - 4) + 10 = 45$$

$$5x - 20 + 10 = 45$$

$$5x = 45 + 10$$

$$5x = 55$$

$$x = 11$$

PROBLEM 4

$$12x - 6 - 2(4x \times 8) = 0$$

$$12x - 6 - 8x - 16 = 0$$

$$4x = 6 + 16$$

$$4x = 22$$

$$x = 5.5$$

Find a common denominator to solve fractions:

PROBLEM 5

$$\frac{x}{3} + \frac{1}{2} = \frac{3}{4}$$

$$\frac{x}{3} + \frac{3}{4} = \frac{1}{2}$$

$$\frac{x}{3} = \frac{(2 \times 3) - (4 \times 1)}{8}$$

$$\frac{x}{3} = \frac{6 - 4}{8}$$

$$\frac{x}{3} = \frac{1}{4}$$

$$x = \frac{3}{4}$$

Simple Geometry

The following formulas and concepts are used to solve simple problems in geometry. They are used frequently in biomechanics:

Supplementary angles. A line intersected by another line forms two angles that equal 180 degrees when added together:

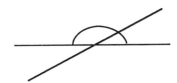

Alternate angle. When two parallel lines are intersected by a third line, the angles on opposite sides of the intersecting line are equal:

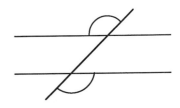

Sum of the angles. All the angles of a triangle added together equal 180 degrees.

Outer angle. An angle outside a triangle equals the two opposite inside angles:

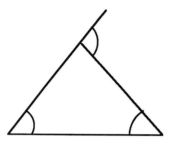

Right triangle. A right triangle has one angle of 90 degrees. This designation is specified by a boxlike marking in the 90-degree right angle.

Pythagorean theorem. In a right triangle, the horizontal and vertical sides are multiplied by themselves and when added together equal the diagonal hypotenuse multiplied by itself. The hypotenuse is generally assigned the letter c:

$$c^2 = a^2 + b^2$$

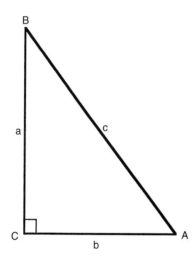

PROBLEM 6

In the following parallelogram, ABCD, side a is 5 cm and side b is 8.5 cm. Angle A is 40 degrees. Line e divides the parallelogram into two equal triangles. Line f divides ABC into two right triangles. The values of the angles in each right triangle include the following:

Angle A (intervening angle) = 40 degrees

Angle A (bisected) = 20 degrees

Angle B (alternate angle) = 140 degrees

Angle B (bisected) = 70 degrees

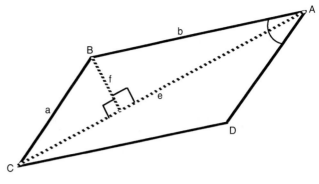

$$20 + 70 + 90 = 180 \text{ degrees}$$

PROBLEM 7

In the right triangle on the following page, ABC, side a is 4 cm and side b is 3 cm. The following solution determines the length of side c:

$$c^2 = a^2 + b^2$$

$$c^2 = 4^2 \text{ cm} + 3^2 \text{ cm}$$

$$c^2 = 16 \text{ cm} + 9 \text{ cm}$$

$$c^2 = 25 \text{ cm}$$

$$c = 5 \text{ cm}$$

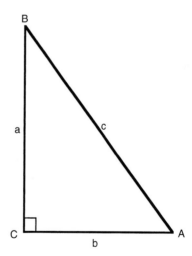

Basic Trigonometry

Trigonometry uses the ratio of known angles to known sides in triangles to determine the values of unknown sides and angles. Through the use of trigonometric functions these values can be determined with very little information. Imaginary triangles in space, on land, or between body parts can produce numerical values for distances and forces that often cannot be measured.

Trigonometric functions were determined by ancient civilizations and were used in the building of pyramids. They are used today to compute the distances of stars and other astronomic objects. Understanding their derivations is a complex mathematical feat. As with the pyramids themselves, they are easier to accept as wonders of nature; understanding why they work is a difficult process.

Sines, *cosines*, and *tangents* are names given to fixed ratios of angles to sides in right triangles. Use sines and cosines when given the value of the hypotenuse and a side or a side and an angle of a right triangle. Use tangents and cotangents when given the value of two sides or a side and an angle of a right triangle. Scientific calculators have these ratios built into their memory chips. A table of sines, cosines, tangents, and cotangents can be found in Appendix E.

Sine. In a right triangle the sine of an angle is the ratio of the opposite side to the hypotenuse:

$$\sin A = \frac{a}{c}$$

Cosine. In a right triangle the cosine of an angle is the ratio of the adjacent side to the hypotenuse:

$$\cos A = \frac{b}{c}$$

Tangent. In a right triangle the tangent of an angle is the ratio of the opposite side to the adjacent side:

$$\tan A = \frac{a}{b}$$

Cotangent. In a right triangle the cotangent of an angle is the ratio of the adjacent side to the opposite side:

$$\cot A = \frac{b}{a}$$

PROBLEM 8

In the following right triangle, ABC, side *a* is 4 cm, and side *c* is 8 cm. How large is angle *A*:

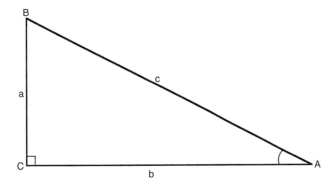

Because the values of side *a* and the hypotenuse are given, use sines to solve this problem:

$$\sin A = \frac{a}{c}$$

$$\sin A = \frac{4 \text{ cm}}{8 \text{ cm}}$$

$$\sin A = 0.5$$

$$A = 30 \text{ degrees}$$

PROBLEM 9

In the following right triangle, ABC, the hypotenuse is 12 cm and angle *A* is 15 degrees. How long are the sides?

Because the hypotenuse is given and the values of both sides are needed, use sines and cosines to solve this problem:

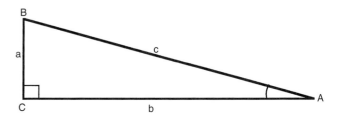

$$\sin A = \frac{a}{c}$$

$$\sin 15 \text{ degrees} = \frac{a}{12 \text{ cm}}$$

$$a = 12 \text{ cm} \times \sin 15 \text{ degrees}$$

$$a = 12 \text{ cm} \times 0.259$$

$$a = 3.11 \text{ cm}$$

$$\cos A = \frac{b}{c}$$

$$\cos 15 \text{ degrees} = \frac{b}{12 \text{ cm}}$$

$$b = 0.966 \times 12 \text{ cm}$$

$$b = 11.59 \text{ cm}$$

Supplementary angle. When one line intersects another, two supplementary angles are formed. The sines of both supplementary angles are equal to each other:

$$\sin A = \sin (180 \text{ degrees} - A)$$

The cosine of one angle is equal to the negative cosine of the other angle:

$$\cos A = - \cos (180 \text{ degrees} - A)$$

Sines and cosines can be used when working with triangles that are not right triangles:

Sine theorem. Two angles and an opposite side or two sides and an opposite angle can yield the values for the rest of any triangle because sides are proportional to the sines of their angles:

$$\frac{a}{\sin A} = \frac{b}{\sin B} = \frac{c}{\sin C}$$

Cosine theorem. Three sides or two sides and an adjacent angle can yield the values of the rest of the triangle because of the relationships between them:

$$a^2 = b^2 + c^2 - (2\ bc \times \cos A)$$

PROBLEM 10

In the following triangle, ABC, side *b* is 6.0 cm, side *c* is 9.0 cm, and angle *A* is 60 degrees. From this information, side *a* can be determined:

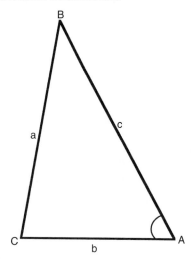

Because two sides and an adjacent angle are given, use the cosine theorem to solve this problem:

$$a^2 = b^2 + c^2 - (2\ bc \times \cos A)$$

$$a^2 = 6^2\ cm + 9^2\ cm - [2(6\ cm \times 9\ cm) \times \cos A]$$

$$a^2 = 36\ cm + 81\ cm - (108\ cm \times 0.5)$$

$$a^2 = 63\ cm$$

$$a = 7.9\ cm$$

Trigonometric Functions

DEGREES*	SINES	COSINES	TANGENTS	COTANGENTS	
0	.0000	1.0000	.0000		90
1	.0175	.9998	.0175	57.290	89
2	.0349	.9994	.0349	28.636	88
3	.0523	.9986	.0524	19.081	87
4	.0698	.9976	.0699	14.301	86
5	.0872	.9962	.0875	11.430	85
6	.1045	.9945	.1051	9.5144	84
7	.1219	.9925	.1228	8.1443	83
8	.1392	.9903	.1405	7.1154	82
9	.1564	.9877	.1584	6.3138	81
10	.1736	.9848	.1763	5.6713	80
11	.1908	.9816	.1944	5.1446	79
12	.2079	.9781	.2126	4.7046	78
13	.2250	.9744	.2309	4.3315	77
14	.2419	.9703	.2493	4.0108	76
15	.2588	.9659	.2679	3.7321	75
16	.2756	.9613	.2867	3.4874	74
17	.2924	.9563	.3057	3.2709	73
18	.3090	.9511	.3249	3.0777	72
19	.3256	.9455	.3443	2.9042	71
20	.3420	.9397	.3640	2.7475	70
21	.3584	.9336	.3839	2.6051	69
22	.3746	.9272	.4040	2.4751	68
23	.3907	.9205	.4245	2.3559	67
24	.4067	.9135	.4452	2.2460	66
25	.4226	.9063	.4663	2.1445	65
26	.4384	.8988	.4877	2.0503	64
27	.4540	.8910	.5095	1.9626	63
28	.4695	.8829	.5317	1.8807	62
29	.4848	.8746	.5543	1.8040	61
30	.5000	.8660	.5774	1.7321	60
31	.5150	.8572	.6009	1.6643	59
32	.5299	.8480	.6249	1.6003	58
33	.5446	.8387	.6494	1.5399	57
34	.5592	.8290	.6745	1.4826	56
35	.5736	.8192	.7002	1.4281	55
36	.5878	.8090	.7265	1.3765	54
37	.6018	.7986	.7536	1.3270	53
38	.6157	.7880	.7813	1.2799	52
39	.6293	.7771	.8098	1.2349	51
40	.6428	.7660	.8391	1.1918	50
41	.6561	.7547	.8693	1.1504	49
42	.6691	.7431	.9004	1.1106	48
43	.6820	.7314	.9325	1.0724	47
44	.6947	.7193	.9657	1.0355	46
45	.7071	.7071	1.0000	1.0000	45
	COSINES	SINES	COTANGENTS	TANGENTS	DEGREES*

*Note: With angles above 45 degrees, use the headings that appear at the bottom of the columns.

Commonly Used Formulas in Biomechanics

Length (Unmeasurable Elements)

When one angle and one side are known or when the hypotenuse of a right triangle is known, the following equations can be used to determine the unknown value:

$$\sin A = \frac{a}{c} \text{ for an angle and an opposite side}$$

$$\cos A = \frac{b}{c} \text{ for an angle and an adjacent side}$$

When two sides of a right triangle are known, the following equations can be used to determine the unknown value:

$$\tan A = \frac{a}{b}$$

$$\cot A = \frac{b}{a}$$

When two angles and an opposite angle or two angles and an opposite side of any triangle are known, the following equation can be used to determine the unknown value:

$$\frac{a}{\sin A} = \frac{b}{\sin B} = \frac{c}{\sin C}$$

When three sides or two sides and an adjacent angle of any triangle are known, the following equation can be used to determine the unknown value:

$$a^2 = b^2 + c^2 - (2 \, bc \times \cos A)$$

Force (Linear Motion)

$$F \quad = \quad m \quad \times \quad a$$
Force   Mass   Acceleration (Gravity)

Force Equilibrium

$$\sum F = 0 \text{ (The sum of all forces equals 0.)}$$

or

$$\sum F_x = 0 \text{ (All horizontal forces equal 0.)}$$

and

$$\sum F_y = 0 \text{ (All vertical forces equal 0.)}$$

TORQUE (ROTARY MOTION)

$$T \quad = \quad f \quad \times \quad ma$$
Torque   Force   Moment arm

MOMENT EQUILIBRIUM

$$\sum M = 0 \text{ (The sum of clockwise and counterclockwise torque equals 0.)}$$

or

$$EFA \quad \times \quad EMA \quad = \quad RFA \quad \times \quad RMA$$
Effort force   Effort moment arm   Resistance force   Resistance moment arm

STRESS (PRESSURE)

$$S \quad = \quad f \quad \div \quad t \quad \times \quad \omega$$
Stress   Force   Tissue length   Tissue width

WORK

Lifting work can be determined with the following formula:

$$L \quad = \quad (m \times g) \quad \times \quad h \quad \times \quad r$$
Lifting work   (Mass × Gravity)   Height lifted   Number of repetitions

Carrying work can be determined with the following formula:

$$C \quad = \quad (m \times g) \quad \times \quad d \quad \times \quad F$$
Carrying work   (Mas × Gravity)   Distance   Number of repetitions

Biomechanical Analysis of Function

The philosophical basis of OT practice states that "Man is an active being whose development is influenced by the use of purposeful activity."[3] This is a short statement, but every OT student learns quickly that the words *purposeful activity* evoke lengthy discussion. Activity analysis helps OT practitioners understand whether an activity is purposeful and has therapeutic value. Through activity analysis the practitioner gains an appreciation of the activity's components and characteristics, which differentiate the therapeutic value of one activity from another. This begins the process that ultimately leads to the therapeutic use of occupation.*

An important consideration in the therapeutic use of activity is the determination of the need for adaptation to facilitate task performance. A full understanding of the individual's abilities and limitations is needed. This is possible only through comprehensive biomechanical analysis, which ensures identification of the real problems to be addressed in the adaptive process. Thus the subsequent problem-solving process is correctly focused. As Parham[5] suggested in her discussion of problem setting, inadequate time spent identifying the appropriate problem to solve can render even brilliant problem solving useless.

Successful adaptation that facilitates an individual's involvement in purposeful activity requires problem setting first. Problem setting includes the identification of priority aspects of a patient's need to receive intervention. Not only must the specific focus of intervention be sorted out from various presenting problems, but the problem-setting process also must occur at a deeper level—specification of the musculoskeletal segment most responsible for activity dysfunction. In this process, which is the essence of biomechanical analysis, the dysfunctional link is tagged, and problem solving leading to adaptation begins.

Background of Biomechanical Analysis

Let us review the basic models from which biomechanical analysis was developed. Reed[7] describes three different biomechanical models—reconstruction, orthopedic, and kinetic. Each model adheres to the assumption that function resulting from voluntary muscle contraction and control (and dysfunction resulting from a lack of

the same) depends on muscle strength, joint range of motion, and physical endurance. Although the reconstruction model suggests the use of voluntary movements in academic and vocational activities, the orthopedic approach more specifically addresses differential treatment of pathological conditions. The kinetic model differs from both in its attention to the analysis of motion during activities and the adjustment of strategies on the basis of the analysis. This model suggests a specific methodology for analysis of motion. The kinetic model is elaborated in the text *Occupational Therapy Principles and Practice*,[4] which was written in collaboration with our profession's founder, William Rush Dunton, Jr.

As our professional emphasis has moved toward greater accountability through the quantification of information, observation analysis has been refined and augmented by methods employing electromyographic (EMG) measurements. Basmajian and De Luca[2] and Trombly and Cole[11] have used EMG measurements to describe specific muscle activity in the hand. These studies have provided valuable information to help the practitioner better understand motion and the agonists responsible for motion in activity performance.

Analyses such as these represent the most accurate methods for absolute determination of muscle activity during function. OT practitioners should use documented studies based on these technical methods whenever possible. However, not every movement in every activity used in the clinic has been studied; studies of normal individuals cannot be directly applied to injured individuals who, in adjusting to their pathological conditions, have developed compensatory movements. Even in its less than absolute nature, biomechanical analysis through activity observation remains a necessary practice.

As a result of time constraints or the belief that analysis can be done intuitively and briefly while setting up the activity, many OT practitioners do not routinely perform biomechanical analysis. The examples that follow suggest that prior biomechanical analysis in each task would have yielded better judgment by the OT practitioner and more effective treatment for the client.

In the use of a deltoid assist in a tabletop activity, the goal is to strengthen the external shoulder rotators to facilitate greater ease in self-feeding. The upper extremities are positioned in 90 degrees of shoulder abduction, and the weights of the assist are moved up and down as internal and external rotation bring the hands to and from

---

*Modified from Greene D: A clinically relevant approach to biomechanical analysis of function, *Occup Ther Pract* 1(4):44-52, 1990.

the table. However, this arrangement actually resists internal rotation and assists external rotation and therefore does not strengthen the intended motion.

Another example is in the use of a mobile arm support to allow self-feeding for an individual who exhibits an inability to bring the hand to the mouth. This individual has adequate shoulder external rotation and elbow flexion but an absence of shoulder abduction and weak wrist extension. Because of the weakness in wrist extension, the individual is unable to maintain grasp and, because of wrist drop, cannot fully elevate the hand to the mouth through external shoulder rotation.

When the arm is placed in the mobile arm support, the individual still cannot self-feed because the real problem—weak wrist extension—is ignored. Meanwhile, external shoulder rotation is possible without the device. With the identification of the real problem, intervention with a simple wrist cock-up splint proves a more successful strategy.

Thus even some of the simplest solutions require reasoning skills beyond simple matching of equipment with common problems. Schön[9] suggests that as the emphasis of intervention shifts more toward technical skills, we may find that problem solving is made more difficult by a narrow application of theory. We, as OT practitioners, must strengthen our ability to reason out solutions based on the uniqueness of a patient's symptoms, which is fully illustrated through biomechanical analysis.

Review of Terms

Biomechanical analysis leads to ideas and terms that require definition. The terms associated with biomechanical analysis are used frequently in daily practice, but a clear definition is necessary for universal application.

Force, as defined by Soderberg,[10] is the action or effect of one body on another (for example, a skeletal muscle acting on a bony segment). The muscle that produces the force responsible for the motion is known as the *agonist*, or *prime mover*. Although muscles often generate force affecting the skeletal system, gravity[6] is a force not produced by a muscle. Gravity is unique in its constant effect, which is to pull a body or bony segment toward the center of the Earth, or straight down in general terms. A gravity-assisted motion is one that occurs even in the absence of muscle contraction. Yet muscular forces are important even in this type of motion because gravity-assisted motions usually are controlled by contractions of muscles that typically perform the motion opposite the one observed. Thus for example, the elbow flexors are the active group in gravity-assisted elbow extension, as in the controlled lowering of the hand from the mouth to the table.

However, elbow flexors that contract to extend the elbow make sense only in the context of muscle contraction.

Although a muscle typically shortens during contraction (concentric contraction), contraction performed against an external force of adequate magnitude to prevent motion results in a contraction with no appreciable change in muscle length (isometric contraction). If the external force exerted on a segment overcomes the muscular force attempting to move the segment in the opposite direction, a lengthening (eccentric) contraction occurs. This is the case in the previous example, in which gravity-assisted elbow extension is controlled by eccentric contraction of the elbow flexors.

A Usable Methodology

Biomechanical analysis has widespread application in the various specialties of OT practice, from handling and positioning of the infant to adaptation and activity design of the adult population. We can use a universally familiar task to demonstrate biomechanical analysis. (Figures G-1 and G-2 are examples of the method used to record the observations made during the task's performance.) The task is donning socks in a seated position, crossing the lower extremities to allow easier access to the foot. This task can be difficult, especially in the older population. Careful analysis that considers the common problems associated with the older client reveals specific steps of great difficulty that can be made easier.

This analysis begins as the OT practitioner observes one joint at a time to establish whether the joint moves into and is held in a position other than its anatomical position. The OT practitioner then develops questions regarding this motion and position. If the motion is cyclic and returns the segment to the original anatomical position, as in shoulder flexion and extension in moving the hand to place an object on a tabletop, only the motion is considered because no position is held. Finally, the practitioner determines whether the motion involved (and any resulting position held) is repetitive or occurs only once in the total performance of the activity. All entries on the form (see Figures G-1 and G-2) are brief, often composed of one-word answers. They are designed to mimic an actual practitioner's notations.

For the purposes of the present discussion, only the analysis of specific segments that present problems is described in detail on the sample forms. The segments discussed include the intervertebral joints, glenohumeral joint, joints of the hand, and hip joint. In the actual clinical setting, the choice can be made as to whether all musculoskeletal segments or only specific ones are analyzed.

INTERVERTEBRAL JOINTS

As the subject reaches to place the sock on the foot, the OT practitioner observes flexion. This description is briefly stated on the form (see Figure G-1). Nothing else

SEGMENT		INITIAL MOTION			HOLDING POSITION			
MOTION/ POSITION OBSERVED	% ROM	RESISTED OR RAPID	GRAVITY ASSISTS/ RESISTS	AGONIST GROUP/ CONTRACTION TYPE (CON OR ECC)	RESISTED	GRAVITY EFFECT	ISOMETRIC AGONIST	REP
V FLEX Reaching for foot	50%	No	Assists	Extensors/ECC	No	Promotes flexion	Extensors	No
V EXT Returning from flexion	N/A	No	Resists	Extensors/CON	N/A			
V L-ROT Turning to reach right foot	<50%	No	No	Left rotators/CON	No	None	Left rotators	No
S PRO Reaching forward	>50%	Slight resistance at end	Slight assist	Protractors/CON	Slightly	Little if any	Protractors	No
S RET Pulling sock	N/A	Resisted	N/A	Retractors/CON	N/A			
GH FLEX Reaching forward and placing sock	<50%	No	Resists	Flexors/CON	No	Promotes extension	Flexors	No
E FLEX Positioning- Pulling sock-	<50% 50%	No Resisted	Resists N/A	Flexors/CON Flexors/CON	No N/A	Promotes extension	Flexors	No

FIGURE **G-1**

Analysis of motion involving the vertebral joints, scapula, and glenohumeral and elbow joints. *ROM,* Range of motion; *CON,* concentric; *ECC,* eccentric; *REP,* repetition; *V FLEX,* vertebral flexion; *V EXT,* vertebral extension; *V L-ROT,* vertebral left rotation; *S PRO,* scapular protraction; *S RET,* scapular retraction; *GH FLEX,* glenohumeral flexion; *E FLEX,* elbow flexion; *N/A,* not applicable.

concerning placement of the sock on the foot (for example, the wrist position) is addressed at this time. Also, no other vertebral position is recognized.

As the practitioner considers next the percentage range of motion, the extent of flexion is approximately 50%. (An estimate is sufficient.) The anatomical position is assumed to be 0% and the full extent of flexion normally possible, 100%.

Next, the OT practitioner considers the nature of the flexion to determine whether the movement is performed rapidly or against resistance. (Resistance is external resistance directed in the opposite direction of the movement and in addition to the effect of gravity.) A motion performed rapidly or against resistance is generally a result of a contraction of the anatomical agonist. Vertebral flexion does not occur rapidly or against resistance.

However, with enlargement of the abdomen or decrease in vertebral flexibility, the individual may encounter resistance to vertebral flexion. The agonist (flexors) is thus identified on the basis of this determination regardless of the effect of gravity. In this case the question regarding the effect of gravity is preempted.

If the individual does not encounter resistance, the vertebral flexion observed is assisted by gravity. In fact, gravity may be considered the prime mover after a slight initial burst of flexor activity. As stated clearly by Rosse and Clawson,[8] "When the prime moving force is generated not by muscle but by gravity, the movement will be controlled, paradoxically, by muscles capable of producing the converse movement, that is, by the antagonists." Therefore the flexion is the result of eccentric contraction of the vertebral extensors. Identification of

SEGMENT		INITIAL MOTION			HOLDING POSITION			
MOTION/ POSITION OBSERVED	% ROM	RESISTED OR RAPID	GRAVITY ASSISTS/ RESISTS	AGONIST GROUP/ CONTRACTION TYPE (CON OR ECC)	RESISTED	GRAVITY EFFECT	ISOMETRIC AGONIST	REP
MCP FLEX Holding sock	50%	No	N/A	Flexors/CON	Yes	N/A	Flexors	No
MCP EXT Opening hand	>50%	No	N/A	Extensors/CON	N/A			
IP FLEX Holding sock	<50%	No	N/A	Flexors/CON	Yes	N/A	Flexors	No
IP EXT Opening hand	50%	No	N/A	Extensors/CON	N/A			
CM#1 ABD Opening hand	50%	No	N/A	Abductors/CON	N/A			
CM#1 ADD Holding sock	<50%	No	N/A	Adductors/CON	Yes	N/A	Adductors	No
OPP Opening hand; holding sock	100%	No	N/A	Abductors, flexors, opponens/CON	Yes	N/A	Adductors, flexors, opponens	No
H FLEX Crossing legs Leaning forward	>50% >50%	No No	Resists Assists	Flexors/CON Extensors/ECC	N/A⟶ No	Legs are crossed Promotes flexion	N/A Extensors	No
H E-ROT Crossing legs	>50%	No	Resists	External/CON /rotators	N/A⟶	Legs are crossed	N/A	

FIGURE **G-2**
Analysis of motion involving the metacarpophalangeal and interphalangeal joints, thumb carpometacarpal joint, and hip joint. *ROM,* Range of motion; *CON,* concentric; *ECC,* eccentric; *REP,* repetition; *MCP FLEX,* metacarpophalangeal flexion; *MCP EXT,* metacarpophalangeal extension; *IP FLEX,* interphalangeal flexion; *IP EXT,* interphalangeal extension; *CM#1 ABD,* thumb carpometacarpal abduction; *CM#1 ADD,* thumb carpometacarpal adduction; *OPP,* opposition; *H FLEX,* hip flexion; *H E-ROT,* hip external rotation; *N/A,* not applicable.

the vertebral extensors as agonists provides the basis for the understanding that an individual's inability to move slowly into vertebral flexion may be the result of dysfunction in the vertebral extensors.

Identification and characterization of the movement are not enough if the movement leads to a position the individual must hold during the activity. In the example of the donning of socks, the individual holds vertebral flexion as the sock is positioned and put on the foot. The effect of gravity is to attempt to continue the flexion. Therefore the isometric agonist is the extensor group, which contracts to resist gravity's flexion tendency.

Finally, as the individual dons the sock, the OT practitioner observes only one flexion motion of the vertebral column for each sock donned.

With identification and analysis of vertebral flexion completed, the OT practitioner views each possible

movement in each segment in order. Vertebral extension is observed when the subject returns from the flexed position. Percentage range of motion is not applicable because this motion is considered a return motion (from flexion to the anatomical position). If a fixed deformity prevents an individual from returning to full vertebral extension, the limitation is documented on the left side of the form with a descriptor such as "lacking 20%" if desired.

Extension is not resisted (by any force in addition to gravity) or performed rapidly, but gravity resists the motion. Therefore the movement is a result of the concentric contraction of the extensor group. Because extension results in the assumption of the anatomical position, no further characterization is necessary other than documentation that this movement, like vertebral flexion, is not repetitive.

The OT practitioner observes slight rotation to the left and right in donning the right and left socks, respectively. Only left rotation is considered in this discussion because the same discussion applies to the right side.

Left rotation is less than 50%. It is not performed rapidly, nor is it usually a movement against resistance in this activity. As in vertebral flexion, however, decreased vertebral flexibility may result in at least some resistance. Although difficult to assess, the ease with which the individual performs the motion is a good indication of the degree of resistance.

Rotation is performed in the gravity-eliminated plane in the anatomical position, but in this activity it is performed in a forward-flexed position. Nevertheless, the counterbalancing effect of the two upper extremities neutralizes the effect of gravity. Without gravity's influence, the left rotator group performs and holds left rotation. Increased resistance resulting from decreased flexibility results in a stronger contraction of the same group; in either case a concentric contraction moves into position and an isometric contraction of the same group holds the position.

GLENOHUMERAL JOINT

Glenohumeral function flexion is apparent as the individual moves the sock toward the foot and places it on the foot. It is less than 50% and occurs slowly against gravity only. The agonist group is the flexor group, which contracts concentrically. As the individual holds the position, again only gravity resists and the isometric agonist is the flexor group. This segment and movement (shoulder flexion) often limits the older population as they dress the lower extremities. Biomechanical analysis can help OT practitioners determine whether this is the weak link in the chain.

METACARPOPHALANGEAL, INTERPHALANGEAL, AND CARPOMETACARPAL JOINTS

Because of their relatively small mass, the digits are negligibly affected by gravity, yet the percentage of time they move and hold positions against resistance is great. Therefore in the consideration of joints distal to the wrist, gravity's effect is ignored and performance against resistance and rapidity of motion receive greater emphasis.

The position of the hand in holding the sock requires partial metacarpophalangeal and interphalangeal flexion (see Figure G-2). In this case, metacarpophalangeal and interphalangeal flexion initially occurs against little resistance as the individual flexes the digits into position to hold the sock. The flexor group contracts concentrically. Flexion does occur against resistance because some strength of grip is required to hold the sock and pull it onto the foot. The isometric agonist is the digit flexor group. The motion is not repetitive.

The carpometacarpal thumb joint is abducted as the individual moves the thumb into position to receive the sock. Abduction is not held, however, because on receiving the sock, the adductors contract concentrically and thus the thumb grasps the sock through a slight adduction movement. A slightly adducted position is maintained in part through an isometric contraction of the adductors as the individual pulls the thumb into a pinch, holding the sock between the thumb and the stable post provided by digits 2 through 5.

The description of the thumb as it grasps the sock is confusing. The thumb has moved into a partially adducted position but remains slightly abducted from the palm. Nevertheless, this position is maintained as a consequence of the powerful thumb adductors' contraction against a stable post, the semiflexed, statically positioned fingers. Imagine what would happen if the abductors were activated to hold the desired degree of abduction. The sock would fall because contraction of the abductors generates thumb motion from the palm, a direction in which no stable post is present. Thumb abduction would obliterate grasp.

HIP JOINT

Limitation in hip function (specifically flexion, adduction, and external rotation) often solely prohibits independent function in donning of the socks. An extreme amount of hip flexion is required (for example, nearly 100% in the right lower extremity when donning the right sock) in the combination of sitting, forward bending, and crossing one lower extremity over the other. This extreme often may be responsible for the difficulty many individuals experience. Any lack in hip flexibility is resistance to the individual's attempt to flex the hip when trying to gain access to the foot. Thus many individuals fail to don socks if they do not first stretch to warm the muscles.

Summary

To facilitate function, we, as OT practitioners, must make comparisons between an individual's ability or disability and the demands of an activity through biomechanical analysis. As we become more skillful in performance observation and analysis, we can better interpret and apply the specific and accurate measurements we make, heightening the quality of OT intervention.

In the previous method, the OT practitioner skillfully observes movement using an organized worksheet to characterize performance one joint at a time. Planning of strategies for rehabilitation and adaptation allows the practitioner to use this analysis to develop a more contextual knowledge. Additionally, more objective documentation paves the way for more meaningful and accountable communication with clients, professionals, and third-party payors.

REFERENCES

1. American Occupational Therapy Association: Minutes of the representative assembly, *Am J Occup Ther* 33:785, 1979.
2. Basmajian JV, De Luca CJ: *Muscles alive: their functions revealed by electromyography,* ed 5, Baltimore, 1985, Williams & Wilkins.
3. Crepeau EB, Cohn ES, Boyt Schell BA: *Willard and Spackman's occupational therapy,* ed 10, New York, 2003, Lippincott Williams & Wilkins.
4. Dunton WR Jr, Licht S: *Occupational therapy principles and practice,* ed 2, Springfield, Ill, 1957, Charles C Thomas.
5. Parham D: Toward professionalism, *Am J Occup Ther* 41: 555-561, 1987.
6. Rasch PJ: *Kinesiology and applied anatomy,* ed 7, Philadelphia, 1993, Lea & Febiger.
7. Reed KL: *Models of practice in occupational therapy,* Baltimore, 1984, Williams & Wilkins.
8. Rosse C, Clawson DK: *The musculoskeletal system in health and disease,* New York, 1980, Harper & Row.
9. Schön D: *The reflective practitioner,* New York, 1983, Basic Books.
10. Soderberg GL: *Kinesiology: application to pathological motion,* ed 2, Philadelphia, 1997, Lippincott Williams & Wilkins.
11. Trombly CA, Cole JM: Electromyographic study of four hand muscles during selected activities, *Am J Occup Ther* 33:440-449, 1979.

Synopsis of Characters

This appendix contains brief descriptions of each character in alphabetical order by first name. These characters evolved from compilations of many individuals the authors have known. Any similarities to real people, living or dead, remain purely coincidental.

Alex Fecteau's first-grade teacher wanted him evaluated by the OT because he walked "funny," fatigued easily, and did not participate in playground games. The school therapist discovered that Alex suffered from generalized muscle weakness, with an increased severity in the proximal muscle groups. The therapist urged his family to seek further medical help. Because Alex's family did not have medical insurance, the school social worker helped them locate a clinic, where a pediatrician diagnosed Alex with Duchenne-type muscular dystrophy.

The school therapist developed alternative playground activities to accommodate Alex's needs and explained the progressive course of Duchenne's dystrophy to the school's staff members. Alex was excused from running laps, which could cause him debilitating fatigue rather than help him build muscle strength.

Bernice Richards, a nightclub singer with C5 quadriplegia, was injured in a motor vehicle accident. Fortunately, Bernice stayed in the spinal cord unit of the rehabilitation center for more than 6 months. During that time staff discovered she had some sparing of her left wrist extensor muscles. Bernice left the hospital driving her own van. Her former employer and loyal fans raised money to make modifications to the stage and restrooms so she could resume her singing career. As a performer, Bernice always cared deeply about her appearance and insisted on learning to apply her own eyeliner before she left rehab.

Crystal Turner, a 4-year-old girl with Down syndrome, came to the outpatient clinic with her parents to learn some activities that would stimulate her gross and fine-motor development. Despite her low muscle tone, she eagerly tried most activities and attempted to keep up with the older children.

Donna Nelson waited tables in the city's most popular Italian restaurant to work her way through college. During her sophomore year, Donna had to take a leave of absence to learn how to manage her recently diagnosed bipolar disorder. Because her job provided much-needed tip money, maintaining upper-body strength became an important component of her psychiatric hospitalization. She resumed college and returned to work after a semester off. Donna planned to continue her education with a master's degree in occupational therapy.

Eduardo Ybarra came to the hand therapy clinic as an outpatient after sustaining a radial nerve injury from a power saw while making his son a Christmas present. Eduardo's injury occurred at home, so he received no industrial compensation from the furniture factory where he worked as a cabinetmaker. Eduardo's health insurance covered his surgery and enough therapy to restore some function in his hand, although not enough for returning to cabinetry. Fortunately, vocational rehabilitation enabled him to take some courses at the local community college. Eduardo is uncertain and depressed about his job possibilities, but he has continued to do some woodworking at home and plans to teach his sons this craft.

Fred Jackson has had rheumatoid arthritis for about 20 years. He came to the hand clinic after undergoing surgery to replace the metacarpophalangeal joints in his hand. The aerospace engineering company where he worked for 30 years underwent a merger that forced the employees to change medical insurance plans. The ensuing confusion disrupted Fred's hand rehabilitation and his surgical results turned out less than he had expected.

Fred's disappointment and anger sometimes made him seem difficult in the clinic. As part of his job, Fred designed many tools for use in the weightlessness of space. Once the OT staff got to know him, they took advantage of his knowledge about biomechanics. He often kept staff and clients enthralled with his stories about astronauts and practical aspects of the space program.

George O'Hara, a middle-aged man with mental retardation of unknown etiology, came to the outpatient clinic for some general reconditioning after a hospitalization for pneumonia. George lived in a group home and worked in a shop that recycled metal scraps. The generalized weakness that followed his 2-week hospital stay caused him to refuse to dress himself or push the carts of metal scraps at work. He resumed both these activities with a little coaching after he had regained some strength and endurance during rehabilitation in a skilled nursing facility.

Henry Isaacs, a 70-year-old grocer, broke his wrist and hip when he slipped on the ice while shoveling the sidewalk in front of his store. After his hip replacement surgery, Henry spent a short time at Maple Grove Skilled Care Facility. While there, he beat all the OT staff members at checkers. Henry took classes in joint protection principles to reduce his risk of developing carpal tunnel syndrome on his return to the grocery store.

Iris Clark, a housewife and mother of three children under age 6, cut her hand on a broken glass while washing dishes. She severed the A1 and A2 tendon sheaths. Though her hand injury and its surgical repair seemed straightforward, her course of rehabilitation proved more complicated due to multiple sclerosis. Because cooking was an essential job function, the OT staff included a kitchen evaluation as part of her treatment. During the time it took for her right hand to fully recover function, they made sure that she could do all the necessary tasks at home.

Jason Black, a third grader with cerebral palsy, worked with OT practitioners at school and in the community clinic. School OT practitioners communicated his needs to those treating him in the clinic so that his new wheelchair would enable him to sit comfortably all day in a classroom. The OT practitioners in his school also coordinated his other needs for adaptive equipment, and he became much more successful feeding himself at mealtimes and using his augmentative communication device.

When OT staff members explained that Jason became fatigued halfway through the cafeteria lunch, the school staff began feeding him the rest of his meal. This increased his energy level, which led to better attention and participation in the afternoon. Jason no longer needed an afternoon nap, cried less often, and responded more actively to his classmates' attentions. Last month, classmates voted Jason the best student in his class, and he got to take home the class mascot, a plush toy wildcat.

Karen Wu fractured her right third metacarpal bone while attempting a maneuver she had seen in a televised ice-skating competition. Although Karen's subsequent efforts and practice helped her to complete the stunt, she avoided telling her mother about the injury and did not get prompt medical attention. By the time Karen received a referral to the hand clinic, tendon adhesions had limited motion in her right middle finger.

At first, Karen refused to wear the recommended extension splint, but the OT staff members finally convinced her that serious athletes always listen to their trainers. Karen decided to approach hand rehabilitation with the same determination she used in skating. With this new perspective Karen redefined herself as an athlete receiving sports medicine, and found it easier to explain to her classmates why she needed to wear her splint.

Linda Valdez visited the OT clinic after she was diagnosed with rheumatoid arthritis. Linda worked as a secretary in a law office and was active in her church as an organizer of the clothing and food banks that served the homeless. On weekends, children and grandchildren gathered at Linda's house to eat and provide each other with material and social support.

The OT staff members taught Linda important joint protection and energy conservation principles and helped her fit them into her busy life. Despite her abilities to delegate and organize, Linda still experienced some of the joint destruction that accompanies rheumatoid arthritis. Over the years, the OT staff members supported Linda through some losses and assisted her in finding creative ways to continue her roles as matriarch and community organizer.

Mary Smith spent her whole life taking care of her family and house until she had a right-side cerebral vascular accident at age 67. Mrs. Smith's family described her as a cheerful lady who always put up seasonal decorations and loved to putter around in her garden. They had difficulty adjusting to the weepy, fearful "old woman" she became after her stroke, and found it increasingly unpleasant to spend time with her. Depression complicated Mary's recovery process, and she required maximum assistance with almost all activities on her arrival at Maple Grove Skilled Care Facility. OT staff members used some gentle rocking and swinging motions to stimulate her vestibular system and concentrated on reducing her fear of falling during transfers.

As she regained more confidence in her sitting balance, Mary took a more active part in self-care and also joined some gardening and cooking groups in the facility. The OT staff members encouraged Mary's family members to learn transfer techniques, after which her family decided they could safely take Mary out on day trips.

Nancy Grant, an occupational therapy student, spent considerable time working in the computer lab as part of her studies. The OT department had several students complain of aches and pains they attributed to long hours in front of computer screens, so the university contracted with the on-campus agency that did job-site analysis and injury-prevention education. Nancy's workstation needed few modifications, but during the injury-prevention education sessions, she learned that her body mechanics at home also contributed to her lower-back pain. She implemented a number of the OT practitioners' recommendations and reduced her level of discomfort working in the lab.

Olivia Xiong attended the same occupational therapy program as Nancy. Although the computer workstations met Nancy's height requirements, Olivia's height caused her to assume postures that contributed to upper-back pain. The OT consulting agency helped the university make a number of modifications to Olivia's workstation, which eliminated her pain.

Paul Zimmerman, a dermatologist with an expanding practice, developed chronic lower-back pain aggravated by positions he had to assume during medical procedures. The OT practitioner gave him a number of suggestions to modify his workstations and equipment. He incorporated these suggestions during office and clinic renovations. The modifications reduced Paul's discomfort and allowed him to stand longer, making several new surgical procedures available to his clients.

Quentin Keller, a retired farmer, came to Maple Grove Skilled Care Facility after a left-side cerebral vascular accident made it impossible for him to live at home alone. Quentin led an independent and active lifestyle before his cerebral vascular accident and had a great deal of difficulty adjusting to his speech and mobility losses. He came to the attention of the OT staff after several falls. Nursing staff had identified several areas over his sacrum as high risk for the development of decubitus ulcers. Nursing staff hoped that the OT department might give him a cushion and lap tray to solve both these problems.

Instead the OT staffers placed Quentin in a shorter wheelchair with an easy-release, 45-degree seat belt and spent several sessions showing him how to transfer from his wheelchair. Quentin could move around the facility more easily and stopped falling. A firm seat and cushion added to Quentin's comfort, and the skin over his sacrum regained its former integrity. He continued to visit the OT department, particularly when he smelled cookies baking.

Raul Estrada, a young man with a developmental disability, recently began working in the same metal-recycling facility as George O'Hara. Raul complained of back pain and refused to go to work. The OT practitioners consulting with Raul's group home decided to visit his job site to determine the root of the problem. They made a number of suggestions to modify the work site and reduce the employees' risk of injury. Raul began some alternative job tasks and back-strengthening exercises while staff modified the job site. Eventually, Raul took pride in the amount of metal he could move around the facility with ease.

Spiros Prasso injured his back on a construction job. His rehabilitation program included several weeks in the work-hardening clinic. Spiros spent time in general strength training and learned proper body mechanics to do his job safely. Spiros returned to work on modified duty but eventually resumed full-duty work on construction sites.

Tony Adams, a 7-year-old boy, became the unwitting victim of a neighbor firing his gun on the Fourth of July. A stray bullet entered Tony's back between the C4 and C5 ventral rami and partially paralyzed Tony's left scapular muscles. Tony had difficulty lifting anything with his left hand and tended to neglect using the left arm, causing overall atrophy. Tony's mother was more concerned about his nightmares, recent bad grades, and bad-behavior reports from school.

Tony's mother took a second job to try to earn enough money so that she and her son could move from the trailer park where the accident had occurred. This left Tony in the care of a 12-year-old cousin. OT staff tried to show Tony's mother and his cousin some games they could play to strengthen Tony's trapezius and other compensatory muscles, but little follow-up care took place at home. The OT staff contacted the OT practitioner who worked in Tony's school in an effort to maintain some continuity of care after his discharge from the clinic.

Vincent Pearson, a retired postal worker, had some residual loss of intrinsic hand muscles after he recovered from Guillain-Barré syndrome. Vincent learned many compensatory movements and had the good fortune to have a wife willing to take care of all the household chores. Vincent continued to read the newspaper and explore the Internet, two of his favorite activities.

Wendy Dabdoub packed fruit for a large mail-order company. Her job involved repetitive movements, and the winter holiday season meant longer hours and incentives to increase the amount of boxes packed each day. Wendy started the new year with tingling and paresthesia in both hands. Friends urged Wendy to undergo surgery for her carpal tunnel syndrome and leave work on disability. Her employer urged her to give therapy a chance before jumping into surgery.

Wendy's fear of hospitals gave her the extra motivation to try therapy. She learned about the causes of carpal tunnel syndrome and found that rest and antiinflammatory medications helped ease her symptoms. OT practitioners performed a job-site analysis and gave the mail-order company an inservice on the prevention of carpal tunnel syndrome. Wendy's employer instituted warm-up and stretch breaks as part of each employee's work day. Wendy returned to work symptom-free without surgery. The company achieved a 25% reduction in disability costs related to carpal tunnel syndrome in those departments using regular stretch breaks.

Xavier Morales had both legs amputated above the knee during a tour of duty in Vietnam. When he returned to the states the Veteran's Administration hospital fitted him with prostheses and Xavier learned to walk using a cane. Xavier preferred his wheelchair for mobility and became active in local wheelchair athletics. He continued to use his prostheses when making sales presentations for his auto parts company. Over the years, Xavier developed quite a wheelchair collection—one for work, one for basketball, and a third for tennis. His community named Xavier "Man of the Year" for his work with the Paralympics and his counseling of Vietnam veterans. Xavier's collection of spare chairs and parts helped other men and women with disabilities get started in the wheelchair sports that he said "saved his life."

Yasmeen Harris, a 10-year-old girl, severed her right median nerve when she crashed through a glass storm door while playing tag with the neighborhood children. The nerve healed well, but she had residual paralysis for about 4 months while the nerve regenerated. During that time, Yasmeen used a hand-based opponens splint decorated with flower decals to give her a functional hand grip.

Zachary Larson, a 12-year-old boy, crushed his right ulnar nerve when he fractured his elbow while skateboarding. The surgeon had to cut damaged tissue and stretch the nerve to reattach it. Zachary had a lot of discomfort and resented having to wear a bivalve splint for almost a year after his injury. He developed passably legible handwriting with his left hand and learned to hit a baseball using his left arm alone. After his recovery, Zachary became an asset as a switch hitter for his high school baseball team.

Overview of Muscle Anatomy

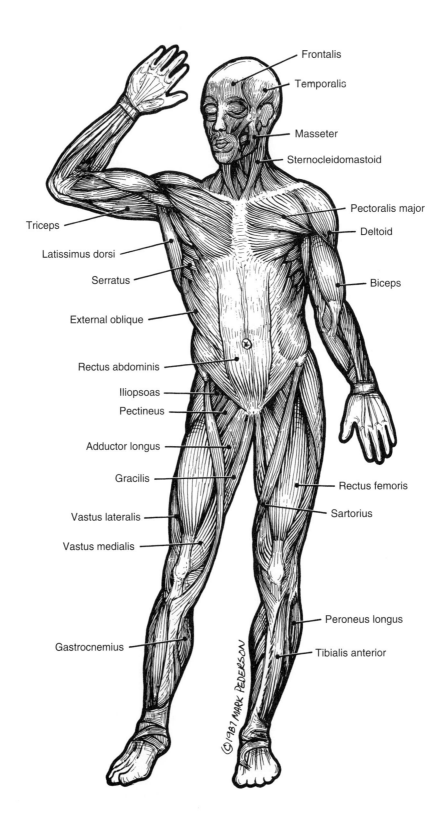

Frontalis

Temporalis

Masseter

Sternocleidomastoid

Pectoralis major

Triceps

Deltoid

Latissimus dorsi

Serratus

Biceps

External oblique

Rectus abdominis

Iliopsoas

Pectineus

Adductor longus

Gracilis

Rectus femoris

Vastus lateralis

Sartorius

Vastus medialis

Peroneus longus

Gastrocnemius

Tibialis anterior

© 1987 MARK PEDERSON

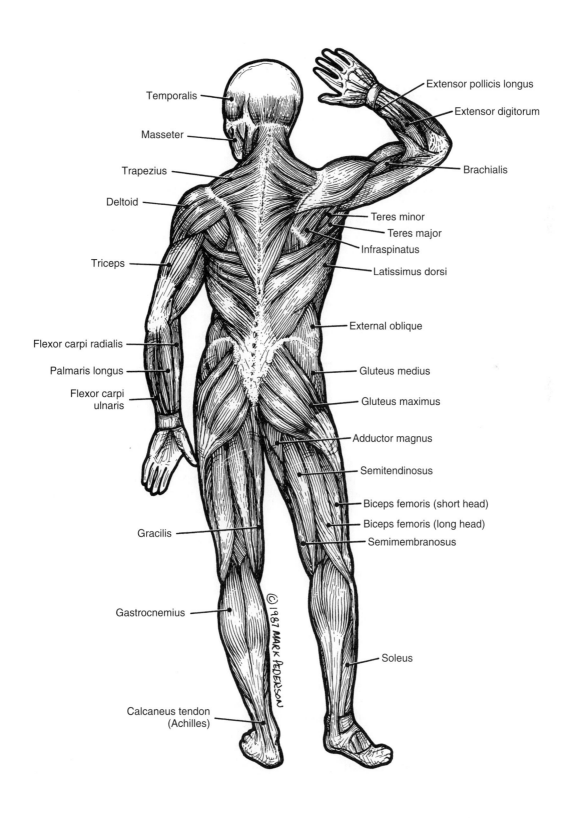

Temporalis

Masseter

Trapezius

Deltoid

Triceps

Flexor carpi radialis

Palmaris longus

Flexor carpi
ulnaris

Gracilis

Gastrocnemius

Calcaneus tendon
(Achilles)

Extensor pollicis longus

Extensor digitorum

Brachialis

Teres minor

Teres major

Infraspinatus

Latissimus dorsi

External oblique

Gluteus medius

Gluteus maximus

Adductor magnus

Semitendinosus

Biceps femoris (short head)

Biceps femoris (long head)

Semimembranosus

Soleus

© 1987 MARK PEDERSON

Working Models of the Fingers and Wrist

Biomechanical models can be valuable tools for teachers and students. They present opportunities for hands-on manipulation. Creating those models provides teachers and students alternative ways to learn. The two models in this appendix have been used in class laboratory settings and hospital teaching programs.

Please keep the following points in mind as you create these models:

- The models are designed to demonstrate mechanical principles and are not intended to be anatomically accurate. For example, the finger model includes metacarpophalangeal (MCP) and interphalangeal (IP) joints. In the model all three joints appear as simple hinge joints to demonstrate movement in one plane only.
- Follow the plans but avoid becoming consumed with measurements. Cut the bony segments generally proportional to the anatomical structures they represent. (For example, the metacarpal bone is longer than the proximal phalanx, which is slightly longer than the middle phalanx, and so on.)
- Be prepared to revise the model. Models often do not "work" the first time. Problem solving around these design details is valuable. For example, place the eyelet pulleys in the approximate positions shown in the diagram at the end of the appendix. After working with the finger model, you may need to move one or two of these eyelets to adjust the relationship of the force (string) with respect to the joint axis.

Please keep the following few items in mind as you use the completed model:

- Orient yourself with the anatomical aspects of the model. For example, the finger model includes the following structures, all of which should be identified before you try to operate the model:
  1. Metacarpal shaft and MCP joint
  2. Proximal, middle, and distal phalanges and proximal and distal interphalangeal joints
  3. Flexor digitorum profundus, extensor digitorum communis, and lumbrical
- As part of your orientation, pull one tendon (string) at a time. Identify what it represents by function and position. For example, if you pull on a string and it flexes the finger, identify this string as the flexor digitorum profundus according to (1) its function in flexing *all* the finger joints, (2) its insertion on the distal phalanx, and (3) its anterior relationship to the side-to-side axes of the MCP and IP joints.
- The model is intended to demonstrate biomechanics; anatomical details have been simplified.

Finger Model

The finger model is a single finger unit including the metacarpal and phalanges (Figure J-1). The metacarpal shaft is anchored to the mounting board, and the proximal, middle, and distal phalanges are free to flex and extend. The model is constructed to allow movement (flexion and extension) in one plane only—the plane of the mounting board.

SUPPLIES

You need the following tools and equipment to build the finger model:

1. 12 to 15 small (½-inch) screws to attach the leather hinges to the metacarpal and phalanges
2. 8 to 10 small eyelet screws to serve as pulleys for tendons
3. 3½-inch × ½-inch squares of leather for hinges (heavier than suede, about ¹⁄₁₆-inch to ⅛-inch thick)
4. 24 inches of soft but strong flexible nylon cord to make tendons
5. Small scrap of ⅛-inch or thinner thermoplastic material
6. A ½-inch × ½-inch board for bony segments (3-, 2.5-, 2-, and 1-inch long pieces for the metacarpal, proximal, middle, and distal phalanges, respectively)
7. A 10-inch × 10-inch piece of ¼-inch-thick plywood for the mounting board
8. 2 screws (about ¾ inch long) to anchor the metacarpal bone onto the mounting board

CONSTRUCTION

Follow these directions, using the diagram of the finger model in this appendix as a guide:

Drill the proper-size holes for the ½-inch screws and attach the bony segments end to end (in order) using

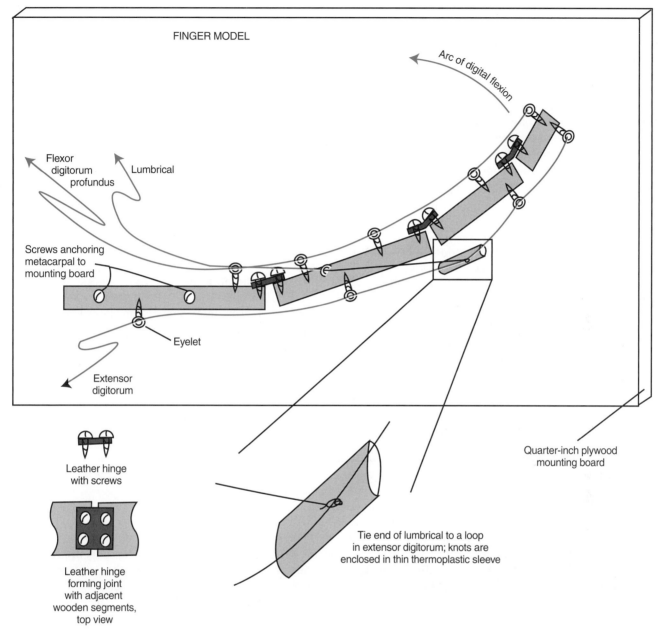

FIGURE **J-1**
Finger model.

the leather hinges and ½-inch screws. Note that the closer together you attach the wood pieces, the less hyperextension of these segments is possible. If you want to show hyperextension (for example, at the MCP joint to demonstrate MCP hyperextension accompanying intrinsic minus hand), attach the leather hinge so that a {1/8}-inch gap remains between the metacarpal and the proximal phalanx.

After "articulating" the segments, drill holes and place the eyelet pulleys according to the illustration. Next,

attach the metacarpal bone to the mounting board as shown. Finally, attach the strings. (Use three different colors to demonstrate the different functions.) Tie strings to the most distal eyelet on the volar side and on the dorsal side, representing the flexor digitorum profundus and extensor digitorum, respectively. Pass each string through the eyelets as shown. Attach the lumbrical string as shown in the inset illustration.

Try it a few times. Remember, the lessons involved in fine-tuning the model are as valuable as any. Students must remember that the best thing about models is that they seldom work correctly in the beginning. They demonstrate all the things that can go wrong, things we often take for granted in normal function.

USE OF THE FINGER MODEL

You can demonstrate a normal digital sweep into extension or flexion by pulling on the appropriate strings. Remember, only with the combination of the lumbrical and flexor digitorum profundus does normal flexion occur. You also may need some lumbrical pull at the end of extension depending on how the MCP joint is constructed.

PATHOLOGICAL PROCESSES

You also can demonstrate a number of pathological conditions with the finger model. A shallow digital sweep, as in the case of intrinsic paralysis, can be shown as follows:

1. Place an empty soda can directly in front of the metacarpal shaft so that it touches the shaft.
2. Pull on the flexor digitorum profundus only and notice the shallow sweep. The tip of the distal phalanx pushes the can from its position (what would be the palm) instead of flexing around the diameter of the can. (You may have to shift the can slightly proximally or distally to ensure the finger demonstrates the effect described.)
3. Extend the digit again and move the can back into place. This time, exert the initial pull on the lumbrical to begin the sweep with the MCP joint (instead of the more distal joints). As the finger begins flexing around the can, initiate a pull in the flexor digitorum profundus simultaneously with the lumbrical. As flexion continues, you must give the lumbrical some slack to allow the flexor digitorum profundus to flex the IP joints. The end result of this combined effort is to produce a deeper digital sweep around the can, allowing the finger to grasp the can.

You also can demonstrate joint contractures by placing sticky-back, hook-and-loop Velcro across any joint. Attach sticky-back hook Velcro to the bony segments (wood) on either side of the leather hinge. Bridge the gap with loop Velcro. Velcro on the flexor side simulates a flexion contracture and limits joint extension. Notice that the joint is limited in active and passive extension, but you can still actively flex the joint.

Using the model, you also can differentiate joint contraction from tendon adhesion. Set another finger model up with sticky-back hook Velcro wrapped around the flexor tendon in front of the metacarpal shaft. Place sticky-back loop Velcro along the front side of the metacarpal shaft in a place where the flexor tendon can be attached via the Velcro. Partially flex the finger using the flexor digitorum profundus. While holding it flexed, push the tendon against the metacarpal shaft to "form" the adhesion. Notice that simultaneous extension of the MCP and IP joints is limited. Passively flexing any joint distal to the adhesion creates slack in the flexor tendon, allowing previously limited joints to be passively extended. Notice also that adhesion prevents active flexion.

Remember that tendon adhesion, unlike joint contracture, demonstrates (1) lack of active motion in the same direction as the tendon adhesion (for example, flexion movement for a flexor tendon adhesion) and (2) limited simultaneous passive motion in the opposite direction of the adhesion in joints distal to the adhesion (for example, extension movement for a flexor tendon adhesion). Joint contracture exhibits limited passive motion in the opposite direction (for example, MCP extension limited by MCP flexion contracture) but no limitation in active motion in the same direction (for example, active MCP flexion with MCP flexion contracture).

Wrist and Finger Model

The wrist and finger model is a model with a wrist, a single working finger similar to the finger model, and a stable thumb post onto which the finger can pinch (Figure J-2). Like the finger model, all movements are limited to one plane. The one forearm bone represented is anchored to the mounting board, and the wrist and proximal, middle, and distal phalanges are free to flex and extend.

SUPPLIES

You need all the supplies previously listed for the finger model (minus the lumbrical parts) and the following additional supplies to construct the wrist and finger model:

1. 8 small (1/2-inch) screws to attach the leather hinges at the wrist
2. 2 to 4 small eyelet screws to serve as pulleys for tendons
3. 2 1/2-inch × 1/2-inch squares of leather for wrist hinges
4. 24 inches of soft but strong flexible nylon cord to use as wrist flexor and extensor tendons
5. A 1/2-inch × 1/2-inch board 8 inches long for the forearm bone
6. A 1/2-inch × 1/2-inch board 1 inch long for the carpal bone of the wrist
7. A 10-inch × 20-inch piece of 1/4-inch plywood for the mounting board
8. 2 screws (about 3/4-inch long) to anchor the forearm bone onto the mounting board

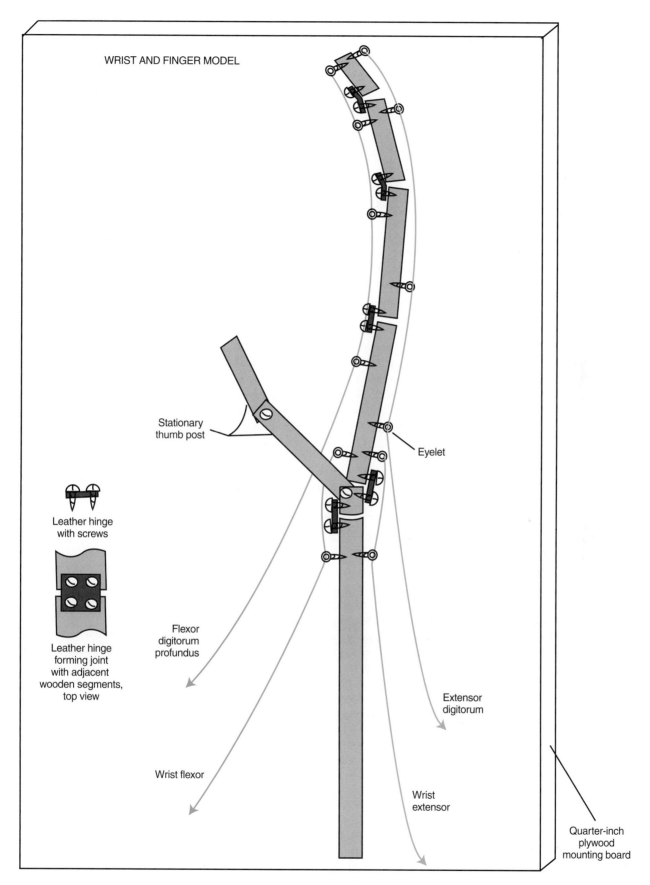

WRIST AND FINGER MODEL

Stationary
thumb post

Eyelet

Leather hinge
with screws

Leather hinge
forming joint
with adjacent
wooden segments,
top view

Flexor
digitorum
profundus

Extensor
digitorum

Wrist flexor

Wrist
extensor

Quarter-inch
plywood
mounting board

FIGURE J-2
Wrist and finger model.

CONSTRUCTION

Follow these directions, using the diagram of the wrist and finger model in this appendix as a guide:

Drill the proper-size holes for the ½-inch screws and attach the bony segments end to end (in order) using the leather hinges and ½-inch screws. Note that the closer together you attach the wood pieces, the less hyperextension of these segments is possible. If you want to show hyperextension (for example, at the MCP joint to demonstrate MCP hyperextension accompanying intrinsic minus hand), attach the leather hinge so that a {⅛}-inch gap exists between the bony segments. For the wrist, follow the illustration and place one hinge dorsally and the other volarly. This allows the wrist to both flex and extend.

After "articulating" the segments, drill holes and place the eyelet pulleys according to the illustration. Next, attach the forearm bone to the mounting board as shown. Finally, attach the strings. (Use four different colors to demonstrate the different functions.) Tie strings to the most distal eyelet on the volar side and the dorsal side, representing the flexor digitorum profundus and extensor digitorum, respectively. Tie strings to the eyelets on the volar side and the dorsal side of the metacarpal, representing the wrist flexor and extensor. Pass each string through the eyelets as shown.

Try it a few times. Again, anticipate some fine-tuning. The lessons involved here are valuable, just like those of the finger model.

USE OF THE WRIST AND FINGER MODEL

You can demonstrate normal wrist extension and flexion by pulling on the appropriate strings. You also can differentiate wrist and finger muscle functions. Most important, you can demonstrate the need for wrist extensors to stabilize the wrist when the long finger flexors such as the flexor digitorum profundus contract to perform grasp. Pulling the flexor digitorum profundus without the wrist extensor results in simultaneous wrist and finger flexion, which creates active insufficiency of the finger flexors and failed grip. This occurs in radial nerve damage.

Active insufficiency is demonstrated on this model. Measure the excursion necessary for the flexor digitorum profundus to flex the three finger joints from full extension to full flexion. (You must hold the wrist in a neutral position manually to prevent the finger flexor from flexing the wrist.) Record this number as the excursion of the finger flexor. Return all the finger joints into extension, and while stabilizing the fingers in extension with one hand, pull the wrist into flexion via the flexor digitorum profundus. Measure the excursion required for the finger flexor tendon to flex the wrist only. Now free the finger and continue pulling on the flexor tendon only through the distance of the remaining excursion. After exhausting the excursion of the flexor digitorum profundus, you should see the wrist in flexion and the fingers partially flexed. No firm grip or pinch to the thumb post is possible unless the flexor tendon is pulled through more excursion.

The model also can demonstrate passive insufficiency. Passively extend the finger of the model, holding the wrist in a neutral position. Hold the finger fully extended and pull the slack from the flexor digitorum profundus. Place a marker or tie a knot in the flexor tendon to prevent it from passing through the most proximal pulley, which would simulate that this muscle has been stretched to its maximum length. Now attempt passive simultaneous finger and wrist extension and notice how the tightness in the flexor tendon prevents full simultaneous finger and wrist extension.

Tenodesis grasp is probably the most important demonstration this model provides. Passively place the wrist and fingers in partial flexion. Take up the slack in the flexor digitorum profundus and hold the flexor down on the mounting board to prevent it from being pulled distally. Pull the wrist extensor while holding down the flexor tendon and watch the wrist extend and the finger flex. (The finger flexes without pulling the flexor tendon proximally.) Holding down the flexor simulates a shortened finger flexor from either lack of stretch or tenodesis surgery. If you attempt wrist extension without holding the flexor onto the board, wrist extension occurs with very little finger flexion.

Learning Objectives

Many students rely on old test questions to study for exams. (In some medical and graduate programs, students become collectors and actually make deals about these tests. You hear statements like, "I have the 1967 edition, but I'm missing the last page. Would you trade my complete 1985 Exam II for the last page of the 1967 test?") Although we do not advocate studying from available exam questions to the exclusion of studying the original text material and course lecture notes, asking and answering one another's questions can be a helpful study tool.

The learning objectives in this appendix serve as study guides for each chapter in the book. In many cases, instructors develop multiple-choice test questions directly reflecting the content emphasized in a course's learning objectives. More directly, students can change each objective into a question when they study for essay or short-answer exam formats.

Chapter 1

- Define *kinesiology* and identify the three physical sciences that contribute to it.
- Describe why kinesiology is considered a narrow approach to movement.
- Identify the basic belief on which OT practice is based.
- Identify the factors influencing individual performance that become clear when movement is viewed within the context of activity.
- Briefly describe and differentiate the mechanistic and transformative philosophies.
- Briefly describe and differentiate the reconstructive, orthopedic, and kinetic models of practice.
- Describe the value of the rehabilitation model as a guide to kinesiologic thinking.

Chapter 2

- Describe the major skeletal movements in terms of planes (surfaces on which the movements occur) and axes (around which the movements are centered).
- Demonstrate the three types of muscle contraction and describe how the two muscle attachments move in each.
- Define *excursion* and describe its effect on muscle length.
- Differentiate the agonist, antagonist, and synergist in a description of muscle action.

- Demonstrate correct use of the terms used to communicate various muscle grades (words and numbers).
- Describe the use of a goniometer to measure joint range of motion and differentiate active and passive joint ranges of motion.
- Provide one-line definitions of the various italicized terms under the section titled "Medical Diagnoses Affecting Movement."
- Differentiate scalar and vector quantities in terms of their measurements.
- Differentiate mass and weight and identify which of the two also is described as force.
- Describe normal force and compare it with shear force.

Chapter 3

- Describe one way in which gravity influences motor development.
- Demonstrate how the center of gravity is approximated.
- Perform the brief calculations and measurements necessary in the identification of an object's center of gravity.
- Determine the center of gravity of the entire body based on the segmental centers of gravity.
- Convert an object's mass (in kilograms) to its weight (in newtons), illustrating how mass is converted to force through the multiplication of mass by the constant for the acceleration of gravity.

Chapter 4

- Provide examples of each of Newton's three laws.
- Describe the conditions of force equilibrium when an individual is seated (at rest) in a chair.
- Demonstrate the three types of muscle contraction and describe the movements of the two muscle attachments in each.
- Describe the effect of excursion on muscle strength in a concentric contraction.
- Describe what is meant by the excursion requirements of movement at a joint.
- Describe what happens to a muscle when its antagonistic motion occurs.
- Describe the change in distance between the origin and insertion of a muscle in a concentric contraction and how this differs from that in an eccentric contraction.

- Describe what happens to the origin and insertion of a flexor muscle when the joint is pulled into extension by an outside force.
- Identify and briefly describe an example of each type of external force described in the chapter.
- Define and differentiate *force magnitude, force orientation,* and *internal (muscular) force direction.*
- Differentiate the determinants of muscle force and excursion.
- Explain how forces are combined through addition and subtraction to determine the resultant force in a tug-of-war game.
- Explain both the parallelogram and polygon methods for the combination of multiple forces when two individuals push a cart.

Chapter 5

- Differentiate rotary and linear motion based on (1) the velocity of points in a bar moving in a line versus in a circle and (2) the orientation of the bar.
- Describe the difference in the effect of the amount of force used in linear versus rotary motion.
- Provide a synonym for the term *torque.*
- Identify factors used in the determination of linear and rotary equilibrium.
- Identify the angle of pull at which all the muscle's force is used for the rotary movement of the joint.
- Identify the angle of pull at which the moment arm is the longest.
- Identify which moment arm produces the strongest movement.
- Provide everyday examples of each lever system.
- Explain why most musculoskeletal levers are class III levers.
- Explain how changing the force's angle of pull and the muscle length affect the tendency of the force to rotate the lever at the joint.
- Identify the lever and axis of various musculoskeletal segments.

Chapter 6

- Differentiate between open- and closed-chain hip movements.
- Describe the relationship between lumbar curve and hamstring length.
- Describe the three basic pairs of movements and the nature of vertebral column movement.
- Describe the normal and pathological curves of the vertebral column.
- Explain the effects of unilateral and bilateral contractions of vertebral muscles.
- Explain how movements differ in direction and plane according to the relationship of the force to the axis.

- Describe movements and muscle functions in the trunk that relate to and accompany upper-extremity movements.
- Describe how the trunk remains balanced against the downward pull of gravity.
- Describe the relationship between head and neck position and the force the position exerts on the cervical intervertebral disks.
- Explain the relationship between rotary force (extension) and compression force during activation of the back extensors.
- Explain the role of pelvic stabilization in seating.
- Describe the basic biomechanics of one common restraint system.

Chapter 7

- Describe the joints of the shoulder complex and the elbow in terms of their classifications and degrees of freedom, including the plane and axis associated with each degree of joint freedom.
- Differentiate scapular from glenohumeral movement.
- State the major movements and movers of the shoulder complex.
- Describe how arrows are used to demonstrate the analysis of muscle forces affecting the shoulder and elbow.
- Describe the scapular movement and stabilization that accompany glenohumeral movement.
- Describe the separate contributions of scapular rotation and glenohumeral abduction to shoulder abduction when an individual raises the hand above the head.
- Explain the main effect of the deltoid compared with that of the supraspinatus in early glenohumeral abduction.
- Explain the biomechanical basis for shoulder subluxation.
- List the various roles of the rotator cuff muscles.
- Describe how manual muscle testing is an example of an isometric torque curve.
- Describe how manual muscle testing is an example of equilibrium of torques.
- Describe how the biceps long head can "become" an abductor of the glenohumeral joint.
- List the combination of joints necessary for flexion and extension and pronation and supination of the forearm.
- Describe how the use of the biceps in elbow flexion can depend on the forearm's position.
- Explain the role of the biceps in supination.
- Describe the contribution of the wrist joint to forearm pronation and supination range of motion.

Chapter 8

- Describe the differential effects of the major wrist flexors in terms of their functions of wrist flexion with deviation and wrist extension with deviation.
- Identify the strongest function, based on moment arm, of each wrist flexor and extensor.
- Describe how synergistic actions of wrist flexors and extensors yield balanced wrist ulnar and radial deviation.
- Describe the various imbalances at the wrist resulting from radial, ulnar, and median nerve damage at the level of the elbow.
- Explain the basic functions of the extrinsic and intrinsic musculature of the hand.
- Describe the balancing effect of the intrinsics on the long digital extensors.
- List in sequence the intrinsic and extrinsic muscles involved in opening and closing of the hand.
- Describe the effects of ulnar and median nerve damage in opening and closing of the hand.
- Describe the various prehension patterns of the thumb.
- Describe the effects of median and ulnar nerve damage on prehension.
- Identify which grasps require the thumb (and in what capacity) and which do not.
- Describe the differential functions of the thumb carpometacarpal, metacarpophalangeal, and interphalangeal joints.
- Describe the differential uses of the thenar and intrinsic thumb adductor muscles in wide versus narrow grip-span grasps that use the thumb.

- Describe the pathokinesiology of ulnar drift, boutonniere, bowstringing, wrist drop with grip failure, and intrinsic minus hand.
- Differentiate between joint contracture and tendon adhesion, using differential movements of adjacent joints to create slack.
- Explain the basis of tenodesis grip (tendon action) and explain tenodesis using the concept of passive insufficiency.

Chapter 9

- List and describe the four factors in stability and identify the missing stability factor in an unstable situation.
- Describe the stability problem of an individual with recent bilateral lower-extremity amputations as the individual attempts to move a wheelchair.
- Identify the stability risks associated with recliner wheelchairs.
- Demonstrate a safe wheelchair-to-bed standing pivot transfer, identifying both the original and the new bases of support.
- Describe lower-extremity movements in the sagittal and frontal planes during normal gait.
- Describe the muscle activity responsible for the movements in the sagittal and frontal planes during normal gait.
- Describe two compensations that an individual with weak hip abductors can use during unilateral stance.

Glossary

Abduction. Movement in a joint that brings the distal segment farther from the midline of the body

Acromioclavicular joint. A small synovial joint at which the clavicle articulates with the acromion process of the scapula

Active insufficiency. A condition in which shortened agonist muscles cannot move all possible joints through their full available ranges of motion

Adduction. Movement in a joint that brings the distal segment toward the midline of the body

Adductor brevis. One of the muscles in the hip adductor group that originates from the pubis and inserts along the linea aspera of the femur

Adductor group. Six muscles—the adductor magnus, adductor brevis, adductor longus, gracilis, obturator externus, and pectineus—that act primarily to adduct the thigh

Adductor longus. The most anterior muscle of the adductor group; originates from the pubis and inserts along the linea aspera of the femur

Adductor magnus. The largest of the adductor group of muscles; originates from the ischium and pubis and inserts linearly along the entire medial femur, with some fibers reaching to the tibial collateral ligament

Afferent nerves. Nerves that carry impulses from the body to the central nervous system

Agonist. A muscle that acts as the primary mover for a specific joint motion

Amphiarthrodial joint. A cartilaginous articulation between two or more adjacent bones that permits limited motion only

Antagonist. A muscle that opposes the agonist for a specific joint motion

Aponeurosis. Any fascial thickening where muscle fibers attach

Atlas. The first cervical vertebra

ATP. Adenosine triphosphate ($C_{10}H_{16}N_5O_{13}P_3$); stores large amounts of energy for various biochemical processes, including muscle contraction through its hydrolysis to ADP ($C_{10}H_{15}N_5O_{10}P_2$)

Autonomic nervous system. A system of efferent nerves and nerve fibers that allow the central nervous system to control organs and glands

Axis. *Physics:* The pivot point for an arc of motion or rotation *Anatomy:* The second cervical vertebra

Balance point. That part of a body upon which a force may act while the body remains in equilibrium

Ballistic movement. Strong, rapid contraction with movement completed primarily through momentum

Base of support. The amount of contact area that a body resting on a surface assumes

Belief. Mental acceptance and conviction in the truth, actuality, or validity of a particular tenet or body of tenets accepted by a group of people

Biceps femoris. One of the hamstring muscles that originates on the pelvis and proximal femur and inserts onto the head of the fibula and lateral tibia

Biomechanics. The science of internal and external forces acting on a living body

Bipennate muscle. A muscle whose fibers converge from opposite sides to attach onto a central tendon, like a feather

Body. A generic term in physics referring to a complete and entire mass or collection of material that is distinct from other masses

Camber. Tilting of wheels from a vertical position to make them more maneuverable

Carpal tunnel syndrome. Compression of the nerves, arteries, and veins that pass through a narrow anatomical compartment formed by the carpal bones and the flexor retinaculum (see page 120, A Closer Look Box 8-1)

Center of gravity. The balance point in or near a body located where the resultant force of the gravitational forces on the body's component particles acts

Center of gravity height. How high a body's center of gravity lies in relation to the surface upon which it stands

Center of gravity projection. A downward extension of the body's center of gravity outside the confines of the body itself

Center of rotation. The central point about which rotary motion occurs

Circumduction. Rotary movement that uses a combination of movements in various planes and involves more than one axis

Closed-chain movement. Movement that occurs at the proximal end of an extremity because the distal end is stabilized (see page 81, Figure 6-11, *B*)

Cocontraction. When agonist and antagonist muscles contract simultaneously to stabilize a joint

Compressive force. A normal force that pushes tissue surfaces closer together

Concentric contraction. Energy-expending process that results in shortening of the muscle fibers

Contracture. A condition in which skin, connective tissue, or muscle becomes shorter in its resting state and consequently limits movement

Coxa valga. A bowlegged appearance caused by an angle of more than 125 degrees between the head and neck and the shaft of the femur

Coxa vara. A knock-kneed appearance caused by an angle of less than 125 degrees between the head and neck and the shaft of the femur

CVA. Cerebral vascular accident, or stroke, caused when bleeding or clotting in the brain results in damage to surrounding neural tissue

Dens. A toothlike protuberance (odontoid process) of the axis on which the atlas rests

Diarthrodial joint. A joint in which a fluid-filled space occurs between two or more articulating bones, allowing freedom of motion

Displacement. Movement in a direction such that an object travels a quantifiable distance, for example, 60 miles north

Distensibility. Expansion or dilation inherent or caused by force experienced within tissue

Dorsal aponeurosis. A triangular-shaped widening of the extensor digitorum tendon over the metacarpophalangeal joint; serves as an attachment for intrinsic muscles; also known as the *extensor expansion, extensor hood,* or *dorsal hood*

Dorsal hood. See *dorsal aponeurosis*

Eccentric contraction. Energy-expending process that results in lengthening of the muscle fibers

Efferent nerves. Nerves that carry impulses from the central nervous system to the body

Elasticity. The inherent property of material to return to its original form or state after deformation

Epiphyseal plates. Centers of cartilaginous growth within bones

Equilibrium. The condition of an object at rest or in unaccelerated motion when acted on by two or more forces so that the resultant of all forces acting on it is zero ($\Sigma F = 0$) and the sum of all torques ($\Sigma T = 0$) about any axis is zero

Equilibrium of torques. The condition of an object in which all tendencies for rotation equal zero ($\Sigma T = 0$)

Erector spinae. Deep back muscles that run parallel to the vertebral column and consist of three major divisions—the spinalis (spine to spine), longissimus (transverse process to transverse process), and iliocostalis (rib to rib)

Eversion. A movement that rotates the sole of the foot from the midline of the body; associated with forefoot pronation

Excursion. The full extent that a muscle's fibers can elongate and shorten

Extension. Rotary movement at a joint that brings the skeletal segments farther from one another

Extensor digitorum longus. A pennate muscle originating on the lateral condyle of the tibia and the upper two thirds of the fibula, its tendon splitting into four tendons that insert onto the lateral four toes

Extensor expansion. See *dorsal aponeurosis*

Extensor hallucis longus. Originates on the midfibula and inserts at the base of the distal phalanx of the great toe

Extensor hood. See *dorsal aponeurosis*

External abdominal oblique. One of four paired abdominal muscles; lies just lateral to the rectus abdominus and attaches medially onto the pelvis and the aponeurosis of the abdomen and laterally onto the ribs

External torque. A tendency toward rotation produced by forces outside the body

Factors in stability. The factors that determine whether individuals maintain balance—center of gravity height, base of support, center of gravity projection, and weight

False ribs. Five pairs of bones that lie inferior to the true ribs and articulate posteriorly with the vertebrae; have no bony anterior articulation

Fascia. Fibrous connective tissue that envelops, separates, or binds together muscles

Fast-twitch muscle fiber. Contains lower concentrations of myoglobin and predominates in muscles that contract rapidly for limited amounts of time

First-class lever. The axis of motion lies between opposing forces of effort and resistance (see Table 5-1 on page 63)

Flexion. Movement at a joint that brings the skeletal segments closer to one another

Flexion moment. A tendency to rotate that results in flexion

Flexor hallucis brevis. Originates on the plantar surface of the cuboid bone and inserts onto the base of the phalanx of the great toe

Flexor retinaculum. Fascia (also known as the *transverse carpal ligament*) that stretches from the hook of the hamate and pisiform bones to the scaphoid and trapezium and forms the fibrous "roof" of the carpal tunnel

Force. A vector quantity with the capacity to do work or cause physical change, such as acceleration of a body in the direction of its application

Frame of reference. Sources of existing philosophy, theory, practice, knowledge, or research findings that are used by an individual or a group to determine how they judge, control, or direct action or expression

Friction. A force that resists movement when two bodies are in contact

Fusiform muscle. A cylindrical muscle in which all the fibers run parallel to one another from origin to insertion

Gait cycle. The normal walking pattern from the time one extremity makes contact with the ground until it swings and contacts the ground again

Ganglia. Collections of nerve-cell bodies that lie outside the central nervous system

Gastrocnemius. One of three muscles that comprise the triceps surae; originates on the medial and lateral condyles of the femur and inserts at the tendo calcaneus onto the calcaneus bone

Gemellus inferior. Originates on the ischial tuberosity and inserts onto the tendon of the obturator internus

Gemellus superior. Originates on the ischial spine and inserts onto the tendon of the obturator internus

Genu valga. A knock-kneed appearance caused by a pathological process of the knee, resulting in outward projection of the distal tibia

Genu vara. A bowlegged appearance caused by a pathological process of the knee, resulting in inward projection of the distal tibia

Glenohumeral joint. Synovial joint at which the head of the humerus articulates with the glenoid fossa of the scapula

Gluteus maximus. Heavy, coarse muscle that pads the ischial tuberosity; originates on the sacrum, coccyx, and ilium and inserts on the femur and iliotibial tract

Gluteus medius. A muscle lying beneath the gluteus maximus that originates on the ilium and inserts onto the greater trochanter of the femur

Gluteus minimus. A muscle lying beneath the gluteus medius that originates on the ilium and inserts onto the greater trochanter of the femur

Goniometer. An instrument used to measure joint angles of motion

Gracilis. One of the hip adductor group of muscles; originates on the pubis and inserts as a tendon onto the medial tibia

Gravitational attraction. The natural phenomenon of attraction between massive bodies so that all smaller masses around a larger mass are pulled toward the center of the large mass

Gravity environment. The natural force of attraction exerted by a celestial body, such as Earth, upon objects at or near its surface, tending to draw them toward the center of the body

Hamstrings. A group of muscles—the semitendinosus, semimembranosus, and biceps femoris—that comprise the back of the thigh; originating from the ischial tuberosity and inserting onto the proximal tibia

Hypertonia. Increased muscle tone or activity

Hypotonia. Less-than-normal muscle tone or activity

Iliacus. Originates on the pelvis and joins with the psoas major to form the iliopsoas tendon, which attaches to the lesser trochanter of the femur

Iliopsoas. Two muscles—the iliacus and psoas major—that originate on the pelvis and lumbar spine and insert as one tendon onto the lesser trochanter of the femur

Iliotibial tract. Fibrous fascia into which a number of muscles insert; runs down the lateral side of the thigh and blends into the joint capsule at the knee

Initial contact. The part of the gait cycle at which the heel makes contact with the ground

Initial swing. The part of the gait cycle at which the toes rise off the ground

Internal abdominal oblique. One of four paired abdominal muscles; lies just inferior and deep to the external abdominal oblique and attaches medially onto the lower ribs and laterally onto the pelvis

Internal torque. A tendency toward rotation produced by forces inside the body

Interossei. Seven small muscles of the foot or hand that originate on adjacent sides of the metatarsals or metacarpals and insert onto the extensor hood mechanism of the hand and the lateral side of the proximal phalanx and joint capsule

Intervertebral disk. A cartilaginous structure that lies between adjacent vertebral bodies in the spine

Intrinsic minus. Metacarpophalangeal hyperextension with incomplete interphalangeal extension caused by weakness of the intrinsic muscles in the hand (see page 18, Figure 2-6; page 132, Figure 8-10; and page 132, Figure 8-11)

Inversion. A movement that rotates the sole of the foot toward the midline of the body; associated with supination of the forefoot

Isometric contraction. Energy-expending process in which the length of the muscle fibers does not change

Joint force. The internal reaction force acting on contact surfaces when a joint is subjected to external loads

Kinesiology. Scientific study of the active and passive structures involved in movement

Kinetic model. Analysis of activity in terms of anatomy, physiology, pathology, and kinesiology to restore function via adaptive equipment or compensatory exercise techniques

Kyphosis. An exaggerated convexity in the thoracic curve of the spine

Labyrinthine reflexes. Motor responses caused or affected by the position of the head and consequently the effect of gravity acting on the inner ear (labyrinth)

Law of acceleration. Newton's second law of motion; states that forces are the product of a body's mass and its acceleration, or $F = ma$ (see pages 44 through 45)

Law of action-reaction. Newton's third law of motion; states that if a force acts on an object and that object remains stationary, an equal force must be acting on the object in the opposite direction (see pages 45 through 47)

Law of inertia. Newton's first law of motion; states that a body at rest or in motion remains so unless acted on by an outside force (see page 44)

Lever arm. The rigid structure that spans the distance from an applied force to its center of motion, also known as the *moment arm of the force*

Leverage. Mechanical advantage produced by the length of the lever arm

Loading. The part of the gait cycle in which the body's weight is shifted onto the lower extremity in contact with the ground

Longitudinal arch. A palmar arch that curves from the wrist to the fingertips, with its apex at the row of metacarpal heads

Lordosis. An exaggerated concavity in the lumbar curve of the spine

Lumbricals. Four small muscles of the foot or the hand that originate on the flexor tendons and insert onto the extensor hood mechanism of the digits

Manual muscle testing. A highly structured procedure of positioning and hand placement used to determine the degree of muscular weakness resulting from disease, injury, or disuse

Matter. A substance made up of atoms and molecules that exists as a solid, liquid, or gas

Mechanical advantage. The ratio of the output force produced to the applied input force, which is usually related to the length of the lever arm (see pages 60 through 61)

Mechanistic. Understanding of the world as a mechanism, especially a tendency to explain phenomena by reference to physical or biological causes only

Midstance. The part of the gait cycle in which body weight is supported by the lower extremity in contact with the ground

Midswing. The part of the gait cycle in which the leg is lifted off the ground and moves forward into terminal swing

MMT. Manual muscle testing

Model of practice. A unique means by which assumptions are organized and arranged to guide study and action within a profession

Moment arm. The perpendicular distance from an applied force to its axis of motion; also known as *lever arm*

Multijoint muscle. A muscle that crosses two or more joint axes, producing motion in more than one joint

Myoglobin. The primary source of oxygen in muscle tissue; has a higher affinity for oxygen than hemoglobin in the blood

Newton. The metric unit of force required to accelerate a 1-kg mass 1 m/sec^2

Normal force. A force directed perpendicularly toward or from a surface area

Nucleus pulposus. Jellylike tissue that can be found at the center of intervertebral disks that absorbs forces on spinal segments

Obturator externus. One of the adductor group of muscles; originates on the pubis and ischium and inserts onto the greater trochanter

Obturator internus. Originates on the ischium and perineal fascia and inserts onto the greater trochanter of the femur

Open-chain movement. Movement that occurs at the distal end of an extremity because the proximal end is stabilized (see page 81, Figure 6-11, *A*)

Orthopedic model. Use of anatomy, physiology, pathology, and kinesiology in the design of restorative activities for specific muscle and joint problems

Pascal. The metric unit used to measure stress in materials, where 1 Pa = 1 N/m^2

Passive insufficiency. A condition in which a multijoint muscle prevents full movement of joints in the opposite direction

Pectineus. One of the adductor group of muscles; originates on the pubis and inserts onto the lesser trochanter of the femur

Pelvic obliquity. Asymmetry of the pelvis in the frontal plane in which one side lies higher than the other in a resting position, usually due to pathological conditions of muscle shortening or bony deformities (see page 90, Figure 6-27)

Pelvic rotation. Asymmetry of the pelvis in the horizontal plane in which one side is anterior to the other in a resting position, usually due to pathological conditions of muscle shortening or bony deformities (see page 91, Figure 6-28)

Pelvic tilt. The angle of the pelvis in the sagittal plane in relationship to the spine

Pennate muscle. A muscle whose fibers originate on a bone and insert along the length of a tendon, like a feather

Percentile weight. The percentage assigned to body segments (such as the forearm or thigh) that represents the proportion of that segment to total body weight (see Appendix B)

Peroneus brevis. Originates on the lower two thirds of the fibula and inserts onto the dorsum of the fifth metatarsal

Peroneus longus. Originates on the lateral condyle of the tibia and the upper two thirds of the fibula and inserts onto the plantar surfaces of the cuneiform and base of the first metatarsal

Peroneus tertius. A partially separated portion of the extensor digitorum longus that originates on the lower fibula and inserts onto the base of the fifth metatarsal

Philosophy. A system of motivating concepts or principles used to critique and analyze fundamental beliefs as they are conceptualized or formulated

Piriformis. Originates on the sacrum and inserts onto the greater trochanter

Point of application. The exact place on a lever on which a force acts

Pound. A term, originating in England, for the unit of force equal to the weight of a standard 1-lb mass, where the local acceleration of gravity is 32.174 ft/sec²

Preswing. The part of the gait cycle in which the heel lifts off the ground

Psoas major. Originates on the lumbar spine and joins with the iliacus to form the iliopsoas tendon that attaches to the lesser trochanter of the femur

Quadriceps femoris. A muscle whose four distinct parts usually are considered as four separate muscles—the rectus femoris, vastus lateralis, vastus medialis, and vastus intermedius

Radial deviation. Movement of the hand or fingers toward the thumb and away from the midline of the body (in anatomical position); also known as wrist abduction

Rate of acceleration. The average rate at which final velocity (v) changes from initial velocity (u) with respect to time (t), or $a = (v - u)/t$; free-falling bodies under the influence of terrestrial gravity fall with an average rate of acceleration equal to approximately 9.81 m/sec² (1 m = 32 ft)

Reconstruction model. Use of voluntary activities that are graded and adapted to specific muscles and joints to restore physical function after illness or injury

Rectus abdominus. The most superficial layer of four paired abdominal muscles; attaches to the sternum superiorly and the pelvis inferiorly

Rectus femoris. One part of the quadriceps femoris that originates on the anterior inferior iliac spine and inserts onto the patella

Resultant force. A single force that is the sum of two or more forces with different orientations and a common point of application

Rotary motion. Movement in a circular arc around an immovable line or axis

Rotation. Joint movement around a longitudinal axis in a horizontal plane

Rotator cuff. Four muscles—the supraspinatus, infraspinatus, teres minor, and subscapularis—that secure the head of the humerus in the glenoid fossa of the scapula and help stabilize the glenohumeral joint

Sacrum. Five fused vertebrae at the caudal end of the spinal column

Sartorius. A long strap muscle originating on the lateral pelvis and inserting onto the medial surface of the tibia just below the knee joint

Scalar. A quantity, such as mass, length, or speed, defined by its magnitude and lacking direction

Scapulohumeral rhythm. Simultaneous glenohumeral and scapular movements that together produce full shoulder abduction and flexion

Scapulothoracic joint. The articulation between the scapula and the thorax (chest wall) that contributes about one third of shoulder motion as it repositions the glenohumeral joint; technically not a "joint"

Scoliosis. A pathological S-shaped curve of the spine that occurs in the frontal plane

Second-class lever. Lends mechanical advantage to the force of effort, which lies farther from the axis of motion than the force of resistance (see Table 5-1 on page 63)

Segmental centers of gravity. The balance point in a segmental portion of the body, such as the forearm or thigh

Semimembranosus. One of the hamstring muscles that originates on the ischial tuberosity and inserts onto the posterior medial surface of the tibia

Semitendinosus. One of the hamstring muscles that originates on the ischial tuberosity and inserts via an aponeurosis onto the upper, medial surface of the tibia

Shear. Forces that operate in tangential or parallel directions to an object's surface

Slow-twitch muscle fiber. Contains higher concentrations of myoglobin and predominates in postural muscles that must work for prolonged periods without becoming fatigued

Slug. A British unit of measurement for a mass that is accelerated at a rate of 1 ft/sec^2 when acted on by a 1-lb force (1 slug equals 32 lb in Earth's gravity, where a 1-lb force accelerates at 32 ft/sec^2)

Soleus. One of three muscles that form the triceps surae; originates on the proximal tibia and fibula and inserts as the tendo calcaneus onto the calcaneus bone

Spasticity. Extreme hypertonicity of muscles exhibited as resistance to movement and increased reflexes

Stance phase. The part of the gait cycle from the point at which the heel makes contact with the ground to the point at which the heel rises above the ground in preswing

Sternoclavicular joint. A small, freely moveable synovial joint at which the clavicle articulates with the sternum

Sternocleidomastoid. Most prominent anterior neck muscle originating on the sternum and proximal clavicle and inserting onto the mastoid process of the skull

Stress. A vector quantity found within the material on which forces act and measured by division of the amount of force by the amount of tissue, for example, N/m^2

Stroke. See CVA

Subluxation. Displacement or partial dislocation of joint components

Swing phase. The part of the gait cycle in which the toe leaves the ground, accelerates into midswing, and decelerates into terminal swing

Synarthrodial joint. An immobile fibrous interface between two or more bones

Synergy. Muscles acting together to produce specific movements

Tangential. A force that operates superficially on an object's surface; also known as a *shear force*

Temporomandibular joint. The synovial joint at which the jaw articulates with the skull

Tendency to rotate. The ability of a force to cause rotation; also known as *torque* (see pages 60 through 61)

Tendinitis. Inflammation of the tendon and its muscular attachments

Tenodesis grasp. Passive tension present in the finger flexors caused by wrist extension because of passive insufficiency of the finger flexor tendons

Tenodesis release. A condition in which wrist flexion causes passive stretching of the extensor digitorum communis to allow sufficient finger extension to release objects held in the hand

Tenosynovitis. Inflammation of the tendon sheath

Tensile. Forces that pull tissues apart

Tensile force. A normal force that pulls two surfaces apart

Tensor fascia lata. A muscle that originates on the iliac crest of the pelvis and inserts onto the iliotibial tract just below the greater trochanter

Terminal stance. The part of the gait cycle in which body weight shifts onto the inside of the foot in preparation for preswing

Terminal swing. The part of the gait cycle in which the swing's momentum is slowed in preparation for initial contact

Third-class lever. Allows resistance to be moved at great speed and through great distance because the force of resistance lies farther from the axis than the force of effort (see Table 5-1 on page 63)

Tibialis anterior. Originates on the lateral condyle and upper two thirds of the tibia and inserts onto the medial sides of the cuneiform and the base of the first metatarsal

Tibialis posterior. The deepest muscle of the leg; originates on the lateral and posterior surface of the upper tibia and the posterior tibia and inserts onto the plantar navicular and cuneiform

Torque. The tendency of a force to cause rotation, as determined by the product of its force and distance from the axis of motion (moment arm), $T = F \times MA$

Torque-angle curve. A curve documenting the amount of torque needed to bring a joint into different positions or joint angles (see pages 142-145 and Figures 8-22, 8-23, 8-24 and 8-25)

Tracts. A bundle of nerve fibers with a common origin, termination, and function; convey impulses within the central nervous system

Transformative. Understanding of the world as a dynamic system in which change is a constant opportunity for evolution and diversification

Transverse arch. A palmar arch that curves from the radial to the ulnar side of the hand, with its apex near the head of the third metacarpal

Transversospinalis. Deep back muscles that run upward and medial to the spinal column and consist of three major divisions—the semispinalis (transverse process below to spinous process above), multifidus (in the furrow between spines and transverse processes), and rotatores (transverse process below to lamina above)

Transversus abdominis. The deepest of four paired abdominal muscles; fibers run horizontally from the ribs and vertebral fascia to an aponeurosis at the midline of the abdomen

Triceps surae. Three muscles—the gastrocnemius, soleus, and plantaris—that form the calf of the lower leg

True ribs. The seven pairs of bones that articulate posteriorly with the vertebrae and anteriorly with the sternum to form the rib cage

Ulnar deviation. Movement of the hand or fingers toward the little finger and closer to the midline of the body (in anatomical position); also known as *wrist adduction*

Ulnar drift. A pathological condition occurring when the extensor digitorum communis tendon slips to the ulnar side of the metacarpophalangeal joint

Vastus intermedius. A part of the quadriceps femoris that originates on the upper two thirds of the femur and inserts onto the other tendons of the quadriceps and the joint capsule of the knee

Vastus lateralis. A part of the quadriceps femoris that originates from the joint capsule of the hip and inserts onto the patella and the lateral joint capsule of the knee

Vastus medialis. A part of the quadriceps femoris that originates on the proximal femur and inserts onto the patella and the medial joint capsule of the knee

Vector. A force or an influence that can be described completely by magnitude and direction

Velocity. Displacement that occurs over a specific amount of time, for example, 60 miles per hour

Weight. A force (equal to the product of the object's mass and the acceleration of gravity) representing the attraction of a body to Earth or another celestial body

Work. The transfer of energy to a body by the application of a force that moves the body in the direction of the force; calculated through multiplication of the force by the distance through which the body moves and expressed in joules, ergs, and foot-pounds

Index

M

LAB MANUAL FOR KINESIOLOGY:

Movement in the Context of Activity

Table of Contents

INTRODUCTION

LINKS TO LABS

BRIEF GUIDELINES FOR ROM AND MMT

BIOMECHANICAL ANALYSIS LAB

COMPETENCY CHECK SHEET FOR TRANSFERS

COMPETENCY CHECK SHEET FOR ROM/MMT

TABLE OF MOTIONS AND MUSCLES TO PALPATE FOR MMT PRACTICAL EXAMS

ADDITIONAL LAB: MMT TO DETERMINE NEUROLOGICAL LEVEL IN SPINAL CORD INJURY

INTRODUCTION

The textbook relies on a thorough prerequisite knowledge of anatomy from previous courses. The helpfulness of these laboratory activities depends upon a basic familiarity with kinesiology and biomechanics as presented in the text. Before beginning to explore the laboratory activities in this manual, read the following questions to assess your current level of understanding. Mark those questions for which you are unsure of the answer and look for the answers in future chapters and labs:

- What happens to the proximal and distal attachments (origin and insertion; O and I, respectively) of a muscle when that muscle contracts in a concentric (shortening) contraction?
- In a shortening contraction what determines whether the insertion moves toward the origin or vice versa?
- How do you determine the location and orientation of an axis?
- What is the best view (from the front, side, or top) for drawing a bone as it rotates around an axis in a specific motion?
- If in a concentric contraction the distance between O and I of a muscle decreases, what happens to this same distance when the muscle undergoes an eccentric contraction?
- What happens to the O and I of a flexor group when the joint is pulled into extension by some other force? (This is another way of asking the above question—right?)
- "Active insufficiency" is a term used to describe a muscle that is insufficient to adequately perform its funcion even though it is actively contracting. What are the two ways in which it is "insufficient"?
- What are the joint positions in which the various multijoint muscles (biceps, long finger flexors) experience active insufficiency?
- "Passive insufficiency" is a term used to describe a muscle being maximally stretched. What is "insufficient" in passive insufficiency?
- What are the joint positions in which the various multijoint muscles (biceps, long finger flexors) experience passive insufficiency?

LINKS TO LABS

These labs were constructed to be accomplished by working in groups of four or five people, following the directions for each station, and working through the activities. Completing the sheets titled "TURN THIS IN" for each lab helps to ensure that you will receive pertinent, individually directed feedback.

Keys to the Labs can be found on the CD-ROM.

LAB	TEXT REFERENCE	KEY
Lab 1. Kinematic Chain, Human Musculoskeletal Movement, Shoulder Model of Joint Movement	Chapters 1-3	Lab 1 Key
Lab 2. Stability, Balance, Wheelchairs, Minimum Assist Transfers	Chapter 3	Lab 2 Key
Lab 3. Overview of ROM and MMT	Chapter 2; Motion CD	Lab 3 Key
Brief Guidelines for ROM and MMT	Motion CD	See Motion CD
Lab 4. Accessory Joint Motions/Muscle Excursion/ Active and Passive Insufficiency/ Maximum Assist Transfers	Chapters 2-4	Lab 4 Key
Lab 5. Torque and Equilibrium Conditions	Chapter 5	Lab 5 Key
Lab 6. Head, Neck, and Trunk: Curves, Movements, Measurements, Muscles	Chapter 6	Lab 6 Key
Labs 7 and 8. Shoulder Complex: Scapular Movement, Differential Functions of Scapular and Glenohumeral (GH) Muscles, Differential Functions of Supraspinatus and Deltoid in GH Abduction	Chapter 7	Lab 7 and Lab 8 Keys
Lab 9. MMT and ROM of Shoulder/Elbow and Forearm: Torque Range of Motion	Chapter 7	Lab 9 Key
Lab 10. Wrist and Hand: Synergistic Function of Wrist Extensors and Finger Flexors	Chapter 8	Lab 10 Key
Lab 11. Torque Range of Motion/Intrinsic Function/Tenodesis Grasp/Pulleys/Review of ROM Limitations	Chapter 8	Lab 11 Key
Lab 12. Prehension Patterns/Intrinsic Function and Digital Sweep/Tenodesis Grasp	Chapter 8	Lab 12 Key
Lab 13. Positioning in a Wheelchair	Chapter 9	Lab 13 Key
Biomechanical Analysis Lab	Chapter 9	BMA Lab Key
Competency Check Sheet for Transfers	Chapter 3	No key
Competency Check Sheet for ROM/MMT	See Motion CD	No key
Table of Motions and Muscles to Palpate for MMT	See Motion CD	No key
Additional Lab: MMT To Determine Neurological Level in SCI	See Motion CD	No key

LAB 1. KINEMATIC CHAIN, HUMAN MUSCULOSKELETAL MOVEMENT, SHOULDER MODEL OF JOINT MOVEMENT

Please read the information on this sheet carefully and reread it at each station. It is written as a guide to your activities during lab. Complete and turn in any sheets titled "TURN THIS IN" to obtain individually focused feedback on your level of understanding of the material.

STATION: KINEMATIC CHAIN

Study the mobile arm support by moving it around. Start with only one segment attached to the joint on the wheelchair. At this station do not sit in the wheelchair and do not try to use the device yet. The idea is to study this traditional rehabilitation device in its most fundamental sense—a simple kinematic (or joint) chain. Build the chain and observe how the motion changes as you add more segments and joints.

TO DO:

For each chain how would you describe the movement in terms of freedom of movement of the end of the chain—"degrees of freedom" of the chain? [Does the end of the chain move only in an arc, on many arcs (i.e., along a surface), or on many surfaces?]

Chain 1: Proximal arm only with one joint located at the chair upright.

Chain 2: Proximal and distal arms with two joints (at the chair and connecting the two moving segments).

Chain 3: Proximal and distal arms and arm trough, three joints in all [at the chair (1); connecting the two segments (2); end of the distal arm, under the trough (3)]. What is responsible for the increase in freedom in the chain as you add more segments?

STATION: HUMAN MUSCULOSKELETAL MOVEMENT

Study your own upper extremity as a kinematic chain. Perform elbow and shoulder flexion to bring food (or drink) to your mouth (self-feeding pattern).

TO DO:

Identify the "joints" and "segments" that make up the chain (starting with the GH joint most proximally and ending with the wrist joint; consider the radioulnar joints together).

Identify the movements.

Try it with two people and see how it differs, and, if you can, describe how they differ in terms of joints used and amount of motion at each joint:

LAB 1: TURN THIS IN

NAME: _____

STATION: MODEL OF SHOULDER JOINT

(1) Articulate the glenohumeral joint model (using the axis provided) so that an abduction movement is possible.
Is it possible for the segment ("humerus") to move anywhere but in one plane? What is the plane for this movement?

(2) Disassemble and rearticulate so that flexion is possible. Compare the different flexion motions possible by placing the axis into the different holes in the glenoid.
How are these motions different, even though each is flexion?
(HINT: How do the planes of flexion/extension differ?)

(3) Considering this model,
what is your conclusion about what dictates the plane in which motion occurs, comparing abduction to flexion and one type (plane) of flexion to another?

LAB 2. STABILITY, BALANCE, WHEELCHAIRS, MINIMUM ASSIST TRANSFERS

STATION: WHEELCHAIR WHEELIES

WITH A WATCHFUL PARTNER:

Sit in a wheelchair (w/c) **AFTER** doing the following:

- remove leg/footrests
- remove armrests (if removable)
- position partner behind you with his/her hands on the handles

With your feet hanging toward the ground, push the rear wheels forward with your hands just enough to raise the front casters slightly off the ground—all this with your partner's hands on the handles, ready to catch the chair if it goes too far—**IT WILL** a few times. If unable to lift the front, have your partner slowly tilt you back (front casters in the air) and then try to balance the chair. If you sense you are going too far back, pull backward on the wheels (handrails) as if to back up. If you are falling forward (front casters moving toward the ground again), push the rear wheels (handrails) forward; this will put you "back in flight."

Try this for about 5 minutes and then switch roles.

Answer the following questions:

1. Identify the projection of the center of gravity when on all four wheels and when on the rear (large) wheels only:

- all four wheels

- rear wheels, during wheelie

2. In terms of factors of stability, why is a wheelie so hard to achieve/maintain?

STATION: TRANSFERS

Use the "Fundamental Steps of a Transfer," a wheelchair, and a transfer belt, and attempt both (1) sliding board transfer and (2) stand pivot transfer with your partner. When you are the person being transferred, you should have good balance and strength (especially trunk control) but need directions from your partner. Make sure that you do all steps, including removing parts from the chair and positioning the chair. Perform each role: therapist and client.

For each kind of transfer, describe the transfer in terms of base of support and projection of the center of gravity.

In general, approach this with a helping mentality, not an "I-am-about-to-do-this-for-you" mentality. Realize that given the proper instruction and a pace that is not too fast the individual being transferred can probably do much of the work. In any case, this is the goal.

FUNDAMENTAL STEPS OF A TRANSFER

1. Be sure that both you and the person being transferred are oriented, informed, and ready.

2. Instruct the client to move slowly and take their time; you will offer support as needed. Moving fast in any kind of assisted transfer usually implies things are on the verge of being out of control.

3. **LOCK THE CHAIR!!**

4. Loosen the seat belt and remove it; remove any part of the chair that can possibly get in the way, because it will and usually in the middle of the hardest part of the transfer! Attach the transfer belt.

5. In all transfers (other than dependent transfers and transfers in which specific precautions are being followed as in the care of someone who has had a total hip arthroplasty [THA]), have the person move toward the front edge of the seat and balance their weight directly over their hips. (Where are you trying to get the center of gravity to fall, and with respect to what?)

6. Have the person lean forward to **BEGIN** to shift their weight toward the new base of support (feet) even if this will be temporary, as in a sliding board transfer. At this point you must be ready with your knees bent and **BACK STRAIGHT** to assist in moving the center of gravity projection forward and onto the transitional base of support. You should begin to use your weight as much as possible (leaning back while holding onto the transfer belt or other appropriate handling spots) to offer assistance **ONLY AS NEEDED.**

7. Now the critical step: where movement really begins and falls occur. **COUNT** to three (or something agreed upon) and **WORK TOGETHER;** have the individual come to a stand or at least get their center of gravity forward, with your assistance as necessary. Encourage slow movements: staying in control. Depending on their weight-bearing ability, the upright position (standing on the transitional base of support) is a good place to pause and determine if things are under control.

8. If the person cannot fully weight-bear or cannot bear weight at all, this pause does not exist, and the move to the transitional base of support and then to the target surface (i.e., the bed in a w/c-to-bed transfer or the toilet in a w/c-to-toilet transfer) all happens in one smooth, graceful motion. Whether you paused or continued, encourage an easy transfer down to the surface. (You are aiming for a nice control of gravity's force through what kind of contractions of which muscles at the knees and hips?) **EVALUATE** your work together immediately, while the transfer is clear in both of your minds.

STATION: WHEELCHAIR STABILITY (INSTABILITY) WITH LOSS OF LOWER EXTREMITIES

Again get in a wheelchair **WITH YOUR PARTNER SPOTTING YOU BY HOLDING ONTO THE PUSH HANDLES.**

Attempt a fast start by pushing hard on the rear wheel rails.

Do this again; this time remove the footrests and fold your legs crossed in the seat so that they no longer hang down. Attempt a fast start, making sure your partner is in place.

What happened the second time: legs folded?

LAB 2: TURN THIS IN

NAME: _____

STATION: WHEELCHAIR STABILITY BASED ON FRONT CASTER POSITION

Wheel around in the chair and pull up to a spot. Stop without backing up first, and lock the chair. With your feet in the footrests and your partner in front of you, lean forward, bringing your chest to your knees as if to reach for something dropped onto the floor in front of you.

What happens as you lean forward?

Now wheel around again. This time stop, back up about 4 feet, and then stop and put the brakes on. Now lean forward as you did before, with your partner in place.

What happens as you lean forward this time?

What accounts for the difference in stability of the chair while leaning forward?
(HINT: Think about front-to-back dimensions of the base of support in each case.)

Therefore what is the general rule for coming to a stop if you intend to lean forward?

LAB 3. OVERVIEW OF RANGE OF MOTION (ROM) MEASUREMENT AND MANUAL MUSCLE TESTING (MMT)

Before working with the motion CD, work through the following lab exercises.
  I. Review: What is AROM and why do we measure it (via goniometry)? What is PROM and why do we measure it? What is the most meaningful measure of ROM? Why is muscle strength measured (via MMT)?
  II. Muscle strength is measured by judging how much resistance is applied against a contracting muscle group: contracting to produce and hold a movement.

GRADE	SAME AS	RESISTANCE
Normal	5/5	"Max" and may "break" contraction (Who has larger MA??)
Good	4/5	"Moderate"
Fair	3/5	Gravity; must have full AROM
Poor	2/5	Gravity eliminated (or minimized); full AROM
Trace	1/5	No motion; palpable contraction

NOTICE:

Grades 3 and 4 are given based on AROM even though this is a muscle strength test. Grades 1, 2, and 3 are the most reliable grades. "Gray areas" are indicated with a "+" or "−" next to each grade.

DEMONSTRATION:

For testing elbow flexors, the individual moves 90% of full range against gravity; this condition is designated not quite "Fair" (always test for "Fair" first by having the individual move against gravity).
If the individual is unable to move completely against gravity as in this case, the next step is to eliminate the resistance of gravity. (NOTE: This assumes you have established PROM is possible, thus ruling out joint restriction as the reason for the lack of full range against gravity.) If full AROM is observed with gravity eliminated, score "Poor." (Had full AROM against gravity been observed, you would know the strength is at least "Fair" and would then give resistance to determine either "Good" or "Normal.")
   So the basic procedure is as follows: (1) give command; (2) simultaneously palpate the muscle if there is a question about its activity (might be substituting); (3) if full AROM, apply resistance to the moved segment (segment distal to the joint of motion, e.g., humerus for shoulder flexion) at the end of motion in the direction opposite motion; (4) simultaneously stabilize the segment proximal to the joint of motion (scapula for shoulder flexion); (5) grade based on feel of resistance or observation of AROM in case of "Fair"; (6) in case of incomplete AROM in the test for "Fair," move the joint through full PROM to rule out joint pathology, *then* test for "Poor" by positioning in the gravity eliminated position. If PROM is incomplete **DO NOT** grade the muscle strength as "Fair" or "Poor" since through PROM you have established the lack of ROM in the test for "Fair" was due to joint limitation and not to weakness. In this case of limited PROM, apply resistance at the end of the observed AROM and grade accordingly.

Do you think you understand? Try answering these questions:

When testing strength on an individual who cannot be freely moved, think about alternatives to the standard procedure, based on logic. For an individual with spinal cord injury (SCI) who must be tested seated upright in a chair:

Can you test for "Fair" ("F") elbow flexion, shoulder flexion, shoulder abduction?

Can you test "F" for elbow extension?
(HINT: How could you position the shoulder for the elbow to extend against gravity?)

Shoulder internal rotation?

THINK: Shoulder internal rotation in upright sitting with the shoulder abducted to 90 degrees and elbow flexed to 90 degrees, fingers pointed forward occurs *with* gravity and requires NO strength. The test for "Fair" shoulder internal rotation requires positioning prone, shoulder abducted to 90 degrees, elbow flexed to 90 degrees, forearm and hand hanging over the side of the table. This allows internal rotation to occur against gravity. If this position is too difficult for the person you are testing and IF you expect normal strength, you can skip the test for "Fair" and jump to testing with applied manual resistance (for "Good" and "Normal" strengths). Do this by having the person perform the movement in the upright seated position, arm adducted and elbow flexed. Even though this test in the gravity minimized plane, apply resistance at the end point of the movement. If the person holds the position as you apply moderate or maximum resistance, score "Good" or "Normal" (depending on whether they held against moderate or maximum resistance). "Poor" and "Fair" grades become irrelevant.

STATION: TRADITIONAL GONIOMETRY ON SKELETON

Use a goniometer to evaluate PROM on the skeleton or on a partner for (1) humeral abduction or (2) elbow flexion and document your results as PROM (i.e., passive range of motion).

    (1) Shoulder (humeral) abduction (from adduction to abduction): _____

    (2) Elbow flexion (from extension to flexion): _____

STATION: PALPATION PRINCIPLES

To palpate is, according to the dictionary, to touch, to examine by the hands. It is to "see" with the hands. Without much experience, we lack the sensitivity to feel and discriminate between different "feels." A few tips help:

- Always have the individual (the "palpatee") relax.

- Gently place your hand(s) on the skin over the structure you are trying to palpate.

- Move your hand(s) in a circular motion, in a sense "looking" for the structure of interest.

- For palpation of a muscle or tendon, have the individual very slightly move in a direction known to require the use of the muscle. Actual movement is not necessary as the thought and slight intention to move will cause a palpable muscle contraction. (Movement will actually make it more difficult to feel the muscle.)

- Immediately following the command to move, have the person relax again. It is the change (from relaxation, to contraction, to relaxation) that will facilitate palpation. In other words, it is difficult to feel one structure among others contraction and relaxation of the muscle fibers defines the structure. Remember, our nervous systems function by differentiating: noticing change. Being aware of constants is much more difficult.

- With all of this in mind palpate the following muscles in association with the movement listed:

MUSCLE	MOVEMENT
Biceps brachii	Elbow flexion; forearm supination while forearm is supported in flexion
Middle deltoid	GH abduction
Lower pectoralis major	GH adduction; GH horizontal adduction
Clavicular head of pectoralis major	GH flexion beginning from 90 degrees of flexion; GH horizontal adduction

STATION: MANUAL MUSCLE TESTING

As an introduction to the CD Motion: Range and Strength, follow the directions in the CD to test the strength in the following muscle groups of a partner. For each go through the procedure for testing grades 5/5 (Normal), 3/5 (Fair), 2/5 (Poor), and 1/5 (Trace). Check off each grade below as you progress. Start with the test for "F" in each case; then move to "N." Then pretend there is weakness (as if the person was unable to move fully against gravity in the Fair test) and test for "P" and "T."

elbow flexors	N	F	P	T
elbow extensors	N	F	P	T

LAB 3: TURN THIS IN

NAME: _____

Answer these general questions about MMT after testing the strength of flexors and extensors according to directions:

What is a general rule for what to stabilize and where to apply resistance?

What is a general rule for testing in terms of which grade to test for first?

What is a general rule for positioning if the grade is apparently below fair (3)?

What is the general procedure for placement of the goniometer? (Simply, how do you orient it?)

STATION: DRAW IT

Draw the fibers of the biceps in their action to flex the forearm at the elbow during a muscle test. The elbow would be held in full flexion. Make sure to begin the arrow at the insertion and direct it parallel to the fibers toward the origin.

Remember, the arrowhead indicates direction; in this case the force pulls its insertion toward its origin. The length of the arrow indicates strength of contraction. Have your arrow represent a force of 100 pounds using the scale 10 pounds = 1 centimeter. Draw curved arrows representing movement of the forearm from its fully extended position into full flexion when the biceps muscle contracts.

BRIEF GUIDELINES FOR ROM AND MMT

The following charts are provided for use as "hints" for goniometry and muscle testing. Their best use is for review after having worked through the Motion CD.

Goniometry: Shoulder–Forearm

JOINT & MOVEMENT	STATIONARY ARM	MOVEABLE ARM
GH Flex & Hyperext	Trunk	Humerus
GH Abd & Add	Trunk	Humerus
GH Hor Abd/Add	Humerus; stays pointing forward after humerus moves (begin with shoulder flexed to 90°)	Humerus
GH Int/Ext R	Inferior to elbow running anterior-posterior (shoulder adducted, arm at side, elbow flexed to 90°)	Forearm
Elbow Flex	Humerus	Forearm (supinated position)
Forearm Sup/Pro	Humerus (shoulder adducted, arm by side, elbow flexed to 90°)	Aligned with pencil held vertical in fisted hand
		Alternate method: Across volar forearm at wrist for supination; across dorsal forearm at wrist for pronation

Strength Testing of Muscle Groups: Shoulder–Forearm

MUSCLE GROUP (& SPINAL SEGMENT)/MOVEMENT	POSITION FOR FAIR TEST	GOOD/NORMAL: APPLY RESISTANCE	STABILIZE
Upper trap (spinal accessory), levator scap (C3-4)/Scap elevation	Upright	Acromion processes	Not necessary
Lower trap (spinal accessory)/ Scap depression	None; position in prone for poor test: shoulder adducted, place hand along side of thigh; lower hand along thigh as if reaching down toward feet	Inferior angle of scapula toward elevation	Not necessary
Middle trap (spinal accessory)/ Scap retraction	Prone, shoulder abducted to 90° and externally rotated, supported on mat; lift hand and UE off of mat surface	Vertebral border and dorsal surface of scapula toward protraction	Not necessary?
Rhomboids (C5), middle trap (spinal accessory)/Scap retraction with downward rotation	Prone, shoulder adducted and int rot, dorsal hand on small of back; lift hand up off of back	Vertebral border toward up rot and protraction	Not necessary
Serratus anterior (C5-7)/Scap protraction (with some upward rotation)	Supine, shoulder flexed to 90°, elbow extended; reach toward ceiling	Proximal humerus toward retraction (toward mat)	Not necessary?
Ant deltoid (C5-6), coracobrachialis (C6-7), Pec major (C5-7), biceps (C5-6)/GH flexion	Upright, humerus adducted; flex only to 90°	Distal humerus toward extension	Proximal to GH joint

MUSCLE GROUP (& SPINAL SEGMENT)/MOVEMENT	POSITION FOR FAIR TEST	GOOD/NORMAL: APPLY RESISTANCE	STABILIZE
Post deltoid (C5-6), latissimus dorsi (C6-8), teres major (C5-6), triceps long head (C7-8)/GH hyperextension	Upright	Distal humerus toward flexion	Proximal to GH joint
Supraspinatus (C5), deltoid (C5-6)/GH abduction	Upright; abduct only to 90°	Distal humerus toward adduction	Proximal to GH joint
Latissimus dorsi (C6-8), pec major (C5-7), teres major (C5-6)/GH adduction	None; position in supine for poor test: shoulder abducted to 90°, move into adduction	Distal humerus toward abduction	Proximal to GH joint
Post deltoid (C5-6)/GH horizontal abduction	Prone, arm over side of mat	Distal humerus toward horizontal adduction	Proximal to GH joint
Pec major (C5-7), Ant deltoid (C5-6)/GH horizontal adduction	Supine, shoulder abducted to 90°	Distal humerus toward horizontal abduction	Trunk/opposite shoulder
Subscapularis (C5-6), latissimus dorsi (C6-8), pec major (C5-7), ant deltoid (C5-6)/GH internal rotation	Prone, shoulder abducted, elbow flexed, forearm hanging down over mat edge	Distal forearm toward external rotation	Humerus
Infraspinatus (C5-6), teres minor (C5), post deltoid (C5-6)/GH ext rotation	Prone, shoulder abducted, elbow flexed, forearm hanging down over mat edge	Distal forearm toward internal rotation	Humerus
Biceps (C5-6), brachialis (C5-6), brachioradialis (C5-6)/elbow flexion	Upright position, shoulder adducted, forearm supinated	Distal forearm toward ext	Anterior humerus
Triceps (C7-8)/elbow extension	If test in upright position, shoulder fully flexed, raise hand above head via elbow extension; if test in prone, shoulder abducted to 90°, forearm and hand hanging over edge of mat, elbow flexed to 90°; if test in supine, shoulder flexed to 90°, extend elbow	Distal forearm toward elbow flexion	Post humerus if shoulder extends; ant humerus if shoulder flexes
Supinator (C6), biceps (C5-6)/forearm supination	Upright, shoulder adducted, holding ball between elbow and side of trunk	Distal forearm toward pronation; try to turn palm down	Not necessary?
Pronator teres (C6-7), pro quad (C8-T1)/forearm pronation	Same as for supination	Distal forearm toward supination; try to turn palm up	Not necessary?

Goniometry: Wrist–Hand

JOINT & MOVEMENT	STATIONARY ARM	MOVEABLE ARM
Wrist flexion/extension*	Radius	2nd metacarpal
Wrist radial/ulnar deviation*	Dorsal mid-forearm; between radius and ulna	3rd metacarpal
MCP flexion (2-5)	Metacarpal; on side or over dorsal surface	Proximal phalanx; on side or over dorsal surface
IP flexion (2-5)	Proximal phalanx (to measure PIP): on side or or over dorsal surface; middle phalanx (to measure DIP): on side or over dorsal surface	Middle phalanx (to measure PIP): on side or over dorsal surface; distal phalanx (to measure DIP): on side or over dorsal surface
Thumb CMC extension ("radial abduction") plane of the palm*	Volar (anterior) radius	1st metacarpal
Thumb CMC abduction; plane 90° to the palm	Radial side of 2nd metacarpal	Dorsal (posterior = back) side of 1st metacarpal
Thumb MCP flexion; plane of the palm	Side or back (dorsum) of 1st metacarpal	Side or back of proximal phalanx
Thumb IP flexion; plane of the palm	Side or back (dorsum) of proximal phalanx	Side or back of distal phalanx

*Measured from a neutral point.

Strength Testing of Muscle Groups: Wrist–Hand

MUSCLE GROUP (& SPINAL SEGMENT)/MOVEMENT	POSITION FOR FAIR TEST	GOOD/NORMAL: APPLY RESISTANCE	STABILIZE
Flexor carpi radialis and ulnaris (FCR, C6-8, & FCU, C6-8)/ Wrist flexion	FAIR: forearm supinated on table, wrist in neutral; flex up away from tabletop; look for balanced flexion; no deviation; if observe stronger tendency toward radial deviation with flexion, ulnar flexor (FCU) is weak; opposite true for radial flexor (FCR). POOR: Forearm on table in neutral pro/supination; flex along tabletop	Thenar and hypothenar eminences together; feel for balanced flexion; no tendency toward deviation either way; if feel stronger tendency toward radial deviation with flexion, ulnar flexor (FCU) is weak; opposite true for FCR	Not necessary; except in Fair test, may have to prevent substitution through pronation
Extensors carpi radialis longus and brevis (ECRL & ECRB, C6-8) and extensor carpi ulnaris (ECU, C6-8)/ wrist extension	FAIR: Forearm pronated on table, wrist in neutral; extend up away from tabletop; look for balanced extension; no deviation; if observe stronger tendency toward radial deviation with extension, ECU is weak; opposite true for ECRL & ECRB. POOR: Forearm on table in neutral pro/supination; extend along tabletop	Dorsum of 2nd and 5th metacarpals: feel for balanced flexion; no tendency toward deviation; if feel stronger tendency toward radial deviation with extension, ECU is weak; opposite true for ECRL & ECRB	Not necessary; except in Fair test, may have to prevent substitution through supination

MUSCLE GROUP (& SPINAL SEGMENT)/MOVEMENT	POSITION FOR FAIR TEST
Flexor digitorum profundus (FDP, C7-T1), MCP, PIP, & DIP flexion (digits 2-5)	May use grasp dynamometer. Or, forearm supinated (palm up), have client flex fingers into palmar crease = FAIR; incomplete ROM doing this = POOR; resist fingertips by pulling out away from palm for GOOD and NORMAL (remember, resist AFTER movement)
Flexor digitorum superficialis (FDS, C7-T1), MCP, & PIP flexion (digits 2-5)	Palm up (forearm supinated) on table, hand held with all but one finger in full extension; have client attempt finger flexion in the one finger: full ROM of MCP and PIP-FAIR; partial ROM-POOR; resist along lateral borders of middle phalanx for GOOD & NORMAL
Extensor digitorum (ED, C6-8), extensor pollicis longus & brevis (EPL & EPB, C6-8), MCP, & IP extension	Palm down on table, extend MCPs, allowing incomplete extension of IPs and briefly pushing distal end of proximal phalanx into flexion ("spring test")
Lumbrical & interossei function (C8-T1)	Have client "make a fist" and then slowly extend their fingers while supporting the dorsum of their hand with your hand so that the MCPs are kept in 90° flexion and the IPs are allowed to extend. Take your hand away and have client try to hold the position = FAIR; inability to hold MCP flexion with IP extension = POOR (or less). Resist on the palmar surface of the fingers, pushing them into MCP extension; ability to hold MCP flexion and IP extension = NORMAL
Abductor pollicis brevis (C6-T1), thumb CMC abduction; this occurs in a plane 90° to the palm	Abduct the thumb away from the palm (full ROM = FAIR; partial ROM = POOR); for NORMAL and GOOD, resist distal end of metacarpal, pushing toward adduction; after abduction movement observed
Flexor pollicis longus (FPL, C7-T1), thumb IP flexion; occurs in the plane of the palm	Stabilize proximal phalanx, observe full IP flexion (FAIR; incomplete ROM for POOR); resist distal phalanx by pushing the pad of the thumb toward extension
Adductor pollicis (AP, C8, T1), thumb CMC adduction	From the abducted position, move the thumb toward the palm (adduction); full ROM = FAIR, incomplete = POOR; resist at the end of the motion, pulling the metacarpal (not the proximal phalanx) into abduction
Opponens pollicis & flexor pol brevis (OP & FPB, C6, T1), thumb opposition	Oppose thumb to little finger; full ROM = FAIR, partial = POOR; attempt to pull apart 1st and 5th metacarpals

STATION: ADDITIONAL MMT HINTS

Additional Explanations for MMT of Wrist Flexion and Extension

Again, the directions for these are often overwhelmingly more complex than necessary. Think about it:

- If someone's ECU is weaker than the other wrist extensors, wrist extension will be accompanied by radial deviation, from the unbalanced action of the ECRL and ECRB. (Refer to Interactive Exercise Figure 8-3.)

- Balanced wrist extension occurs via the ECRL, ECRB, and ECU. Without the ECU, the ECRL and ECRB radially deviate with extension.

Therefore much of the test is observation. To test against resistance, observe extension against gravity (= Fair) and then apply resistance: (1) straight into flexion for all extensors; (2) into flexion and radial deviation to test ECU; and (3) with flexion and ulnar deviation to test ECRL and ECRB.

Additional Explanations for "Finger Interphalangeal Extension"

There is a commonly given test for strength of lumbricals and interossei. The truth is, if there is weakness in these muscles, you know it before you test anything:

Weakness in lumbricals and interossei shows up as hyperextension of MCPs and inability to completely extend the IPs (known as "claw" deformity).

When you see this, it "tells" you there is weakness in both groups if digits 2-5 are affected equally and in the interossei (not necessarily the lumbricals) if only digits 4 and 5 are affected.

You can provide more helpful information by describing the "claw" than by grading the muscle strength.

To formally test, do this:

1. Have the person "make a fist"; then with your hand as a guide to keep the MCPs flexed, ask them to straighten the fingers out to your palm.

2. This places the hand in the "lumbrical position" (which is held ONLY if lumbrical and interossei muscles are functioning). Being able to hold the position = Fair.

3. Resist by pushing the fingertips toward the direction of MCP extension = Normal.

4. Inability to hold the position = Poor.

LAB 4. ACCESSORY JOINT MOTIONS/MUSCLE EXCURSION/ACTIVE AND PASSIVE INSUFFICIENCY/MAXIMUM ASSIST TRANSFERS

STATION: ACCESSORY JOINT MOTIONS

Attempt the four accessory motions on an articulated knee joint. This will work only with a joint you "build" — not with a typical articulated skeleton. "Build" the knee by attaching cords for the medial and lateral collateral, and anterior and posterior crucitate ligaments. Using a good anatomy atlas as a guide, this is easier than it sounds. If you have done well, the knee will have much more joint play in flexion than in extension, the close-packed position of the knee.

Identify, by moving the joint, the loose-packed position.

In the loose-packed position, perform distraction, A/P glide, lateral glide, rotation.

On a partner, using the MCP joint, attempt (carefully) the four accessory motions.

Do this in MCP extension (loose-packed position for the MCP).

Try it in the close-packed position (MCP flexion) and notice the difference.

Are these accessory motions voluntary (active) or passive?

Why is rotation possible at this joint even though by construction it is a two-axis joint, allowing only flexion/extension and ab/adduction?

STATION: ACTIVE AND PASSIVE INSUFFICIENCY

Watch the lab demonstration.

STATION: MAXIMUM ASSIST TRANSFERS

IMPORTANT: Do these only with a lab instructor present to give feedback on body mechanics!! Watch the Movie/Animation first by clicking on: Max Assist Transfer. This shows a maximum assist transfer of a person who has trunk control.

Following the "Fundamental Steps of a Transfer," attempt a sliding board transfer on a partner. This time do the following:

SLIDING BOARD TRANSFER

Tape tubing to your partner's forearm or thigh, simulating either an IV or a catheter. The other end should be hooked onto the wheelchair. In the transfer have your partner extend their knees so their feet are out in front and cannot be used to bear weight: **THIS WILL BE A MAXIMUM ASSIST TRANSFER**. She/he may help in the transfer only by shifting weight but should carry no weight on their lower or upper extremities.

Comments/Self-evaluation (What do you need to work on to do this well and safely?):

SCOOT TRANSFER

Do the same now for a scoot transfer (stand pivot with no real standing phase)—essentially a sliding board transfer without the sliding board. Make sure in this case to get the wheelchair as close as possible to the surface to which you are transferring. Your partner should have his or her feet on the ground and you should lock knees, either with or without the knee belt. Again simulate a moderate to maximum assist transfer: the "client" should bear little if any weight on their lower extremities. (Note: If you simulated an IV with tubing in the first transfer, simulate a catheter in this second transfer.)

Self-evaluation Comments/Self-evaluation (What do you need to work on to do this well and safely?):

Do each of these transfers in a trunk-control and non-trunk-control scenario following the demonstrations of each. Be sure to tend to the catheter/IV—moving the end attached to the chair over to the mat before the transfer.

LAB 4: TURN THIS IN

NAME: _____

STATION: MUSCLE EXCURSION REQUIREMENTS FOR JOINT MOVEMENT

Familiarize yourself with one of the models. These models were built to demonstrate, among other things, the excursion requirements of movement. Identify the mark on each tendon and watch the marks move (one at a time) as you passively move the finger.

(1) Name the tendon with the marker: _____

(2) Pull on the tendon to cause full motion and measure the active excursion necessary for the tendon to perform the COMPLETE MOVEMENT of the finger. (If it is a finger flexor, the flexion movement should begin and excursion measurement should start at a position of full finger extension.) Record the excursion requirement for the motion: _____

(3) Study passive motion excursion requirements of the same tendon. Place the digit in an extreme position (i.e., full finger flexion). Identify the mark on the flexor tendon and measure its movement as the finger is passively moved from full finger flexion to full finger extension. What is the direction of movement in the flexor when finger extension occurs?

(4) What happens if the flexor tendon gets "stuck" on a scar (following healing from trauma) and is unable to glide and move distally during a passive motion in the antagonistic direction (i.e., during extension)?

(5) What happens if the flexor tendon is "stuck" on a scar (following healing from trauma) and cannot move proximally as the muscle contracts and pulls on it to perform its agonistic function?

LAB 5. TORQUE AND EQUILIBRIUM CONDITIONS

STATION: TENDENCY-TO-ROTATE (TORQUE) BASED ON DISTANCE (MA) FROM THE AXIS (CTR)

Use the forearm/elbow model to demonstrate equilibrium of torques.

DIRECTIONS:

(1)   Attach the force gauge (measuring pull of the biceps) to the position closest to the joint. Record how much biceps elbow flexion force is required to suspend the 50-gram weight elbow extension held at the distal end of the forearm with the forearm held at 90-degrees flexion: _____ grams

(2)   Go back to the extended position and reattach the biceps flexion force gauge to the position slightly distal to the original attachment. Again record the biceps flexion force required to suspend the same 50-gram elbow extension weight at 90 degrees of elbow flexion: _____ grams

(3)   Leave the biceps (force gauge) attached but rotate the 50-gram elbow extension weight 180 degrees so the weight (creating an elbow extension tendency) is not held as far out as in conditions (1) and (2) but is closer in toward the elbow. Record the amount of elbow flexion force necessary to hold the weight at 90-degrees elbow flexion: _____ grams

Please reattach the force gauge to the original proximal position and rotate the weight back out to the distal position to prepare the model for the next group.

QUESTIONS:

Why is more biceps elbow flexion force required to balance the 50-gram elbow extension weight when the flexion force gauge (biceps) is inserted close to the joint?

Why is less biceps flexion force required to balance the 50-gram elbow extension weight when the 50-gram extension weight is held closer in toward the elbow?

STATION: EVERYDAY FORCES AND THEIR TENDENCIES

Identify various forces at play (at work?) around the room. For example, think about moving things by sliding them along the floor or pulling up the shades; the force that makes us tired at the end of the day ("I can barely stand up"). List three different forces identified:

1)

2)

3)

In terms of equilibrium of forces, when the shade is pulled up and it stays up, is this equilibrium and if so how is it established—what are the forces involved?

STATION: EFFECT OF THE FORCE OF GRAVITY

Identify various movements of the human musculoskeletal system (and positions held in the human musculoskeletal system) that are caused by the force of gravity.

- In the upright (standing) position, list the resting positions of the shoulder, elbow, and wrist. We would say gravity's effect on the shoulder, elbow, and wrist is:
  shoulder _____ and _____; elbow _____; wrist_____
- In the supine position, with the elbow held just past 90-degrees flexion, revise the list:
  shoulder _____; elbow_____; wrist_____

LAB 5: TURN THIS IN

NAME: _____

STATION: TENDENCY TO CAUSE ROTATION

Using the upper extremity (UE) skeleton, use the different attachment points to attach the line and the force gauge serving as the elbow flexor. In each case, pull on the line and move the forearm (flex the forearm at the elbow joint) through about 90 degrees of motion. Simultaneously, have a partner provide resistance to flexion at the end point of the motion (90 degrees elbow flexion) with a separate force gauge—apply the resistance at the wrist and be sure to apply it at 90 degrees to the forearm in each trial. Pull with the same resistance for each trial—always applied at 90 degrees to the forearm.

As you pull on the flexor, have another partner measure the amount of excursion of the string (muscle) required to pull the elbow into 90 degrees of flexion.

Measure the force required to hold the position at 90 degrees against the partner's resistance.

Measure the moment arm when the joint is at 90 degrees.

Repeat for the other attachments (insertions): measure the excursion required to move the joint from 0 to 90 degrees, the force required to hold the end position, and the moment arm of the force at 90-degrees elbow flexion.

TRIAL	ATTACHMENT	FORCE	MOMENT ARM	EXCURSION
1	#1			
2	#2			
3	#3			
4	#3			NA

Each time begin the effort by repositioning the elbow at the start point (0-degrees flexion).

Now, with the line attached at #3, go back to the starting (0-degrees flexion) position and measure the force needed to begin the motion and the moment arm at the joint position of between 15 and 45 degrees flexion. Record your results in the table.

What is the effect of changing the attachment of the string (muscle)?

Considering trials 1 to 3, what is the relationship between the force needed for movement and the moment arm of the force?

Based on trial 4 compared to trial 3, what can you say about the amount of elbow flexor force necessary for contraction of the muscle early in elbow flexion versus later (around 90 degrees of flexion)?

In summary, what is the relationship between elbow flexion force, flexion moment arm, and excursion of the elbow flexor?

As the flexion moment arm increases flexion force required _____.

As the flexion moment arm increases, excursion of flexor required _____.

LAB 6. HEAD, NECK, AND TRUNK: CURVES, MOVEMENTS, MEASUREMENTS, MUSCLES

STATION: CURVES OF THE VERTEBRAL COLUMN AND BALANCE OF THE COLUMN AGAINST GRAVITY

Using the skeleton of the trunk:

Identify the three normal curves. Which of the three is most superior, middle, and most inferior? Which two are convex anteriorly, and which one is convex posteriorly?

Manipulate the pelvis to demonstrate flattening of the lumbar curve. Which way must the anterior-superior iliac spine (ASIS) be tilted to flatten this curve?

With one person loosely stabilizing the trunk in an upright position, pull on the four muscle groups attached to the trunk to simulate trunk flexion, extension, and lateral flexion to the right or left. Remember that these muscles originate largely from the pelvis. So as you pull on the cords to balance the column or to move it, pull from the origin (see the demonstration). Notice the large MA for flexors and the short MA for extensors.

STATION: MOVEMENTS OF THE TRUNK AND ASSOCIATED UPPER EXTREMITY MOVEMENTS

Using your own bodies, observe in a partner the following motions (watch the demonstrations). For each reach identify the following: (1) elbow and shoulder positions held during the reach; (2) scapular movement and position during and while holding the reach; (3) trunk movement and position during and while holding the reach.

- Reaching forward as far as possible with both arms—putting "everything" into it. In other words, reaching with more than arm's length:
Elbows are _____ ; shoulders are _____ ; the scapula moved through _____ and held it; trunk moved through _____ and held it.

- Reaching directly to the left or right—again, extreme reach:
Elbows are _____ ; shoulders are _____ ; the scapula moved through _____ and held it; trunk moved through _____ and held it.

- Reaching as far as possible with the right arm for an object located to the left of the left shoulder:
Elbows are _____ ; shoulders are _____ ; the scapula moved through _____ and held it; trunk moved through _____ and held it.

STATION: TRUNK MOVEMENTS AND MEASUREMENTS

Movements of the vertebral column are measured in a variety of ways, only one of which is through the use of a goniometer. We will use linear measurements (tape measure) to measure the extent of vertebral flexion, extension, and lateral flexion, and a standard goniometer to measure rotation. Work with a partner and perform the following:

Trunk Lateral Flexion

The subject is standing with feet a shoulder's width apart and then laterally flexes the trunk to the limit of motion. Measure the distance between the tip of the third finger and the floor:_____.

What substitution movements are possible that would invalidate this measurement?

Trunk Extension

Subject is prone (with a pillow under the abdomen, optional for our lab today) with the hands positioned palm down on the mat at shoulder level. The subject then extends the elbows (doing a push-up of the upper trunk), raising the trunk to extend the thoracolumbar spine. Measure the distance between the suprasternal notch and the mat at the extent of motion: _____.

Trunk Flexion

Subject is standing upright, feet a shoulder's width apart, and then flexes the trunk forward to the limit of motion. Measure the distance along the center of the back between the spinous process of C7 and the vertebra between the two iliac crests. Do this by taking one measure before and one after the motion and then subtracting the first from the second: before _____; after _____; difference = _____.

Threats to reliability: **What would cause this measurement to be inconsistent from time to time or to vary because of the person performing the measurement?**

Trunk Rotation

Rotation anterior to the right: Subject is seated and turns so that the shoulders and chest face as far right as possible. Measure the angle between the shoulders (a line drawn through the acromion processes) and a line drawn through the center of both femoral heads: right rotation (rotation anterior to the right) = _____; left rotation (rotation anterior to the left) = _____.

What substitution movements are possible that would invalidate this measurement?

LAB 6: TURN THIS IN

STATION: VERTEBRAL ROTATION ON THE MODEL

Use the box model of the cervical column to study the effect of unilateral and bilateral contractions of the transversospinalis muscle group.

Pull on the left transversospinalis one segment at a time; what happens? How do we communicate this motion? ("Rotation to the left" is not necessarily clear. What side of the box (vertebra) is moving left? Is any side turning to the right?)

Do the same to the right.

Pull on both, simulating a bilateral contraction. What happens? Why? (What motions are canceled yielding the net result?)

LABS 7 AND 8. SHOULDER COMPLEX: SCAPULAR MOVEMENT, DIFFERENTIAL FUNCTIONS OF SCAPULAR AND GLENOHUMERAL (GH) MUSCLES, DIFFERENTIAL FUNCTIONS OF SUPRASPINATUS AND DELTOID IN GH ABDUCTION

STATION: DYNAMIC MODEL OF THE SHOULDER COMPLEX

- Identify the two major muscle groups on the model. What function does each string provide when "contracting" alone? (You may have to provide "active assist" for the motion once you see what the string attempts to perform.)

Scapular motion: _____

Humeral motion at glenohumeral joint: _____

- How much glenohumeral abduction is possible by "contracting" only the glenohumeral abductor?
- What combination of muscle functions and movements is necessary to move the hand to a position above the head?

STATION: TRACKING THE SCAPULA THROUGH UPPER EXTREMITY MOTIONS

Using your own bodies, observe in a partner the following motions (watch the demonstrations):

At rest, seated upright: Have your partner reach with one hand behind the back and up to the level of the scapula. This will cause the scapula to wing and make it easier to find structures. In this position, palpate these structures on your partner:

inferior angle of the scapula
vertebral border of the scapula
scapular spine
acromion

Have your partner return to a resting position and then reach forward as far as possible with one arm, pushing the hand as far out in front as she/he can. Attempt to follow the vertebral border of the scapula and identify this motion of the scapula. (What other term is used for the motion?)

In a resting position: Now have your partner move through complete abduction, bringing their hand high into the air above the head. Palpate the movement of the scapula, paying close attention to the inferior angle.

About how many centimeters did it move?

What is this motion of the scapula? (What other terms have you heard used to describe this motion?)

STATION: REVIEW QUESTIONS ABOUT MMT

GH flexors: How would you test this group if the subject was unable to complete the movement required for a "Fair" (3) or above grade?

GH abductors: What is the position for testing for a grade of "Fair" (3) or better? What is a likely substitution in the case of weakness in this group?

GH internal rotation: What is the direction of resistance applied?

GH extensors: What segment must be stabilized?

Scapular elevation: Could you test this group for a "Normal" (5) grade in a supine position—for someone unable to get up out of bed?

Scapular protraction: How would you test for "Normal" or "Good" strength if the individual was unable to flex the GH joint to assume the test position?

LABS 7 AND 8: TURN THIS IN

NAME: _____

STATION: DYNAMIC MODEL OF DIFFERENTIAL PULL AT GLENOHUMERAL JOINT

Orient yourself to the model:

- Identify the two muscles represented by the three strings.
- Pull on the strings inserting on the lateral humerus (upper third of the shaft). This is the _____, and when acting alone as in this model, what is its primary effect?
- Now pull on the muscle coursing across the superior aspect of the humeral head and inserting on the greater tubercle. This is the _____, and when acting alone what is its function?
- Why do you think the supraspinatus is used early in GH abduction and the deltoid is more important later (and not preferably early in abduction)?

STATION: DRAW IT

(1)   Draw the fibers of the middle deltoid, upper and lower trapezius, and serratus anterior in their actions to abduct the humerus at the shoulder and hold in abduction.

(2)   Draw arrows (vectors) representing forces of these muscles. Make sure to begin the arrow at the distal attachment (insertion) in each case, and direct the arrow parallel to the fibers toward the (proximal attachment) origin. Remember, the arrowhead indicates direction—in this case each force pulls its insertion toward its origin.

(3)   Draw the MA for each force.

(4)   Draw curved arrows representing movement and direction.

LAB 9. MMT AND ROM OF SHOULDER/ELBOW AND FOREARM: TORQUE RANGE OF MOTION

STATION: THINGS TO THINK ABOUT

In comprehensive goniometry and MMT of the shoulder, we must think of the entire complex: GH joint, scapula, and acromioclavicular (AC) and sternoclavicular (SC) joints. Also think about not only GH muscles originating from the scapula and inserting on the humerus (i.e., deltoid, supraspinatus) but also scapular muscles originating on the trunk and inserting on the scapula (i.e., trapezius, serratus anterior).

Also remember we assume a stable origin (proximal attachment) so that a concentric muscle contraction results in movement of the insertion (distal attachment). When this does not happen we see things such as downward rotation of the scapula because of the action of the deltoid and supraspinatus on their origin (scapula). That is, when the upward scapular rotators fail to stabilize the scapula during humeral abduction, we observe downward scapular rotation due to the unbalanced action of the deltoid and supraspinatus.

QUESTIONS:

- When movement at a joint occurs, at what angle of pull is ALL of the force of the muscle being used for rotary motion?

- In terms of angle of pull, where in the motion is the moment arm the longest?

- In terms of moment arm, at what moment arm is the movement the strongest?

- In terms of the "strongest movement" of the musculoskeletal segment, make sure you understand why all of the following statements are the same:

"Elbow flexion is strongest when the joint is at a position of 90 degrees flexed because the flexors have their best angle of pull and the muscle length is good."

"The torque produced by the elbow flexors is greatest at 90-degrees flexion because the moment arm is at its longest length and the actin and myosin overlap is optimal for force production by the muscle fibers."

"The torque produced by the elbow flexors is greatest at 90-degrees flexion because the force of flexion is furthest away from the axis (greatest perpendicular distance) and the actin and myosin overlap is optimal for force production."

- Why does the torque curve not reveal individual tendencies of the biceps and brachialis?

- Another word for the tendency to cause rotary motion is: _____.

STATION: TORQUE RANGE OF MOTION FOR ELBOW EXTENSION AGAINST "TIGHT" ELBOW FLEXORS (MYOSITIC CONTRACTURE)

The big question here is: "How much force is necessary to extend the elbow to a specific position?" The elbow end position is constant, and we are evaluating how much force is required to do passive ROM to this position.

Extend the elbow to the point of 90 degrees of flexion as read on the goniometer. You will start with this "tight elbow" in a position of greater than 90 degrees of flexion and pull toward extension in a position of less flexion, or about 90 degrees. (**VERY IMPORTANT:** Make sure you pull the forearm with the force gauge angled 90 degrees to it.)

How much force is necessary: _____?

For background information, measure the moment arm of the force you are exerting to passively range the elbow: MA = _____.

Go back to the beginning or resting position—about 130 degrees elbow flexion. Start pulling with the force gauge and notice there is little to no resistance in extension in the beginning. This time draw a graph to document the amount of force required from the beginning of this extension motion. Document the resistance as read on the force guage at the elbow positions of 120, 110, 100, and 90 degrees of flexion.

Note: You are starting in flexion and pulling into more and more extension. The elbow measurements are in terms of flexion. Therefore, as you increase extension of the joint, the measurement of the joint should be decreasing degrees of flexion.

FORCE

120   110   100   90

Degrees of Flexion

How would we express this in terms of torque instead of the force value read on the scale; that is, how could you convert each force reading to torque?

STATION: TORQUE RANGE OF MOTION AND ERRORS IN MEASUREMENT

At this station pull the elbow toward extension into a position of 90-degrees flexion. Intentionally pull with the force gauge (1) oriented 90 degrees to the moving segment (forearm) as before and then (2) at an angle much less than 90 degrees, a pull more parallel to the forearm (instead of perpendicular).

How much force was required in trial 1 at 90-degrees pull: _____?

How much force was required in trial 2: _____?

Notice much more force is required to passively range this stiff elbow into extension (from 130 degrees of flexion to 90 degrees of flexion) if the ranging force you exert as the therapist is applied at an angle other than 90 degrees. This less-than-90-degree angle of pull induces a large linear component directed into the joint. This force has nothing to do with extending the elbow and is wasted. That is why it takes more force to do the same job. If you were using torque range of motion as a way to measure stiffness as it is typically used, your measurement would be in error. The greater force needed to range the joint would reflect greater stiffness in the tissues. However, had someone been watching, they would know the tissues had not become stiffer—the therapist measured it wrong!

Therefore, when measuring the force (or torque) required to pull a "stiff joint" to a specific position, you should always direct the force you provide employing an angle of _____ degrees.

LAB 9: TURN THIS IN

STATION: MOCK MMT AND GONIOMETRY PRACTICAL EXAM

With a lab instructor (or fellow student) set up a mock practical exam for ROM and MMT of the shoulder and elbow. For muscle testing, test for and mark all grades even though your "subject" probably has normal strength.

Active Joint ROM (AROM) Measurement:

JOINT	MEASUREMENT
shoulder flexion	
shoulder abduction	
shoulder internal rotation	
shoulder external rotation	
shoulder horizontal abduction	
shoulder horizontal adduction	
elbow flexion	
forearm pronation	
forearm supination	

Muscle Strength Measurement through MMT:

JOINT	MEASUREMENT
shoulder flexion	
shoulder extension	
shoulder abduction	
shoulder adduction	
shoulder internal rotation	
shoulder external rotation	
shoulder horizontal abduction	
shoulder horizontal adduction	
elbow flexion	
elbow extension	
forearm pronation	
forearm supination	

LAB 10. WRIST AND HAND: SYNERGISTIC FUNCTION OF WRIST EXTENSORS AND FINGER FLEXORS

STATION: ISOMETRIC TORQUE CURVE OF FINGER FLEXORS

Use the dynamometer on the second grip-span setting. Attempt three grip efforts, each with the wrist in a different position from full extension to full flexion.

1. Start by having the subject attempt a maximum effort with the wrist in a comfortable amount of extension for grasp; measure this position (_____ degrees extension) and take the grip strength reading from the dynamometer (_____ lb). Label the horizontal axis of the graph with this wrist position measurement as the middle position of the graph and plot the grip strength measurement over this point according to the scale on the vertical axis.

2. Next, measure grip strength with the wrist held in forced full wrist extension and plot this to the right of the center point. (You may have to hold the subject's wrist in this position during the grip effort.)

3. Last, measure grip strength again with the wrist held in full wrist flexion. (You may have to hold the subject's wrist in this position during the grip effort.) Again plot the force of grasp (in pounds) on the Y axis (vertical) and the wrist position on the X axis (horizontal). This wrist position should be to the left of center on the horizontal axis.

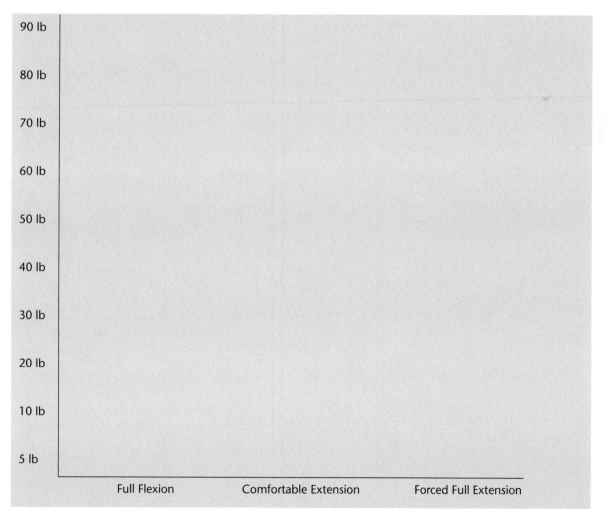

What happens to strength of grasp as the wrist position changes?

What is the specific effect on finger flexors (when grip begins from different wrist positions)?

LAB 10: TURN THIS IN

STATION: BALANCE OF FUNCTION AT THE WRIST

Use the wrist/hand model (holding the ball) to perform balanced wrist extension (against gravity) and wrist flexion (with gravity).

1. Have one person hold the proximal forearm of the model and stabilize it, the same as it would be at 90-degree elbow flexion preparing to lift the ball from the table.

2. With the forearm pronated and the hand holding the ball resting on the tabletop, have another student use the radial and ulnar wrist extensors to lift the ball off the table using wrist extension.

3. Carefully lower the ball down to the tabletop.

What type of contraction in which muscles is performed to lift the ball from the tabletop?

What is the effect of using either the ECRL or the ECU but not both?

LAB 11. TORQUE RANGE OF MOTION/INTRINSIC FUNCTION/TENODESIS GRASP/PULLEYS/ REVIEW OF ROM LIMITATIONS

STATION: MEASURING A STIFF PIP JOINT—TRADITIONAL GONIOMETRY

Working in your group (at least three people) and using a goniometer:

1. Measure how far the PIP of the model can be extended. Be careful not to tear the tissue. (Breaking the model is the same as damaging the client!!) It is important that each group member keeps their measurement a secret from the rest of their group.

   Measurement of PIP joint (extension to flexion): _____

2. Compare your measurement with those of other group members. There will probably be some differences among the measurements.

   What accounts for the differences?

STATION: MEASURING A STIFF PIP JOINT—TORQUE RANGE OF MOTION

Now, as in the previous station, measure PIP extension of the model. This time use a goniometer and a force gauge.

Chart the amount of force necessary to extend PIP to the end of its range.

PIP flexion measurement: _____ (This is the amount of extension lacking in the joint. If you can passively range the joint to 45 degrees of flexion, it is said to lack 45 degrees to full extension.)

Force required: _____grams

Measuring Progress

How can this record become a series of measures charted over time? Fill in the graph with values obtained later that would indicate improvements over a five-week period.

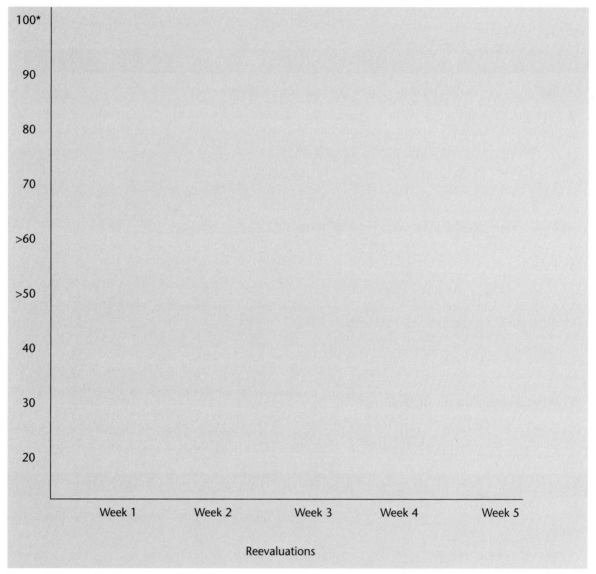

*Degrees 20 through 100 (Y axis) represent the PIP flexion measurement, pulling with a 500-gram force. As with the elbow, document PIP joint measurements in degrees of flexion only. Improvement shows declining numbers as the flexion contracture improves, ranging the PIP joint into more extension (less flexion).

LAB 11: TURN THIS IN

NAME: _____

STATION: WATCH THE VIDEO: INTRINSIC CORRECTION

Movie 8-1: Intrinsic Correction

The tweezers are applied to the tendon of the lumbrical/interosseus. What is the relationship of the force exerted through the hemostats to the MCP joint?

What is the relationship of this force (exerted **THROUGH** the ED tendon) to the PIP and DIP joints? _____

What is the effect of the force exerted through the hemostats:

on the MCP _____

on the PIP and DIP _____

STATION: WATCH THE VIDEO: TENODESIS GRASP

Movie 8-2: Tenodesis Grasp

Watch the video segment in which Skip grasps and raises the telephone receiver to his ear. Notice the grasp.

1. What are at least two requirements for an effective tenodesis grasp?
_____ and _____

How should you perform PROM in someone with a tenodesis grasp (or someone developing a tenodesis grasp)?

(HINT: You could think of this in terms of what not to do; that is, never range the fingers and wrist simultaneously into _____. Do you know why?)

2. Why would you need to perform PROM to the fingers and wrist of someone with a tenodesis grasp?

STATION: LARGE FINGER MODEL

DO TWO THINGS:

1. Measure the amount of excursion required to fully flex the finger (a) with the tendon going through the pulleys and (b) with the tendon taken out of the pulleys.
   a. _____
   b. _____
2. Determine what happens at each joint without the pulleys, especially at the IP joints, as you begin in full extension and pull proximally on the FDP.

STATION: SUMMARY OF LIMITATIONS IN ROM

By now we have explored many reasons why someone's ROM might be limited. Do not forget that some problems limit AROM but not PROM and vice versa. List all of the problems you can remember:

AROM LIMITED	PROM & AROM LIMITED

LAB 12. PREHENSION PATTERNS/INTRINSIC FUNCTION AND DIGITAL SWEEP/TENODESIS GRASP

STATION: EXAMPLES OF PREHENSION PATTERNS (GRASPS)

Look around and find objects that require the following grasps: cylindrical spherical, lateral (also called 3-jaw chuck or key punch), hook, power grasp, scissors tip prehension.

Indicate with a "T" grasps that require use of the thumb in some way.

Indicate with a "T-O" grasps that require thumb opposition.

STATION: SHALLOW DIGITAL SWEEP IN INTRINSIC MINUS HAND

Using one of the finger models (Appendix J, Finger Model), place the container in the circle and attempt to grasp it with the finger. Start with the finger pulled into full extension with the EDC.
    First release the EDC and pull only on the FDP and notice what happens. What happens when you attempt to grasp only with the FDP?

    Next extend the digit again with the EDC, and this time attempt to grasp using the combination of the lumbrical first and then the FDP. What happens with the combination?

STATION: TENODESIS GRASP AND RELEASE

Using the forearm and two-finger hand model (Appendix J, Wrist and Finger Model), determine a way to flex the finger into a grasp around the cup without actively shortening the long finger flexor (without pulling proximally to simulate a contraction). You will need to simulate a shortened length of the finger flexor as would occur over time if the finger was not extended at all joints simultaneously, stretching and maintaining its length. Do this in the following way:

1. Passively range the wrist into flexion and pull the slack out of the finger flexor without flexing the finger.
2. Pinch the finger flexor tendon against the radius to simulate "tenodesis surgery"— shortening the FDP.

Now, think about ways to create tension in the finger flexor without contracting (pulling on) it. It is possible by stretching it across one of its joints. The tension created will then cause motion at other joints even though the finger flexor itself did not actively shorten; remember, you are holding it still.

While holding the finger flexor against the radius as described above, pull on the wrist extensor and watch the finger flex. What was the combination that resulted in grasp (tenodesis grasp)?

LAB 13. POSITIONING IN A WHEELCHAIR

STATION: EVALUATE PROM AND FLEXIBILITY

Evaluate PROM of the hip joints on a partner. For ROM, align the stationary arm with the midaxillary line of the trunk and the moving arm with the femur. The axis of the goniometer should be in line with the hip side-to-side axis for flexion/extension. **PERFORM THIS MEASUREMENT PASSIVELY FLEXING THE HIP WHILE SIMULTANEOUSLY FLEXING THE KNEE.**

Evaluate flexibility—the degree to which PROM is allowed or limited by the muscle resting length (or distal excursion). Again use the goniometer but this time passively **FLEX THE HIP WITH THE KNEE EXTENDED.** Flex the hip only to the point that the pelvis begins to posteriorly tilt (note the flattening of the lumbar area or the posterior movement of the ASIS). Record this hip flexion measurement in the right column of the table below.

DEGREES HIP FLEXION/KNEE FLEXED	DEGREES HIP FLEXION/KNEE EXTENDED

An alternative measurement is to passively flex the hip and knee to 90 degrees. Then while watching the pelvis and holding the hip flexed at 90 degrees, slowly extend the knee to the point where the pelvis begins to posteriorly tilt (or notice flattening of the lumbar curve). (In individuals with very short hamstrings, begin the measurement with greater than 90 degrees of knee flexion.) Note or measure the knee position at the point where the pelvis begins to move. Short hamstrings will stretch early in the knee movement, yielding a knee flexion measurement of, for example, 80 degrees. Long hamstrings will allow the knee to be fully extended (0-degrees knee flexion) without ever moving the pelvis!

STATION: POSITIONING THE SKELETON IN THE UPRIGHT POSITION

Using an articulated skeleton with short hamstrings attached try to position the skeleton in "good sitting position"—trunk supported, pelvis in anterior tilt with no obliquity and no rotation. You will need to evaluate the skeleton either during its positioning or prior to your attempts. Especially look at the PROM of the hips through standard goniometry and FLEXIBILITY evaluations (see previous station). After completing the task, answer the following questions:

What happens to the pelvis when the skeleton is placed into the chair attempting bilateral hip flexion to 90 degrees? [In other words, when you initially place it into the "normal" sitting position (hips/knees at 90-degrees flexion), how does the pelvis position itself?]

Identify four essential components of your "seating system." (This should include specific cushions used for the seating surface and any propping-up cushions. The chair itself is not one of the components.) List additional components if you used them.

STATION: POSITIONING THE SKELETON IN THE RECLINED POSITION

CHAIR	BENEFITS	PROBLEMS
Recliner	(1) Redistributes force …	(1) Introduces shear …
	(2)	(2)
	(3)	
Tilt-in-Space	(1)	(1)
	(2)	(2)

To effectively identify benefits/problems, each student should take a turn getting into each of the two chairs. Make sure the brakes are locked before you are tilted or reclined by a partner in either chair.

Now consider the recliner and tilt-in-space for the purpose of: (1) building tolerance to sitting in an upright position following spinal cord injury (there is usually a problem with orthostatic hypotension); (2) building sitting tolerance in terms of pressure on the ischial tuberosities. How would these chairs be used to build tolerance to the upright position? (Think in terms of a schedule.)

How does placing the trunk at some angle off of the vertical (i.e., 45 degrees) change the amount of force on the ischial tuberosities? [HINT: Beginning of answer = With the trunk reclined or tilted back, the center of gravity projection (representing the weight of the trunk and head) …].

What **UNWANTED** force results from use of the recliner for pressure and position tolerance building that **DOES NOT** result from use of the tilt-in-space chair?

Basic Points to Understand about the Vertebral Column, Pelvis, and Hamstrings in Positioning

- The attachment of the hamstring muscles proximal and distal to the articulation of the femoral head and the pelvic acetabulum results in movement of the origin (pelvis) of the hamstrings with passive movement of the hip and knee—especially in the case of "tight" or shortened (at rest) hamstrings.
- Short hamstrings are associated with posterior pelvic tilt, which due to the attachment between the pelvis and lumbar vertebrae results in flattening or even reversal of the normal lumbar curve (normally convex anteriorly).
- The shorter the hamstrings, the earlier the pelvis will tilt posteriorly in the course of hip flexion, as the hamstrings are stretching in this passive movement—if the knee is prevented from flexing while the hip is flexed. For example, in walking, the hip flexes in swing while the knee is thrown into extension via the momentum of the swing—thus stretching the hamstrings at both joints simultaneously.
- The distance between the ischial tuberosity (origin of hamstrings) and inferior-medial tibial plateau (general insertion of hamstrings):
  — At position of hip and knee extension = 35 cm
  — At position of hip flexion to 90 degrees with knee flexed to 90 degrees = 49 cm
  — At position of 90-degrees hip flexion with the knee fully extended = 55 cm (This position corresponds to "passive insufficiency" for the hamstrings.)
- A pelvis that is oriented in posterior tilt while sitting because of hamstrings that are stretched with the hips and knees in 90 degrees of flexion should be considered "fixed," and the function of positioning would not be to correct this but to accommodate it and allow comfortable sitting. Accommodation is through the use of 90-degree footrests with adjustable foot plates to allow greater than 90-degrees knee flexion in sitting (to allow the hamstrings to slack). Other aspects of intervention may be aimed, meanwhile, at stretching the hamstrings to allow a more functional pelvic position in sitting.
- Other factors resulting in "fixed" positions include joint contractures from soft tissue shortening secondary to long-standing inability to move out of a position.
- An individual with a hip adductor contracture should be positioned allowing "wind sweeping" of the thighs. (With the contracture on the left, the right hip is abducted, left adducted.) Positioning the thighs symmetrically and in neutral ab/adduction results in pelvic rotation, right side rotated anteriorly with a left-sided hip adduction contracture. A contracture in the left hip adductor prevents left hip abduction to neutral. Attempting left hip abduction pulls the pelvis such that the right ASIS moves anteriorly when the left hip is passively forced into abduction; that is, due to the adduction contracture, no abduction occurs; instead you are using the left femur as a lever to rotate the pelvis.
- Pelvic obliquity may occur in the case of a unilateral hip extension contracture that is not accommodated by the seating/positioning system such that, for example, the right posterior thigh (with a right extension contracture) hits the seating surface first in sitting and pushes the right pelvis superiorly when attempting to sit on both buttocks.

BIOMECHANICAL ANALYSIS LAB

Watch the video in lab and perform two separate biomechanical analyses following the biomechanical analysis forms below. In the first column, each of the segments already has been identified. You still need to describe where in the activity the positions or movements are observed AND if both movement and position are observed versus movement only. NOTE: Consider the forearm movement to be a pouring movement and analyze as such.

Analysis 1: Coffee cup grasp using handle
Video Clip: Cup Grasp: Handle

ID AND DESCRIBE MOTION/POSITION	ROM	GRAVITY'S EFFECT	AGONIST GROUP-CONTRACTION TYPE
Forearm supination			
Wrist extension			
Wrist radial deviation			
Thumb CMC abduction			
Index MCP/PIP flexion			

Analysis 2: Coffee cup grasp NOT using handle—hand around cup
Video Clip: Cup Grasp: Cup

ID AND DESCRIBE MOTION/POSITION	ROM	AGONIST GROUP-CONTRACTION TYPE
Thumb CMC abduction—*Is there any thumb CMC abduction?*		
Index MCP/PIP flexion		

Analysis 3: Coffee cup grasp using handle—nerve damage
Video Clip: Cup Grasp: No Problem
Video Clip: Cup Grasp: Nerve Damage

ID AND DESCRIBE MOTION/POSITION	ROM	AGONIST GROUP-CONTRACTION TYPE
Thumb CMC abduction		
Thumb CMC adduction		
Thumb IP flexion		

How is the thumb used—what is the muscle functioning to bring the thumb to the other side of the handle, the side opposite the index finger?

Which nerve is damaged?

Is damage at the level of the wrist or elbow?

Analysis 4: Self-feeding/drinking pattern
Video Clip: Self-Feeding

ID AND DESCRIBE MOTION/POSITION	ROM	GRAVITY'S EFFECT	AGONIST GROUP-CONTRACTION TYPE
Shoulder external rotation			
Shoulder flexion/abduction (scaption)			
Choose another joint you feel is important to analyze in this activity			

COMPETENCY CHECK SHEET FOR TRANSFERS

NAME: _____

DATE OF STAND PIVOT: _____   DATE OF SLIDING BOARD: _____

TRANSFER ASPECT	+ OR –
Correctly position wheelchair	
Clear instructions (Count "1, 2, 3.")	
Lock chair	
Remove safety belt	
Attach transfer belt	
Remove wheelchair parts	
Scoot forward	
Lean forward	
Flex knees to 90 degrees or slightly more	
Stand pivot: client's knees between yours; sliding board placed halfway under bottom using weight shift.	
Assistance given with straight back, bending at knees and hips, stand as close as possible, no twisting of back	
Transfer proceeds unrushed including client sitting on new surface (slow sitting from stand; slow scooting across)	
Individual fully and safely seated on new surface; sliding board out	

COMPETENCY CHECK SHEET FOR ROM/MMT

NAME: _____

Test muscle groups first, beginning with the against gravity test (Fair or 3/5) followed by the gravity eliminated test.

MMT
Correctly position subject (check for Fair and Poor tests)
Clear instructions
Proximal stabilization
Resistance at end of ROM
Resistance on distal segment
Resistance in opposite direction of muscle pull
"What is the purpose of MMT"?
Palpation: Demonstrate palpation at rest, during attempted contraction, and at rest

GONIOMETRY
Goniometer stationary arm proximal
Accurate alignment of goniometer
Clear instructions
Correct reading
Gentle (no bruising!!)

TABLE OF MOTIONS AND MUSCLES TO PALPATE FOR MMT PRACTICAL EXAMS

MOTION	MUSCLE(S)
Elevation/depression	Upper trapezius/lower trapezius or latissimus dorsi
Adduction (retraction)	Middle trapezius and rhomboid major
Abduction (protraction)	Serratus anterior
Shoulder:	
Flexion	Anterior deltoid or pectoralis major
Extension	Posterior deltoid or latissimus dorsi
Abduction	Middle deltoid
Adduction	Latissimus dorsi or pectoralis major
Horizontal abduction	Posterior deltoid
Horizontal adduction	Pectoralis major or anterior deltoid
External rotation	Infraspinatus, teres minor, or posterior deltoid
Internal rotation	Teres major, latissimus dorsi, pectoralis major, or anterior deltoid
Elbow:	
Flexion	Biceps and brachioradialis
Extension	Triceps tendon (just above olecronon)
Forearm:	
Pronation	Pronator teres
Supination	Biceps brachii, supinator
Wrist:	
Extension	ECRB and ECU
Flexion	FCR, PL, and FCU
Digits 2-5:	
Flexion; know tests for FDP (DIP flexion) and FDS (PIP flexion)	FDP palpated at the distal interphalangeal (DIP joint crease)
Lumbricals/interossei:	None
Extension	EDC
Thumb:	
Extension (test MCP or IP)	Extensor pollicis longus or brevis
Flexion (test MCP or IP, but know why these differentiate the FPL from FPB)	Flexor pollicis brevis and longus
Abduction ("palmar abduction" test CMC)	Abductor pollicis brevis
Adduction	None
Opposition	Abductor pollicis brevis and opponens pollicis

ADDITIONAL LAB: MMT TO DETERMINE NEUROLOGICAL LEVEL IN SCI

Work in groups of four. The assignment is to diagnose the neurological level of function in a spinal cord injury scenario. One of two students working together should play the part of the person with the spinal cord injury, according to the guidelines given here. The other two members of the group will plan and carry out the evaluation. You are trying to determine, through MMT, the highest functioning level (according to segmental level) of the spinal cord—this is known as the "neurological level" and is the number used in the statement of the diagnosis, i.e., C5 quadriplegia. This has everything to do with segmental (not peripheral) nerve innervation.

In the section "Brief Guidelines for ROM and MMT" (see pages L-21 to L-28) and in the motion CD muscles are listed with their segmental or spinal nerve innervations. Here is the way to use this information:

- If you test a muscle innervated by C5&6 and it tests 3/5, this "Fair" strength grade is telling you the muscle is not fully innervated.
- If you test another muscle innervated by C6 only or by C6&7 and it is 0/5, the picture becomes clearer that C5 is connected; C6 and higher numbers (anatomically lower levels of the cord) are not.
- Further testing of muscles with C5, C6, C7 innervations confirms the finding.
- Functioning C5 and nonfunctioning C6 were responsible for the first muscle testing 3/5; nonfunctioning C6 and higher numbers are responsible for 0/5 strength in muscles innervated by the higher numbered segments.
- Everything innervated by segments C5 and lower numbers (segments located anatomically higher in the cord) should test 5/5.

SPECIFIC DIRECTIONS:

1. As you administer the MMT exam, fill in the blanks on the evaluation sheet. Test only one side: left or right.
2. After completing the MMT on the "client/patient," go through their guidelines and write the correct muscle grades in the column next to the one you filled out; talk about any discrepancies.
3. Use the corrected muscle grades to determine the neurological level. You should be looking for a level between C5 and C8. Everyone should start high—with scapular movements—and continue proximal to distal in your testing until you begin to consistently find 0/5 strength.
4. IF you are running out of time, evaluate the short list: scapular elevation, GH flexion, elbow flexion, elbow extension, wrist extension, thumb abduction, thumb IP flexion, lumbrical/interosseus function. In this case fill in the rest of the grades from the guidelines.

Group 1 Instructions for Client Team

You should study this chart and be able to "fake" weaknesses according to the following. Your performance should be good enough that the evaluation team can interpret the results without looking at the chart. After the evaluation, each group member should interpret the results. It is best to work **INDIVIDUALLY,** develop your interpretation, and enter it under "Neurological Level." **THEN** discuss the results among all four (or five) members of the group, working together to finalize your opinion. If the group consensus is different from your determination, do not delete your conclusion about neurological level. Instead put the consensus in the next blank and briefly describe why you changed your mind—why the group discussion led to a change in your interpretation about neurological function.

STRENGTH	MOVEMENTS
4 or 5/5	Scapular elevation, depression, retraction
3/5	Glenohumeral (GH) abduction, GH flexion, horizontal abduction, external rotation, elbow flexion, forearm supination
2/5	Scapular protraction, GH extension (hyperextension), GH adduction, horizontal adduction, internal rotation
0/5	Elbow extension, forearm pronation, wrist & finger flexion & extension, thumb opposition, thumb abduction, thumb IP flexion, lumbrical/interossei function

Neurological level: _____

Group consensus about neurological level: _____

Reason for difference in interpretation: What did you fail to consider?

Group 2 Instructions for Client Team

You should study this chart and be able to "fake" weaknesses according to the following. Your performance should be good enough that the evaluation team can interpret the results without looking at the chart. After the evaluation, each group member should interpret the results. It is best to work **INDIVIDUALLY,** develop your interpretation, and enter it under "Neurological Level." **THEN** discuss the results among all four (or five) members of the group, working together to finalize your opinion. If the group consensus is different from your determination, do not delete your conclusion about neurological level. Instead put the consensus in the next blank and briefly describe why you changed your mind—why the group discussion led to a change in your interpretation about neurological function.

STRENGTH	MOVEMENTS
4 or 5/5	Scapular elevation, depression, retraction, GH abduction, GH flexion, external rotation, horizontal abduction, elbow flexion, forearm supination
3/5	Scapular protraction, GH extension (hyperextension), GH adduction, horizontal adduction, GH internal rotation, thumb opposition & abduction (could be 2/5 with this level injury), wrist extension (ulnar side feels weaker = 2/5)
2/5	Forearm pronation, wrist flexion (but ulnar side feels weaker = 0/5), finger extension
0/5	Elbow extension, finger flexion, thumb IP flexion, lumbrical/interossei function

Neurological level: _____

Group consensus about neurological level: _____

Reason for difference in interpretation: What did you fail to consider?

Group 3 Instructions for Client Team

You should study this chart and be able to "fake" weaknesses according to the following. Your performance should be good enough that the evaluation team can interpret the results without looking at the chart. After the evaluation, each group member should interpret the results. It is best to work **INDIVIDUALLY,** develop your interpretation, and enter it under "Neurological Level." **THEN** discuss the results among all four (or five) members of the group, working together to finalize your opinion. If the group consensus is different from your determination, do not delete your conclusion about neurological level. Instead put the consensus in the next blank and briefly describe why you changed your mind—why the group discussion led to a change in your interpretation about neurological function.

STRENGTH	MOVEMENTS
4 or 5/5	Scapular elevation, depression, retraction, scapular protraction, GH abduction, GH flexion, GH extension (hyperextension), GH adduction, GH internal rotation, GH external rotation, horizontal abduction, horizontal adduction, elbow flexion, forearm supination, thumb opposition & abduction (could be 3/5 with this level injury), wrist extension (ulnar side feels weaker = 3/5)
3/5	Elbow extension, forearm pronation, wrist flexion (but ulnar side feels weaker = 0/5), finger extension, thumb extension
2/5	Finger flexion (FDS), lumbrical/interossei function
0/5	Finger flexion (DIP), thumb IP flexion, thumb adduction

Neurological level: _____

Group consensus about neurological level: _____

Reason for difference in interpretation: What did you fail to consider?

Group 4 Instructions for Client Team

You should study this chart and be able to "fake" weaknesses according to the following. Your performance should be good enough that the evaluation team can interpret the results without looking at the chart. After the evaluation, each group member should interpret the results. It is best to work **INDIVIDUALLY,** develop your interpretation, and enter it under "Neurological Level." **THEN** discuss the results among all four (or five) members of the group, working together to finalize your opinion. If the group consensus is different from your determination, do not delete your conclusion about neurological level. Instead put the consensus in the next blank and briefly describe why you changed your mind—why the group discussion led to a change in your interpretation about neurological function.

STRENGTH	MOVEMENTS
4 or 5/5	Scapular elevation, depression, retraction, scapular protraction, GH abduction, GH flexion, GH extension (hyperextension), GH adduction, GH internal rotation, GH external rotation, horizontal abduction, horizontal adduction, elbow flexion, elbow extension, forearm supination, forearm pronation, thumb opposition & abduction (could be 3/5 with this level injury), wrist extension, wrist flexion (but ulnar side feels weaker = 3/5), finger extension, thumb extension
3/5	Finger flexion (FDS & FDP), lumbrical/interossei function, thumb adduction, thumb IP flexion
0/5	None

Neurological level: _____

Group consensus about neurological level: _____

Reason for difference in interpretation: What did you fail to consider?